NOTES ON VETERINARY OPHTHALMOLOGY

NOTES ON VETERINARY OPHTHALMOLOGY

Sheila Crispin MA Vet MB BSc PhD
DVA DVOphthal DipECVO FRCVS

Professor of Comparative Ophthalmology
University of Bristol

Colour pictures
sponsored by

Blackwell
Science

© 2005 by Blackwell Science Ltd
a Blackwell Publishing company

Editorial offices:
Blackwell Science Ltd, 9600 Garsington Road, Oxford OX4 2DQ, UK
   Tel: +44 (0) 1865 776868
Blackwell Publishing Professional, 2121 State Avenue, Ames, Iowa 50014-8300, USA
   Tel: +1 515 292 0140
Blackwell Science Asia Pty Ltd, 550 Swanston Street, Carlton, Victoria 3053, Australia
   Tel: +61 (0)3 8359 1011

First published 2005

Library of Congress Cataloging-in-Publication Data
Crispin, Sheila M.
   Notes on veterinary ophthalmology / Sheila Crispin. – 1st ed.
      p.   cm.
Includes bibliographical references (p.)
ISBN 0-632-06416-1 (pbk. : alk. paper) .
1. Veterinary ophthalmology.   I. Title.

SF891.C75 2005
636.089'77 – dc22

                                                                2004009930

ISBN 0-632-06416-1

A catalogue record for this title is available from the British Library

Set in 9 on 11.5pt Sabon
by SNP Best-set Typesetter Ltd., Hong Kong
Printed and bound in India
by Replika Press Pvt. Ltd Kundli

The publisher's policy is to use permanent paper from mills that operate a sustainable forestry
policy, and which has been manufactured from pulp processed using acid-free and elementary
chlorine-free practices. Furthermore, the publisher ensures that the text paper and cover board
used have met acceptable environmental accreditation standards.

For further information on Blackwell Publishing, visit our website:
www.blackwellpublishing.com

CONTENTS

PREFACE AND ACKNOWLEDGEMENTS

This brief text comprises the ophthalmology notes used to teach the theory of veterinary ophthalmology to generations of veterinary students. They have been expanded to provide a more comprehensive overview for those in general practice with an interest in, but no specialist knowledge of, veterinary ophthalmology. The first section sets out the instruments that are used and the manner in which examination of the eye and adnexa is performed; this is followed by a section on emergencies and trauma that crosses the species. There are then sections that cover general and canine ophthalmology, feline ophthalmology, rabbit ophthalmology, farm animal ophthalmology and equine ophthalmology. The notes conclude with brief appendices on ophthalmic terminology, topical medical preparations, basic principles of anaesthesia and surgery and the cranial nerves innervating the eye and adnexa.

I am indebted to Janssen Animal Health for a most generous donation towards the cost of the colour photographs. I am very grateful to the Photography Unit of the Bristol Veterinary School for many of the photographs taken by Mr John Conibear and Mrs Tracy Dewey and to Mr Nick Crabb for the line drawings. I am particularly indebted to Mr John Mould for the excellent gross and microscopic preparations of the eye.

I wish to acknowledge the major contributions of Professor Dennis Brooks and Dr Andy Matthews to uveitis and glaucoma in the equine section. My past colleagues in the Ophthalmology Unit have given generously of their time and expertise and particular thanks go to Dr David Gould for commenting on early drafts of the manuscript and also to Mr Jim Carter and Mr Rob Lowe for their support. Any errors, however, rest entirely with the author.

My thanks go to many colleagues, in both medical and veterinary ophthalmology, for engendering and stimulating my interest in this fascinating subject.

S. Crispin
2004

ORGANISATIONS

BVA	British Veterinary Association
CERF	Canine Eye Registration Foundation
ECVO	European College of Veterinary Ophthalmologists
ISDS	International Sheep Dog Society
KC	Kennel Club

TERMS

AP	auriculopalpebral
BVD-MD	bovine virus diarrhoea–mucosal disease
CALT	conjunctival-associated lymphoid tissue
CEA	Collie eye anomaly
CT	computed tomography
CNS	central nervous system
CPRA	central progressive retinal atrophy
ERG	electroretinography
ERU	equine recurrent uveitis
EUA	examination under anaesthesia
FB	foreign body
FeLV	feline leukaemia virus
FECV	feline enteric coronavirus
FIP(V)	feline infectious peritonitis (virus)
FIV	feline immunodeficiency virus
GME	granulomatous meningoencephalitis
GPRA	generalised progressive retinal atrophy
GSE	general somatic efferent
GVE	general visceral efferent
HA	hyaloid artery
HDL	high density lipoprotein
IBKC	infectious bovine keratoconjunctivitis
IBR	infectious bovine rhinotracheitis
IL-2	interleukin-2
IOKC	infectious ovine keratoconjunctivitis
IOP	intraocular pressure
KCS	keratoconjunctivitis sicca
KP	keratic precipitates
MRD	multifocal retinal dysplasia
MRI	magnetic resonance imaging
NSAID	non-steroidal anti-inflammatory
NTF	non-tapetal fundus
ONH	optic nerve head
PCR	polymerase chain reaction

PHPV	persistent hyperplastic primary vitreous
PIFM	pre-iridal fibrovascular membrane
PLL	primary lens luxation
PLR	pupillary light reflex
PPM	persistent pupillary membrane
PRA	progressive retinal atrophy
PTF	preocular tear film
RD	retinal dysplasia
RPE	retinal pigment epithelium
RPED	retinal pigment epithelial dystrophy
SARD	sudden acquired retinal degeneration
SCC	squaemous cell carcinoma
SOL	space-occupying lesion
STT	Schirmer tear test
TEME	thromboembolic meningoencephalitis
TRD	total retinal dysplasia
TSCL	therapeutic soft contact lens
TVL	tunica vasculosa lentis
VCTM	viral and chlamydial transport medium

SECTION 1
OPHTHALMIC EQUIPMENT AND EXAMINATION

INSTRUMENTS AND EQUIPMENT

BASIC INSTRUMENTS FOR OPHTHALMIC EXAMINATION

- Penlight (focussing or narrow beam)
- Condensing lens (20D or 2.2 pan retinal®)
- Magnifying loupe or otoscope with speculum removed
- Direct ophthalmoscope
- Schiøtz tonometer

ADDITIONAL INSTRUMENTS

- Finoff ocular transilluminator
- Slit lamp biomicroscope
- Monocular indirect ophthalmoscope
- Binocular indirect ophthalmoscope
- Tonometer (e.g. TonoPen®)
- Gonioscopy lens (e.g. Barkan or Koeppe)

BASIC EQUIPMENT FOR DIAGNOSTIC PROCEDURES

- Ophthalmic stains – fluorescein sodium (1% and 2%) and rose bengal 1%
- Sterile water, sodium chloride 0.9%, Hartmann's solution
- Local anaesthetic for topical use (e.g. proxymetacaine hydrochloride 0.5%, amethocaine hydrochloride 0.5% and 1%)
- Combined local anaesthetic and ophthalmic stain (e.g. proxymetacaine hydrochloride 0.5% and fluorescein sodium 0.25%)
- Local anaesthetic for injection (e.g. lignocaine [lidocaine] hydrochloride 1% and 2%, prilocaine hydrochloride 1%, mepivacaine hydrochloride 2%)
- Mydriatic (e.g. tropicamide 1%)
- Miotic (e.g. pilocarpine hydrochloride 1%)
- Schirmer Tear Test papers
- Kimura spatula or other sterile scraper, e.g. disposable scalpel blade
- Sterile swabs or cytobrushes for sample collection for culture
- Clean, dry, grease-free microscope slides
- Suitable stains for smears, e.g. Gram and Giemsa
- Cotton wool
- Calipers/ruler
- Nasolacrimal cannulae (re-usable sterilisable metal or disposable sterile plastic)
- Sterile syringes and needles

OPHTHALMIC EQUIPMENT AND EXAMINATION

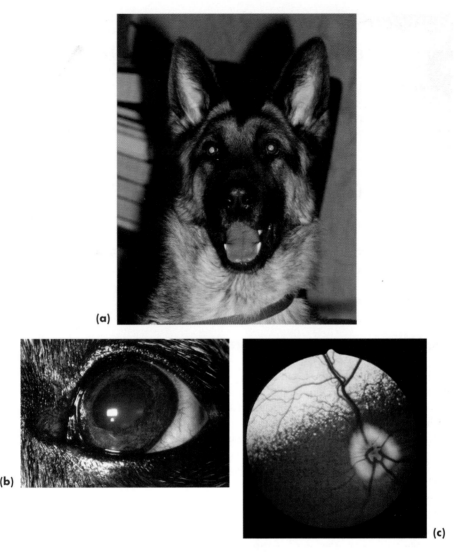

(a)

(b)

(c)

Figure 1.1(a–c)   Normal canine head (a), close up of the eye (b) and ocular fundus (c). A sound knowledge of normal ocular structure and function, together with a logical examination technique, underpins diagnostic ophthalmology.

INSTRUMENTATION

Penlight or other light source

Disposable and non-disposable penlights (Figure 1.2(a)) are available. Focussing ability is desirable, as is a detachable cobalt blue filter. The Finoff ocular transilluminator with halogen illumination and a detachable cobalt blue filter is probably the most useful light source for ophthalmic examination. A Finoff ocular transilluminator can be attached to the rechargeable battery handle of a direct ophthalmoscope (Figure 1.2(b)).

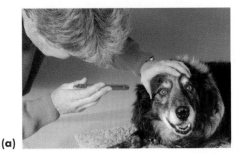 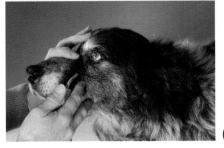

(a) (b)

Figure 1.2 **(a)** Penlight light source. **(b)** A Finoff ocular transilluminator (Welch Allyn) can be used to provide a white light source or a cobalt blue filter can be attached to provide a blue light source.

Technique
- The light source is used on its own or in conjunction with a magnifying lens
- It is better to conduct the examination in the dark, so as to minimise distracting reflections
- The information obtained from light source examination is enhanced when the light is shone from a number of different angles

Magnification
Magnification can be achieved using an otoscope with the speculum removed (Figure 1.3(a)), a convex lens, a loupe (e.g. simple monocular magnifying glass or binocular loupe), a slit lamp biomicroscope or a direct ophthalmoscope (see below). Magnification, combined with a light source, is ideal for detailed examination of the adnexa (eyelids, lacrimal apparatus, orbit and para-orbital areas), anterior segment (anterior part of the globe, up to and including the lens) and posterior segment (lens, vitreous and fundus).
- A slit lamp biomicroscope (Figure 1.3(b)) is an essential purchase for those with a serious interest in ophthalmology, but cost is the major limiting factor for those in general practice
- Both portable and table mounted types of slit lamp are available. The advantages of portable, cordless models for veterinary ophthalmology are obvious

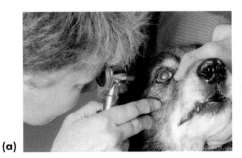 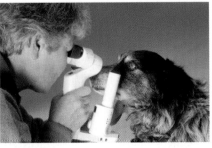

(a) (b)

Figure 1.3 **(a)** An otoscope (Welch Allyn) with the speculum removed provides a simple means of magnification. **(b)** A slit lamp biomicroscope is the best instrument available for examination of the anterior segment.

Lens

- A lens is a device that refracts (bends) light, and the vergence (bending) power is measured in dioptres (D). A convex, magnifying (plus) lens causes convergence of incident light, whereas a concave, reducing (minus) lens causes divergence of incident light.
- The focal length of a lens is directly proportional to its curvature radius, so that a lens of high curvature has a shorter focal length, and is more powerful, than a lens of longer focal length. A strong convex lens (high plus) produces a small, bright image whereas a weaker convex lens (lower plus) produces a larger, less bright image.
- Lenses of 10D or 15D can be used to aid examination of the adnexa and anterior segment. Lenses of 20D–40D can be used for indirect ophthalmoscopy. Lenses of 60D–90D are also available and usually used in conjunction with a slit lamp for fundus examination.

Indirect ophthalmoscopy

Commercially-manufactured monocular and binocular types are available, but are expensive. A penlight, or Finoff transilluminator, and condensing (convex) lens may be combined to provide an inexpensive means of performing monocular indirect ophthalmoscopy and this is probably the technique of choice for those in general practice.

Monocular indirect ophthalmoscopy
Optics

- If a convex (plus) lens is held in front of the eye, an aerial image of the fundus can be seen. This technique is known as indirect ophthalmoscopy, because the examiner is not observing the fundus directly.
- The image obtained is virtual, inverted, reversed left-to-right and magnified. The field of view (the area of the fundus that can be seen at any one time) is greater, albeit with less magnification, than can be obtained with a direct ophthalmoscope. Dilating the pupil will enlarge the field of view, irrespective of whether indirect or direct ophthalmoscopy is used.
- Indirect ophthalmoscopy is useful when the ocular media are opaque as it provides better penetration of partially-opaque eyes than direct ophthalmoscopy. It is not affected by major refractive errors in the patient's eyes.

Equipment

- Penlight: Any type of penlight or transilluminator, or even a small torch with narrow beam of light, will be adequate. The light source should be bright. Focussing ability is valuable, but not essential.
- Indirect lens and penlight (Figure 1.4(a)): In most domestic mammals, a 2.2 pan retinal® lens (Volk) or a 20D convex lens are the most versatile. The pan retinal® 2.2 is particularly valuable as it combines magnification of 2.68× – nearly that of the 20D lens (image magnification 3.13×, field of view 46°), with a field of view of 56° – almost that of a 30D lens. A 30D lens (image magnification 2.15×, field of view 58°) or 40D lens (image magnification 1.67×, field of view 69°) may be used if the eye or pupil is relatively small (e.g. puppies).

- Indirect lens and slit lamp biomicroscope: A 60D lens (image magnification 1.15×, field of view 68°) and a 90D lens (image magnification 0.76×, field of view 74°) are valuable for examination of small eyes and pupils, but their use may be regarded as specialist because they are best used in conjunction with slit lamp biomicroscopy.
- Commercially-manufactured monocular indirect ophthalmoscopes (lens and light source in one instrument) are also available and have the advantage that they are simple to use and the image viewed is upright (Figure 1.4(b)). Models of this type are useful for the widely varying conditions under which ophthalmoscopy is performed in large animal ophthalmology.

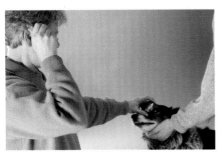

(a)

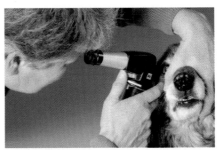

(b)

Figure 1.4 Indirect ophthalmoscopy. The technique is performed in the dark and is most rewarding when the pupil is dilated. **(a)** Monocular indirect ophthalmoscopy using a condensing lens and penlight. **(b)** Monocular indirect ophthalmoscopy using an American Optical monocular indirect ophthalmoscope. **(c)** Binocular indirect ophthalmoscopy using a Keeler all pupil model.

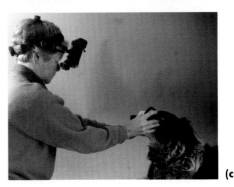

(c)

Technique using penlight and condensing lens
- Mydriasis (tropicamide 1%) is required for complete examination
- A darkened room is necessary for proper examination
- The condensing lens is held between forefinger and thumb, some 2–8 cm from the patient's eye and it is usual to steady the hand holding the lens by resting the little finger and ring finger against the animal's head
- The light source is held close to the observer's head; the observer–patient distance is approximately 50–75 cm
- The observer's eye, the light source, the lens and the patient's pupil should all lie in the same axis. It is easier to achieve this in small animals if the person holding the animal's head elevates the nose slightly

- The lens can be held close to the eye initially and then gradually moved away from the eye until the image fills the lens. The correct distance of the lens from the eye is soon learned

Binocular indirect ophthalmoscopy
- The technique is as for monocular indirect ophthalmoscopy, but with the advantage that the examiner has a free hand, as the ophthalmoscope is head mounted, so that it is easier to position the patient (Figure 1.4(c))
- Spectacle models are probably most comfortable for extended use, but there are many models available
- Binocular indirect ophthalmoscopy has the real benefit of stereopsis (i.e. depth perception) and many models also incorporate a teaching mirror
- Cost is a limiting factor

Direct ophthalmoscopy
The correct choice of instrument is crucial and it is better to purchase a well-designed, robust ophthalmoscope that will last for years, rather than compromise on quality. It is sensible to purchase a model that can be used with other devices, such as the Finoff transilluminator and otoscope.

Optics
- The image obtained is real (examined directly), erect and magnified; the field of view is small, at only some 6°
- The instrument's optical properties are affected by refractive errors in the patient's eyes

Equipment
- A suitable instrument has an on/off switch and rheostat, a lens magazine and lens indicator window, a range of apertures (e.g. large and small diameter round, round with graticule, slit beam) and both white light and red-free (green) light
- The lens range is approximately +30D (magnifying lenses) to −30D (reducing lenses). Most of the reducing lenses are not needed in veterinary ophthalmology
- A darkened room is needed for detailed examination
- Mydriasis (tropicamide 1%) is helpful, as it will increase the field of view

Distant direct ophthalmoscopy (Figure 1.5(a,b))
Technique
- Distant direct ophthalmoscopy utilises an observer–patient distance of 25–40 cm and usually a 0 setting.
- The direct ophthalmoscope is ergonomically designed to provide a close 'orbital fit' for the examiner and should always be held as close to the observer's eye as possible.
- Spectacle wearers (i.e. those with refractive errors) should remove their spectacles and set the prescription of the relevant spectacle lens in the lens aperture of the direct ophthalmoscope. The observer's eye should be placed as close to the viewing aperture of the ophthalmoscope as possible in order to maximise the field of view.

- Distant direct ophthalmoscopy may be used to compare the direction of gaze and pupil size (symmetry of gaze, symmetry of pupil size). In addition, any opacities present in the ocular media (cornea, aqueous, lens, vitreous) will appear as black forms against the fundus reflex (the reflection from the back of the eye), so this is a useful screening device prior to close direct ophthalmoscopy.
- It is a useful way of distinguishing senile nuclear sclerosis of the lens (concentric dark rings) from cataract (black opacity).
- The colour of the fundus reflex varies according to the colour of the tapetum.

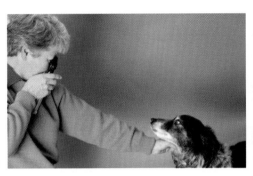 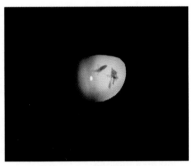

(a)   (b)

Figure 1.5(a,b) Distant direct ophthalmoscopy. With the ophthalmoscope (Welch Allyn) at arm's length from the animal, both the eyes can be viewed simultaneously and compared to check the direction of ocular gaze and the symmetry of pupil size and shape (a). In addition, any true opacities of the ocular media will appear as dark, even black, silhouettes by retro-illumination (b), as illustrated here in relation to lens opacities.

Close direct ophthalmoscopy (Figure 1.6(a,b))

- The direct ophthalmoscope is used for fundus examination (image magnification 15×) as well as to provide a magnified illuminated view of other ocular and adnexal features. Image magnification is markedly reduced (to approximately 2× for external ocular features) as the plane of focus moves anteriorly.
- The slit beam is useful for examination of the anterior chamber if aqueous flare is a possibility and is also helpful when examining the fundus for potential elevations (e.g. retinal detachments, papilloedema) or depressions (e.g. papillary and peri-papillary colobomas).
- Red-free (green) light will enhance contrast. It can help to distinguish resolving retinal haemorrhage from normal retinal pigment and will also allow the depth of conjunctival, episcleral and scleral blood vessels to be more readily differentiated.
- The graticule provides an approximate means of measuring the area of a lesion. When sequential measurements are made it is easiest to compare the lesion with something of fixed diameter, providing it is normal, in order to check whether the lesion is static, enlarging or reducing. The optic nerve head (optic disc) is most commonly used as a fixed reference point for retinal and choroidal lesions.
- It is also possible to obtain approximate measurements of the height and depth of gross lesions by making use of the fact that a difference of focus of one dioptre represents a difference of level of 0.3–0.4 mm.

OPHTHALMIC EQUIPMENT AND EXAMINATION

(a)

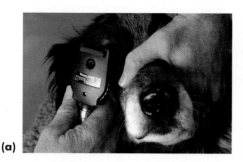

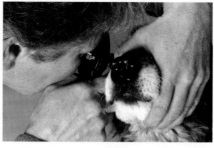

(b)

Figure 1.6(a,b) Close direct ophthalmoscopy. It is sometimes easier to put the ophthalmoscope (Welch Allyn) in the correct position first (a) before attempting to view the ocular fundus (b). Note how close the instrument is to the animal and that the observer's fingers are resting against the animal's head.

Technique
- If the observer is emmetropic (normal vision), a 0 setting is most commonly used when examining the fundus. Spectacle wearers should remove their spectacles and set the prescription of the relevant spectacle lens in the lens aperture of the direct ophthalmoscope.
- It is crucial to keep the light intensity as *low* as possible, especially when the tapetum is highly reflective, as in the normal cat or any animal in which retinal thinning results in hyperreflectivity.
- Note that fundus examination can detect areas that are thickened or raised (appear dull) and areas that are thinner than usual (appear hyperreflective).
- Ideally, the observer's right eye is used to examine the animal's right eye and the observer's left eye is used to examine the animal's left eye.
- The instrument is placed close to the subject's eye and steadied against the animal's head with the middle and ring fingers. The field of view becomes larger as the distance between the observer and subject decreases, so the maximum available field of view is obtained with the observer as close as possible to the subject's eye.
- Fundus examination is straightforward if the ophthalmoscope has been positioned correctly and the light from the instrument is shining through the subject's pupil *before* the observer's eye is brought as close as possible to the viewing aperture. Thus the ophthalmoscope is correctly aligned and in place before the observer attempts to look at the fundus.
- Once the fundus has been examined, the ophthalmoscope can be used for examination of more anterior features, although it is easier to use other magnifying devices (e.g. loupe, otoscope, slit lamp) for examination of the anterior segment. The ophthalmoscope is kept in the same position as before, close to the eye, and the lens diaphragm rotated clockwise in order to move up through the lenses (usually from 0 to +20).
- As the observer increases the strength of the plus lenses, the focus of observation gradually extends anteriorly, so the magnified details of the fundus, vitreous, lens, iris, aqueous, cornea and lids are successively visualised.
- The approximate settings (±5D) required when the ophthalmoscope is placed 2 cm

from the patient are: eyelids and ocular surface +15 to +20; anterior chamber and iris +14 to +12; lens +12 to +8; fundus 0. When the ocular media (vitreous, lens, aqueous humour and cornea) are clear, as in the normal eye, it will not be easy to focus on essentially transparent structures.

EXAMINATION

PROTOCOL

- The protocol seeks to provide a logical order of examination; it is usual to proceed from external to internal, so that the fundus is examined last (Figure 1.7)
- Both eyes and their adnexa should be examined
- Note that whilst the examination protocol is standard not every diagnostic procedure will be required on each patient
- Most ophthalmic examinations in domestic animals are best performed in the minimally-restrained, conscious, non-sedated animal
- Ophthalmic examination can be summarised as 'hands off' in the light, then 'hands on' in the light without any aids other than magnification. Examination in the light is followed by examination in the dark, using first a light source and magnification and second ophthalmoscopy, both indirect and direct
- It is important to make careful drawings of any abnormalities detected: meticulous recording encourages proper examination. Photography is also of value. Sequential recording provides an accurate record of the disease process and response to treatment

OPHTHALMIC EXAMINATION

Animal's Name .... Date of Examination .... Reference Number(s) ....

Owner's Name, Address and Telephone Number ....

....

....

Referring Veterinary Surgeon ....

Species .... Breed .... Age .... Sex .... Weight ....

Primary complaint ....

General examination ....

Ophthalmic examination ....

Diagnosis..

Examination technique: Mydriatic Yes ☐ No☐: Penlight Yes ☐ No☐: Magnification Yes ☐ No☐:
                          Slit lamp biomicroscopy Yes☐ No☐: Indirect ophthalmoscopy Yes ☐ No☐
                          Direct ophthalmoscopy – Distant Yes ☐ No ☐: Close Yes ☐ No ☐

Diagnostic tests: Schirmer Tear Test Yes☐ No☐ STT I right .... left .... [STT II ....]
                          Scrape Yes ☐ No ☐: Swab Yes ☐ No ☐: Culture Yes ☐ No ☐:
                          Impression smear Yes☐ No☐: Cytology Yes☐ No☐: Biopsy Yes☐ No☐
                          Tonometry Yes☐ No☐ IOP right ...... IOP left ...... Gonioscopy Yes☐ No☐
                          Diagnostic imaging .... ERG ··

Ophthalmic examination	Right	Left	Illustrations and comments
Orbit and periorbita			
Eyelids			
Lacrimal system			
Conjunctiva			
Limbus, episclera, sclera			
Cornea			
Anterior chamber			
Drainage angle			
Iris and pupil			
Lens			
Vitreous			
Fundus			
Neurological examination			
Vision			
Palpebral/corneal reflexes			
PLR and related responses			

Figure 1.7 Record of ophthalmic examination. The columns marked right and left eye can be marked with a simple tick (normal) or cross (abnormal) and further comments added under 'Illustrations and comments'. Such examination forms can have diagrams of the eye as part of the form and abnormalities noted can be added to these. However, when different species are examined it is often more accurate to make line drawings of the eye and its abnormalities for each case.

BASIC TECHNIQUE OF PATIENT EXAMINATION

- *Careful observation* of the whole patient (without handling), can usefully be done whilst taking the history
- *Physical examination* of the whole patient
- *Neuro-ophthalmological examination* ± full neurological examination if indicated (see Appendix 4, pp 353–355)
- *Ophthalmic examination* of both eyes and their adnexa

Box 1.1 Basic principles of routine ophthalmic examination

1 Always examine *both* eyes in light *and* darkness and always look *internally* as well as *externally*
2 Under *normal lighting* conditions perform a 'hands off' assessment initially (naked eye) and then a 'hands on' examination of the adnexa and external eye (magnification may be essential)
3 Basic neuro-ophthalmological tests performed in the light: oculovestibular reflex, menace and visual tracking responses, palpebral and corneal reflexes
4 Under conditions of *darkness* check for ocular symmetry and examine the internal eye:
   ○ Symmetry of gaze, pupil size and shape and opacities in the ocular media – distant direct ophthalmoscopy
   ○ Anterior segment (external eye to lens) – light source ± magnification
   ○ Posterior segment (vitreous to fundus) – indirect and close direct ophthalmoscopy
5 Basic neuro-ophthalmological tests performed in the dark: pupillary light reflex, swinging flashlight test, dazzle reflex and visual tracking using a beam of light
6 Perform relevant diagnostic tests (see text) after completing the routine examination
7 If unsure seek advice – do not adopt a 'wait and see' approach

---

Neuro-ophthalmological examination
Vision testing

- Menace response of each eye in turn, with the other eye covered. A threatening gesture should be made, without touching the patient or creating air turbulence in order to elicit a protective blink. The pathway for this learned response involves the optic nerve (II) as the afferent arm, central cerebral and cerebellar interconnections and the facial nerve (VII) as the efferent arm.
- Fixating response associated with visual tracking using, for example, cotton wool balls dropped from a height, or the fine beam of a penlight playing upon surfaces; the latter method is more effective under dim or dark light conditions.
- Visual placing reaction. Small animals can be carried towards an object that they can see, such as a table surface. Normal animals approaching a table in front of them will reach towards the table before their carpal region reaches the edge of the

table. Peripheral vision can be assessed by approaching the table from the side. Large animals can be led towards a kerbstone, step or similar.

- Maze test, for example, negotiating in a strange environment or in a maze constructed of haphazardly placed obstacles under both normal light and dim lighting conditions. Blindfolding allows each eye to be assessed in turn.

Pupillary light reflex (PLR), swinging flashlight test and dazzle reflex

- A bright light shone into one eye causes both pupils to constrict (positive direct and consensual response). The pathway for the reflex is subcortical and involves the optic nerve (II) as the afferent arm and parasympathetic fibres in the oculomotor nerve (III) as the efferent arm. The afferent fibres cross in the optic chiasma and pretectum to influence both oculomotor nerve nuclei. Iris sphincter-muscle function must also be normal for the PLR to be normal. It is usual for initial pupillary constriction to be followed by a slight redilation, this phenomenon is termed 'pupillary escape' and is due to light adaptation of the photoreceptors.
- If the light source is moved rapidly from one eye to the other (swinging flashlight test), a direct response can be observed in the first eye and a consensual response in the fellow eye in the normal animal. The fellow eye will then remain constricted while the light is focussed upon it (direct pupillary response).
- The dazzle reflex provides some indication of retinal and optic nerve function, as well as that of the facial nerve. A bright light (preferably a halogen light source) shone into the eye along the visual axis should elicit a rapid blink. The pathway for the reflex is subcortical and involves the optic nerve (II) as the afferent arm, rostral colliculus, subcortical connections and the facial nerve (VII) as the efferent arm.

Reflex pupillary dilation

If the animal is placed in a darkened room for some 30 seconds, reflex pupillary dilation occurs. The afferent arm is the optic nerve (II) and the efferent arm is reduced parasympathetic tone to the pupillary constrictor muscle leaving the actions of the dilator muscle, which is under sympathetic control, unopposed.

Palpebral and corneal reflexes

These reflexes are used to test sensory innervation to the periocular skin, eyelids (palpebrae) and cornea. The afferent arm is the ophthalmic branch of the trigeminal nerve (V₁) and the efferent arm for the palpebral reflex is the facial nerve (VII) – the normal response is a rapid blink. The efferent arm for the corneal reflex is the facial nerve and the abducens nerve (VI) – the normal response is a rapid blink and retraction of the globe (*retractor bulbi* muscle) with an indirect mechanical effect that causes protrusion of the third eyelid (nictitating reflex).

Oculovestibular reflex

If the animal's head is moved in different directions, both eyes tend to maintain their original direction of gaze. The eyes move slowly in the opposite direction to the movement and then, under the influence of the vestibular system, flick rapidly in the direction of the movement. In normal animals the eyes move in unison and the physiological nystagmus ceases as soon as the head movements stop.

STAGES OF OPHTHALMIC EXAMINATION

Daylight or artificial light (naked eye ± basic magnification)
Adnexa (eyelids, lacrimal apparatus, orbit, para-orbital areas)
- Note eye size, symmetry, position and movement
- Observe and palpate the supra-orbital fossa in horses
- Palpate the incomplete, bony, orbital rim and orbital ligament of cat and dog and the complete, bony, orbital rim of horses and farm animals (e.g. cattle, sheep and pig)
- Check normal blink (adequacy and rate) and protective blink (e.g. menace response and palpebral reflex)
- Check apposition of the eyelids to the globe (so-called 'congruity')
- Note direction of the upper eyelid lashes in dogs, horses and farm animals
- Observe presence, position and size of the lacrimal puncta
- Check for presence of the nasal ostium in horses and cattle
- Check for presence and position of the third eyelid

Globe
- Note the appearance of the ocular surface. In the presence of tear film dysfunction or ocular surface disease there will be disruption of the corneal light reflex (the reflection of a light source on the cornea)
- Decide what diagnostic tests will be needed if the ocular surface is abnormal
- Carry out a brief preview examination of the 'white' of the eye (bulbar conjunctiva, episclera and sclera), limbus, cornea, anterior chamber, pupil, iris and lens

Darkness (light source ± magnification or slit lamp biomicroscope)
- Perform detailed examination of bulbar conjunctiva, episclera and sclera; note colour, thickness, blood vessels and degree of pigmentation
- Examine the limbus, note its definition and degree of pigmentation and the disposition of any blood vessels
- Examine the cornea, note its lustre and clarity, the presence and position (including depth) of any opacities, the presence and depth of any blood vessels; decide whether further diagnostic tests will be required
- In horses, note the grey zones (medial and lateral cornea) which mark the insertion of pectinate ligaments into the posterior cornea
- Observe the depth and transparency of the anterior chamber, note the position and colour of any opacities. Focal illumination from a number of different angles is rewarding
- Examine the filtration angle of cats and horses by direct inspection; in dogs a gonioscopy lens is used for this purpose at a later stage of examination if required
- Note the appearance, position and stability of the iris. Pay particular attention to the pupillary margin and note whether it is regular or irregular in outline, observe the *granula iridica* present in herbivores
- For comprehensive examination of the lens, vitreous and fundus mydriasis is essential and a mydriatic may be applied to the eye once other diagnostic tests have been completed

- Observe the position and clarity of the lens; localise any lens opacities; in old dogs, note whether the pearly grey opalescence of nuclear sclerosis of the lens is obvious to the naked eye
- Examine the vitreous, noting whether any opacities are present

Darkness (direct and indirect ophthalmoscopy)

- Examine the ocular fundus using indirect ophthalmoscopy, followed by direct ophthalmoscopy
- Distant direct ophthalmoscopy is used as a screening method for symmetry of gaze, equality of pupil size and shape, identification of opacities in the ocular media and the distinction of cataract and senile nuclear sclerosis of the lens – cataract appears as a dark, often black, silhouette, while nuclear sclerosis does not
- With indirect and close direct ophthalmoscopy, note the appearance of the optic nerve and immediate peripapillary area, the retinal vasculature, choroidal vasculature, tapetal fundus (when present) and non-tapetal fundus
- If haemorrhage is suspected on fundus examination, use the red-free light option on the direct ophthalmoscope to enhance colour contrast between pigment and haemorrhage
- If depressions or elevations are suspected on fundus examination (e.g. papillary or peripapillary coloboma, papilloedema) the slit beam option on the direct ophthalmoscope can be used to aid confirmation

Order of diagnostic tests

The order in which appropriate diagnostic tests might be performed after initial ophthalmic examination. Those tests placed in parentheses are not performed as part of routine assessment.

- *(Corneal sensitivity measurement)* – This measurement can be approximated by using a fine wisp of cotton wool touched on the cornea from the side, a blink should be elicited.
- *Schirmer tear test* (STT) to check production of the aqueous portion of the tear film: STT I must be performed *before* any preparations are applied to the eye (STT II is less commonly performed). This test is illustrated later in Section 3, pp 96–97.
- *(pH of conjunctival sac)* – A pH paper is placed in the lower conjunctival sac for a few seconds. In normal animals, the pH of the conjunctival sac is on the alkaline side of normal. This is a useful test if chemical injury is known or suspected.
- *Eyelid or conjunctival swabs and scrapes* (may be taken without using local anaesthetic): A pre-moistened (e.g. with culture medium) sterile swab is rolled against the palpebral conjunctiva of the ventral fornix – usually from about the centre of the eyelid medially so that the third eyelid prevents inadvertent corneal damage (Figure 1.8).
- *Corneal scrapes and swabs* require prior application of a topical local anaesthetic, usually proxymetacaine hydrochloride 0.5% (Figure 1.9). It is important to ensure that the whole area is sampled, especially the peripheral part of the ulcer, as this is where organisms may be replicating (Figure 1.10).
- *Smears* can be made using clean, dry, glass slides (similar technique to that for haematology preparations). The slides are air dried, usually fixed in alcohol and then stained (e.g. Gram stain).
- *Fluorescein sodium* is an orange solution that changes to green in alkaline condi-

tions and fluoresces in blue light. Fluorescein should be applied *after* swabs or scrapes have been taken. Fluorescein 1% or 2% is most commonly used to delineate corneal ulcers. A 2% solution is best used to check for aqueous leakage (Seidel test). Topical fluorescein application as part of diagnostic tests is illustrated in Sections 2, 3, 4, 6 and 7.

- *Rose bengal* is a dark red solution which is not widely used in veterinary medicine as it is irritant to the eye. It is a vital stain, and will be taken up by exposed cells with inadequate mucin cover. Rose bengal is of value in the study of ocular-surface disease, dry-eye syndromes and ulcerative keratitis. Topical rose bengal can be used after topical fluorescein and is illustrated in the equine Section 7, p. 289.

- *Tests* that might be used to investigate nasolacrimal drainage include application of fluorescein 1% to demonstrate patency of the nasolacrimal drainage system, cannulation, irrigation, dacryocystorhinography and catheterisation of the whole system.

- *(Tonometry)* – Topical local anaesthetic should be applied to the cornea if the intraocular pressure is to be measured by contact tonometry (e.g. Schiøtz, Mackay-Marg or TonoPen®). The Schiøtz and TonoPen® tonometers are those most commonly used in veterinary practice (Figure 1.11(a,b)).

- *(Gonioscopy)* – In the dog, particularly, the iridocorneal (drainage) angle can only be examined using a gonioscopy lens (specialist procedure). Topical local anaesthetic should be applied to the cornea prior to the procedure.

- *Biopsy samples*, including needle aspirates, would be taken after other routine diagnostic tests (amethocaine hydrochloride, applied for some 30 seconds by direct contact using a cotton-tipped applicator, is normally selected if the sample is to be taken under topical anaesthesia).

- A mydriatic may be applied after routine diagnostic tests and gonioscopy have been completed. Tropicamide 1% takes about 15 minutes to dilate the pupil in adult animals. In dogs and cats the effects last for up to three hours and rather longer than this in most farm animals and horses.

- Any other diagnostic drugs that affect the pupil (e.g. phenylephrine or pilocarpine) should be applied after the ophthalmic examination and once other diagnostic tests have been completed.

- *(Electrophysiological tests)* – The electroretinogram is the most commonly applied test and is used to assess retinal function, especially in cases of sudden blindness or as part of cataract patient assessment (specialist procedure).

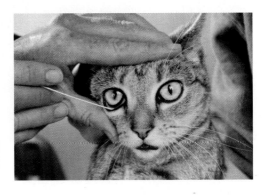

Figure 1.8 Taking a conjunctival swab from the ventromedial conjunctival sac of a cat.

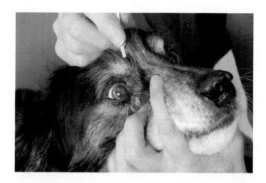

Figure 1.9 Application of topical local anaesthetic to the eye. The hand holding the drops is steadied by resting it on the animal's head.

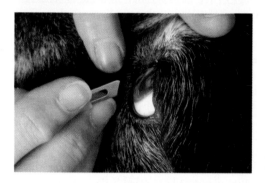

Figure 1.10 The blunt (handle) end of a disposable scalpel blade can be used to obtain a corneal scrape.

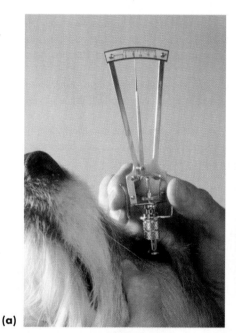

(a)

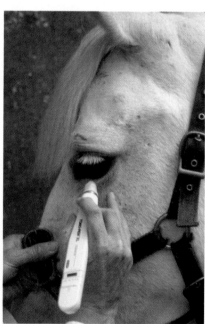

(b)

Figure 1.11(a,b) Tonometry using a Schiøtz tonometer in a dog (a) and a TonoPen® in a horse (b).

Record keeping (Figure 1.7, p. 12)
- Accurate recording (using simple line drawings as part of the clinical record or employing a standard ophthalmic examination form)
- Photography

SECTION 2
OPHTHALMIC EMERGENCIES AND TRAUMA

INTRODUCTION

An emergency is an unexpected event requiring immediate action. In all the examples listed below in Box 2.1, prompt and correct action will offer the best chance of full recovery at least cost to the client. The severity of the situation must be assessed as accurately as possible at the *first examination*, otherwise the best opportunity to restore normality is lost. Management options include *referral* to a specialist veterinary ophthalmologist if the facilities of the practice are inadequate or the expertise of the staff is insufficient to cope with the problem.

Box 2.1 Ophthalmic emergencies

- Acute exophthalmos including globe prolapse (globe prolapse commonest in dog)
- Orbital inflammation – abscess and cellulitis (all species, but commonest in dog)
- Foreign bodies (all species)
- Gross trauma to globe and/or adnexa (all species)
- Complicated corneal ulceration and corneal infection (all species)
- Thermal and chemical injuries (all species)
- Acute uveitis (mainly dog and horse)
- Acute glaucoma (mainly dog, but other species can be affected)
- Sudden loss of vision (all species)
- Sudden onset of ocular pain (all species)

There are some general rules that are common to all species, of which meticulous examination of the eyes and the rest of the animal is the most important, followed by the ability to decide, at an early stage, the most appropriate course of action, including prioritisation of the clinical findings (Figure 2.1(a,b)). Sedation and local nerve blocks are helpful in the assessment of large-animal ocular emergencies and, sometimes, examination under general anaesthesia will be required at an early stage of assessment in all species. Topical local anaesthesia may be a useful adjunct to ocular examination and may also be used to reduce the amount of general anaesthetic required in patients under general anaesthesia, but it should not be used as part of any treatment regime. Systemic analgesia is helpful for both the examination and subsequent management of many ophthalmic emergencies. Indwelling lavage devices will make treatment of large animals with painful eyes very much easier and, certainly, more precise. For periocular and ocular insults in herbivores, and for some deep penetrating injuries in carnivores, prophylactic tetanus treatment should be administered.

When intraocular surgery is required it is assumed that it will be performed under general anaesthesia and a brief resumé of routine general anaesthesia is outlined in Appendix 3. For extraocular and adnexal surgery the anaesthetic techniques that may be selected are mentioned briefly in the text. Similar considerations apply to surgical procedures outlined in other sections of the book.

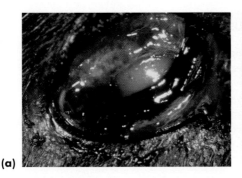
(a)
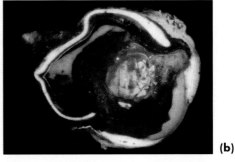
(b)

Figure 2.1(a,b) Gross appearance (a) and section (b) of a ruptured globe (with acknowledgements to J.R.B. Mould).

ACUTE EXOPHTHALMOS (PROPTOSIS)

The differential diagnosis of acute exophthalmos or proptosis (forward displacement of the globe) is not always easy, as the location of the underlying abnormality can be periorbital, orbital or a combination of both and, on occasion, there may also be globe involvement. Causes include trauma, periorbital and orbital infection, inflammation, abscessation and haemorrhage. Rarely, aggressive tumour growth with neoplastic infiltration can also present acutely. The commonest causes of orbital neoplasia are outlined later.

TRAUMATIC GLOBE PROPTOSIS AND PROLAPSE

Traumatic globe proptosis and globe prolapse (dislocation of the globe beyond the plane of the eyelids) are usually the result of direct impact to the eye, orbit or periorbita, but can also be associated with head and neck injuries. Adnexal, subconjunctival and orbital haemorrhage are common accompaniments; the latter may dissect anteriorly beneath the conjunctiva.

Acute proptosis
In cases of acute proptosis, provided that the globe is retained within the orbit and within the plane of the eyelids, treatment is conservative and consists of ocular lubrication to protect the cornea, systemic analgesics and restricted activity. Early application to the periocular region of an ice pack wrapped in a towel may help to reduce periocular swelling. Emergency *tarsorrhaphy* (suturing the upper and lower eyelids together) to provide effective tamponade is sometimes needed if progressive proptosis occurs as a result of, for example, continuing retrobulbar haemorrhage. Possible complications of extensive haemorrhage include an increase of intraocular pressure (IOP) and optic nerve compression because of the high intraorbital pressure.

Globe prolapse (Figure 2.2(a,b))
Globe prolapse is commoner in dogs than other species and in commoner brachycephalic dogs with a shallow orbit. It may sometimes occur if the animal is not handled

properly, especially if the dog is manipulated by the scruff of the neck. The Persian cat is unusual amongst cat breeds in having a relatively shallow orbit. Globe prolapse is rarer and more serious in non-brachycephalic dogs and other species because more force will be required to dislocate the globe from a deeper orbit. The prognosis for normal vision in the long term is always guarded because traction damage to the optic nerve often results in Wallerian degeneration and eventual optic atrophy. Fewer than 50% of dogs retain vision in the long term and in cats almost 100% will be left with a blind eye. Avulsion of extraocular muscles (especially the medial rectus muscle) and nerve damage are common, so the animal is sometimes left with a squint.

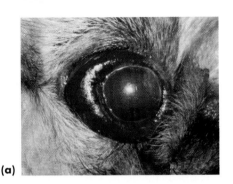 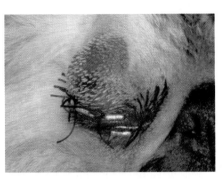

(a)   (b)

Figure 2.2(a,b) Globe prolapse of the right eye in a Pekingese following direct trauma to the head from a kick. The zygoma was also fractured. The clinical presentation of this 'red eye' is a combination of subconjunctival haemorrhage and venous congestion – the latter because the eyelids have gone into spasm behind the globe equator, resulting in impeded venous return (a). Following restoration of the prolapsed globe to the orbit, the lateral canthotomy was closed and the upper and lower eyelids were sutured together (b). Three horizontal mattress sutures of 4-0 silk were laid, with vertical entry through the lower eyelid skin, via the lower and upper eyelid margins and upper eyelid skin, horizontally through hollow silastic tubes and then vertically back to emerge from the lower eyelid skin. The sutures do not penetrate the full thickness of the eyelids. The position of all the sutures should be checked before they are tied, incorporating additional horizontal hollow silastic tubes for each lower eyelid suture. The aim of the temporary tarsorrhaphy is to provide good ocular surface protection whilst ensuring that that the suture tension is spread so that there is no possibility of inadvertent abrasion to the underlying cornea.

Diagnosis of globe prolapse

- This is straightforward and can usually be made from the owner's description
- History may be helpful (e.g. road traffic accidents and fighting) or unhelpful (e.g. genuinely unknown and non-accidental injury)
- Check for and prioritise any other injuries present (i.e. may need to stabilise the patient before attending to the eye)
- Assessment of potential ocular damage (e.g. globe rupture) can be aided by ultrasonography

Treatment

- Speed is of the essence, so the animal should be seen immediately. The owner may be able to prevent further damage, notably corneal and conjunctival desiccation, by gently applying pressure to the region with soft material such as a clean tea towel or cotton handkerchief that has been soaked in water. This action sometimes restores the globe to the orbit in brachycephalic dogs, but the owner should still seek rapid veterinary attention.

- Very soon after prolapse has occurred the eyelids go into spasm behind the equator of the globe making reduction more difficult and adding to the oedema and marked vascular congestion (redness) which are a rapid consequence of this problem (Figure 2.2(a)). Once this situation is reached it may be impossible to reposition the globe without general anaesthesia.

- Provided other injuries permit, and the optic nerve remains intact, general anaesthesia is performed without delay. Following application of ophthalmic ointment with an oily excipient (e.g. fucidic acid gel or chloramphenicol ointment), the eye is repositioned by gently easing the eyelids over the globe (*not* by simply attempting to force the eye back into the orbit). It is often sensible to perform a generous lateral canthotomy before attempting this manoeuvre if swelling is marked. If the globe has been completely dislocated from the orbit and the optic nerve avulsed, then it is better to remove the globe.

- Once the eye is back in the orbit it should be retained in place by temporary tarsorrhaphy (Figure 2.2(b)). The upper and lower lids are sewn together using approximately three horizontal mattress sutures of non-absorbable soft material such as 3-0 to 4-0 silk. These are preplaced so as to avoid contact between the sutures and the globe. Stents, made from, for example, silastic tubing are used to support the horizontal passage of the sutures as they are often under considerable tension. If a lateral canthotomy has been performed it is closed after the tarsorrhaphy has been completed.

- If there are no contraindications, the patient is usually given a single dose of corticosteroid (e.g. dexamethasone) at the time of surgery and a 7–10 day course of systemic antibiotic. The sutures are removed (following topical local anaesthesia) after 14 days. A lateral squint (because of avulsion of the medial rectus muscle) may be obvious at the time of the prolapse, but is more likely to be observed when the tarsorrhaphy is taken down.

ORBITAL INFLAMMATION

The origins of *orbital cellulitis* and *orbital abscess* may be identical, and both can be a cause of proptosis. Orbital cellulitis is typified by diffuse inflammation, whereas a retrobulbar abscess (orbital abscess) is characterised by localised inflammation. Other less common causes of orbital inflammation include acute *inflammation of the lacrimal (dacryoadenitis)* or *zygomatic gland (sialoadenitis)*, acute *masticatory myositis* and acute *extraocular polymyositis*, all of which can present as acute exophthalmos. Dacryoadenitis and sialoadenitis may be associated with infection, in which case a course of systemic antibiotic is indicated. Anti-inflammatory therapy may also be required if the inflammation fails to respond to antibiotics. For acute masticatory myositis and acute extraocular polymyositis, immunosuppressive levels of systemic corticosteroids (prednisolone 2 mg/kg) are indicated initially and then slowly tapered off if there is a positive response.

RETROBULBAR (ORBITAL) ABSCESS

Clinical signs (Figure 2.3)
- Not uncommon; affected animals usually present with unexplained acute onset of ocular discomfort and they may be pyrexic
- A history of previous trauma, including fights and stick injuries, is helpful, but may be separated from the acute onset of clinical signs by days or weeks. Infections of the nose, mouth or sinuses also have the potential to involve the orbit
- Affected animals are often very reluctant to eat and there is invariably severe pain on attempting to open the mouth
- There is often marked conjunctival injection and a mucopurulent ocular discharge. Conjunctival oedema (chemosis) may also be present
- Exophthalmos, which is generally, but not invariably, axial (i.e. there is no associated squint). Ocular motility is usually restricted because of the space-occupying effect of the inflammation
- The third eyelid is prominent

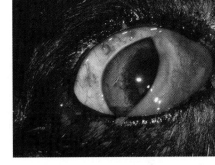

Figure 2.3 Retrobulbar abscess in a dog. Ocular redness, exophthalmos and third eyelid prominence are the most obvious clinical features, although a sparse ocular discharge was also present.

Additional investigations
- It is important to differentiate orbital inflammation from orbital neoplasia (see later)
- Routine haematology may indicate neutrophilia with a shift to the left
- Diagnostic imaging; ultrasonography with or without ultrasound-guided needle biopsy can be helpful. Computed tomography (CT) and magnetic resonance imaging (MRI) are less frequently employed in the diagnosis of inflammatory orbital disease
- Careful examination of the oral cavity under general anaesthesia: redness, a soft, fluctuating swelling or a draining tract behind the last upper molar tooth may be present

Treatment of retrobulbar abscess
- Systemic analgesia will be required while the animal is in pain, whichever course of action is adopted.
- A retrobulbar abscess consists of a localised or loculated abscess that can be treated with a course of broad-spectrum systemic antibiotic (usually for three weeks

minimum) in all species. A combination of cephalexin (effective against aerobic bacteria) and metronidazole (effective against anaerobic bacteria) is normally selected.

- Abscess drainage is an alternative in *carnivores*, but *only* if there is obvious redness and a fluctuating swelling or a draining tract behind the last upper molar tooth. The animal is anaesthetised (an analgesic premedicant is sensible) and positioned with a head down tilt. A cuffed endotracheal tube (uncuffed e/t tube in the cat) is passed and the pharynx is packed with damp gauze bandage that can be secured to the endotracheal tube. The abscess is drained immediately posterior to the last upper molar tooth. A small nick is made in the mucous membrane with a scalpel and the actual probing of the region is best done with fine haemostats; sharp instruments should be avoided. Success is indicated when free drainage is established and pus or serosanguinous fluid is released. The material should be subjected to a smear for cytology, as well as culture and sensitivity, so that the correct choice of broad-spectrum systemic antibiotic is made. The wound is left open.

ORBITAL CELLULITIS

Orbital cellulitis is, strictly speaking, diffuse inflammation of structures posterior to the orbital septum, and is most commonly caused by infection. Orbital cellulitis is rare, but can be life threatening because of the proximity of the brain and meninges. Any infection involving the nose, mouth or sinuses has the potential to spread to the orbit, but occasionally there is extension from sites such as the pituitary gland (e.g. pituitary abscess) and *equine* guttural pouch. The most frequently identified causes include puncture wounds of the periorbita and eye, penetrating foreign bodies that migrate from the oral cavity and sinusitis. Actinobacillosis (*Actinobacillus lignieresii*) is a possible infectious cause in herbivores, *cattle* particularly.

Clinical signs
- Similar to those of retrobulbar abscess, but the periorbital swelling is more diffuse and there is often marked swelling of the eyelids and conjunctiva. Ocular motility may be restricted if the inflammation surrounds the globe
- The onset is usually sudden and exophthalmos can be a key presenting sign; third-eyelid prominence is not always present
- Painful and serious
- Pyrexia and anorexia may be present
- Leukocytosis can be marked

Diagnosis
- Diagnostic imaging can be helpful
- Needle aspiration or biopsy is required to provide material for culture and cytology or histology

Treatment of orbital cellulitis
- Any wound should be thoroughly cleaned and debrided; more radical excision may be required if there is a deep penetrating injury or tissue necrosis

- Hot compresses can be helpful
- A course of systemic antibiotic should be given as outlined above for a retrobulbar abscess and, ideally, selected on the basis of culture and sensitivity testing
- Exposed cornea and conjunctiva require protection with a bland ophthalmic lubricant, with or without antibiotic (e.g. chloramphenicol ointment), during the period of globe prominence
- Systemic analgesics will be required for as long as pain persists
- If the cellulitis is a consequence of a deep penetrating injury then prophylactic tetanus treatment should be administered

ORBITAL NEOPLASIA

Orbital neoplasia is an uncommon cause of acute exophthalmos as most types of orbital neoplasia are associated with a chronic time course. There is a wide range of possible tumour types and acute onset exophthalmos is usually associated with highly-malignant and invasive tumours or haemorrhage from such tumours. The origin of primary tumours is likely to be orbital or nasal, the latter invade the orbit via the thin medial orbital wall. Secondary tumours are often multifocal and the orbit is one of a number of sites involved. Multicentric lymphoma is the commonest secondary tumour to involve the orbit and affected *horses*, in particular, can present acutely. If refined diagnostic imaging techniques are not available, referral should be considered.

Diagnosis and differential diagnosis
- The classical signs of an orbital space-occupying lesion may be present (exophthalmos and third-eyelid prominence)
- In addition there may be some or all of globe deviation, resistance to globe retropulsion, vascular congestion, chemosis, ocular discharge, nasal discharge, reduced airflow from the nostrils, epistaxis and intraoral swelling
- Clinical signs may also be more generalised, particularly if the orbital involvement is indicative of metastatic spread
- Diagnostic imaging techniques (radiography, ultrasonography, computed tomography, magnetic resonance imaging) are key to establishing the location and extent of the tumour
- Accurate diagnosis invariably requires histological examination of biopsy material and allows management options to be defined more precisely

Management
- The prognosis for tumours associated with acute onset exophthalmos is guarded to grave
- The major treatment options are surgical removal, radiotherapy and chemotherapy, with or without sacrifice of the eye. The location and extent of most orbital tumours render the retention of a functional eye most unlikely if surgery is undertaken
- Such cases are best referred

FOREIGN BODIES

The majority of foreign bodies are associated with acute onset of ocular pain, ble-pharospasm and lacrimation. The history can be very helpful and careful examination often reveals the source of discomfort.

Clinical approach
- The history from the owner is usually typical and the onset can sometimes be related to specific events, like the last period of exercise or to factors in the animals' environment
- Careful examination of the eye, adnexa and periocular region is crucial
- It is usually sensible to examine the eye following topical application of local anaes-thetic (e.g. proxymetacaine hydrochloride 0.5%)
- In large animals, systemic sedation/analgesia and an auriculopalpebral (AP) nerve block will aid examination
- In some small animals, and occasionally in large animals, the eye is so painful that general anaesthesia should be selected at the outset
- Diagnostic imaging is an important part of clinical assessment (radiography, ultra-sonography and CT scanning)
- Magnetic resonance imaging must *not* be used if there is any possibility of magnetic foreign material (ferrous metals)

Clinical signs
- Acute discomfort, with excessive lacrimation, blepharospasm ± conjunctival oedema are the most common early clinical signs. If the foreign body is not identified and removed then the discharge may quickly become mucopurulent or haemorrhagic.
- The foreign body may be visible. However, if it is not immediately obvious a thor-ough examination of all aspects of the conjunctiva should be carried out, looking carefully under the upper and lower eyelids and beneath the third eyelid (see Section 3, pp 101–109 for the technique). The upper and lower puncta should be inspected. The cornea, limbus and 'white' of the eye should be examined minutely, followed by the internal ocular structures. Magnification is often required, particularly in, for example, small *rodents*.
- If no obvious cause is found then referral should be considered, particularly when the history is suggestive of a foreign body. It is not acceptable to adopt a wait and see approach as foreign bodies can migrate to less accessible sites, including within the eye.

INTRAOCULAR AND INTRAORBITAL FOREIGN BODIES

The history may be helpful, but in many cases there is no history and it is the pres-ence of a relatively innocuous wound to the periocular region or globe, or a change of ocular appearance, that prompts further investigation. Some foreign bodies, typically gunshot, will have penetrated and traversed the globe before they become embedded in the orbit. The entry wound in gunshot injuries is not always obvious in hairy animals and any unexplained periocular or ocular wound should prompt further investigation, including diagnostic imaging (e.g. ultrasonography).

Many foreign bodies are relatively inert (glass, high quality plastic, stone and high-quality alloys such as stainless steel) whereas others (organic material, low-grade plastic, iron, copper and low-quality alloys) are not well tolerated. Gunshot injuries are common in cats (usually non-accidental injury) and gun dogs (usually accidental injury).

Metallic foreign bodies that have travelled at high speed into the eye or orbit will generate a temperature high enough to sterilise the foreign body so that endophthalmitis is less likely (Figure 2.4(a–c)). In contrast, intraocular or orbital organic material may well provoke endophthalmitis or orbital cellulitis. Organic material may reach the orbit or eye directly (e.g. stake injuries from wood) or following migration from other sites, such as the conjunctival sac (e.g. grass seeds).

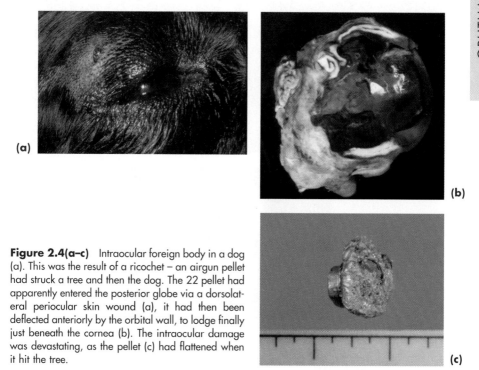

(a)

(b)

Figure 2.4(a–c) Intraocular foreign body in a dog (a). This was the result of a ricochet – an airgun pellet had struck a tree and then the dog. The 22 pellet had apparently entered the posterior globe via a dorsolateral periocular skin wound (a), it had then been deflected anteriorly by the orbital wall, to lodge finally just beneath the cornea (b). The intraocular damage was devastating, as the pellet (c) had flattened when it hit the tree.

(c)

Diagnosis
- History
- The naked-eye appearance is highly variable, ranging from no indication of external damage to complete disruption of the globe
- Comprehensive examination of the periocular region, adnexa and eye
- Diagnostic imaging techniques may include orbital radiography, ultrasound examination and CT scans. MRI may be used to identify non-metallic foreign bodies not identified by the other techniques, but must *not* be used if there is any chance of the foreign body consisting of magnetic foreign material

Management

The assessment and management of these cases requires specialist assistance, unless the eye is beyond repair and painful, in which case it is best removed.

LACRIMAL SYSTEM FOREIGN BODIES

Foreign bodies (FBs) may become lodged in the puncta, canaliculi or nasolacrimal ducts. Investigation is as for lacrimal dysfunction (see later) and should be performed in such a way that the foreign body is not inadvertently flushed into the narrow intraosseous portion of the nasolacrimal duct (Figure 2.5(a,b,c)).

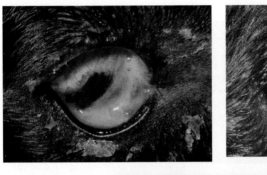

(a)

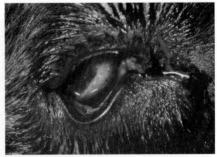

(b)

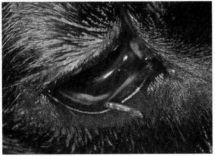

(c)

Figure 2.5(a–c) Foreign body (grass seed) in the upper punctum of a dog. A unilateral profuse mucopurulent ocular discharge is the most striking feature of the clinical presentation (a), but the owner had also reported intermittent haemorrhage. Once the discharge had been carefully cleaned away it was apparent that the haemorrhage was a consequence of the mechanical irritation from a foreign body whose tip can be seen protruding from the upper punctum (b). The grass seed has been removed and the upper punctum and canaliculus cannulated prior to gentle irrigation to remove any remaining small particulate matter via the lower canaliculus and punctum (c).

Treatment

- Visible foreign bodies are grasped with fine forceps and gently extracted from the affected punctum, taking care to ensure that no small particles remain behind. Gentle (retrograde) irrigation usually via the normal, unaffected, punctum with digital occlusion of the lacrimal sac region (to prevent access to the nasolacrimal duct) may be needed to remove detritus from the affected punctum and canaliculus. This is because the foreign body may undergo some disintegration within the affection punctal and canalicular portions of the lacrimal drainage system.

- There is usually no need to provide antibiotic treatment in the management of acute cases. Where a short course of antibiotic treatment is felt to be necessary it is better to supply a solution rather than an ointment or gel.
- Complex cases, particularly those where the foreign body is not visible, may require specialist help and early referral should be considered.

CONJUNCTIVAL FOREIGN BODIES INCLUDING THOSE INVOLVING THE THIRD EYELID

Foreign bodies are a reasonably common source of conjunctival injury and are frequently of an organic nature (seeds, barley awns, wood, etc). The conjunctival sac can accommodate surprisingly large foreign bodies, whereas less spectacular, but usually more traumatic, are foreign bodies, sometimes small in size located beneath the third eyelid (Figure 2.6(a,b)). The rapid onset of conjunctival oedema, especially in cats, can make the task of finding foreign bodies more difficult.

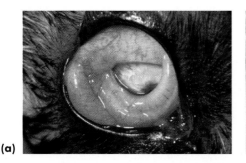 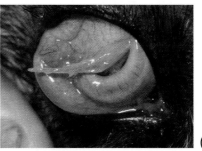

(a)   **(b)**

Figure 2.6(a,b) Foreign body (grass seed) behind the third eyelid of a dog. The owner had been walking through fields with the dog only hours earlier and had noted her pet's acute ocular discomfort during the walk. There were intense pain, blepharospasm and lacrimation and the tip of a grass seed was just visible behind the third eyelid (a). After several applications of topical local anaesthetic the grass seed was removed (b) and the eye checked for additional debris and further damage, neither of which was present.

Treatment
- The foreign body is removed carefully, usually under topical local anaesthesia.
- A short course of antibiotic ointment (chloramphenicol) or gel (fucidic acid) may be needed if there has been conjunctival desiccation or damage and especially if there is any secondary corneal trauma.

CORNEAL FOREIGN BODIES

Clinical signs are similar to those for any acute corneal injury (i.e. pain, blepharospasm and lacrimation), with the foreign body being visible in many instances (Figure 2.7(a–c)). Referral should be considered for complex cases (e.g. deep FBs with risk of ocular damage or collapse of the globe on extraction).

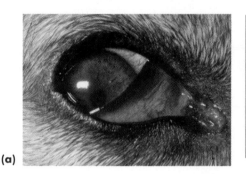

(a)

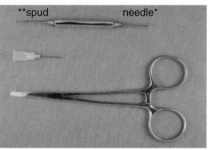

(b)

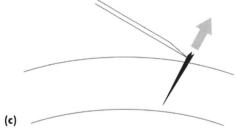

(c)

Figure 2.7(a–c) Corneal foreign body (thorn) in a dog (a). Note that the thorn is of regular shape and does not penetrate the full thickness of the cornea, so it can be removed safely without fear of additional corneal damage or globe collapse. General anaesthesia is not usually required and the foreign-body in this case was removed using a foreign-body needle (b) as illustrated (c) following the topical application of local anaesthetic.

Treatment
- Foreign bodies require removal if they are causing irritation or are capable of causing irritation. Organic foreign bodies are the commonest necessitating this approach.
- Superficial foreign bodies can be removed a few minutes after application of topical local anaesthetic (e.g. proxymetacaine hydrochloride 0.5%) using a foreign-body spud, a surgical spear, or cotton wool wound round the tips of fine mosquito forceps. Patience is required. Flat foreign bodies in particular (e.g. plant material, flakes of metal or paint) can be quite difficult to remove as they become embedded in the superficial cornea where they set up a considerable reaction.
- Foreign bodies that have penetrated the cornea and are accessible are best removed using a 25-gauge needle or a foreign-body needle, inserted at 90° into the protruding tip of the foreign body. The foreign body is removed slowly and carefully in the

direction exactly the reverse of the angle of entry. Whilst it is tempting to attempt to grasp the foreign body with tissue forceps, this may cause it to penetrate more deeply and is better avoided. It is sometimes necessary to undermine corneal foreign bodies with a 15-gauge scalpel blade or a Beaver blade to facilitate removal.

- Advice or referral should be sought for animals with complex foreign bodies (e.g. fish-hooks), intracorneal foreign bodies, those that may also have penetrated the iris ± lens, and those of uneven shape (e.g. some thorns).
- Corneal foreign bodies and micropuncture wounds in general may become the site of a *corneal stromal abscess* (see Section 7, p. 289), especially when organic material is involved. Infection (usually by fungi or bacteria) is an additional complicating factor when there has been a puncture wound or foreign body retention. The history and clinical appearance (white, cream or yellow in colour) may help in reaching a diagnosis. Abscesses often show no tendency to heal, particularly if they are deep, and natural resolution will only occur if the foreign material triggers a vascular response. If topical medical treatment does not bring about improvement and resolution of an abscess, then surgical extirpation is probably the treatment of choice.

TRAUMA

Traumatic injury is common in veterinary ophthalmic practice and there are a variety of causes. The clinical approach is as already outlined for foreign bodies. It is also worth noting that the number of cat-related traumatic ocular injuries has increased in dogs and cats in the UK in parallel with the increase in the cat population.

ORBITAL TRAUMA

Trauma in this region, especially that associated with penetrating injury, can result in direct damage to the blood vessels, nerves and muscles of the orbit. Damage to bone is less common.

Clinical signs
- Pain, blepharospasm and lacrimation are common to most acute insults involving the globe and orbit
- Asymmetry of the head, ± eye, and palpable disruption of normal bony contour if a displaced fracture is present
- Strabismus with or without exophthalmos. Enophthalmos in the acute stage is rare and may indicate globe rupture, major orbital disruption or entrapment of extraocular muscles associated with displacement of bony fragments
- Vision may or may not be affected according to such factors as associated intraocular damage (e.g. intraocular haemorrhage, globe rupture) and the type of extraocular damage (e.g. stretching or avulsion of the optic nerve may have an immediate effect on vision). In some cases, however, the eye and vision are normal
- Other possible clinical signs include epistaxis, crepitus and subcutaneous emphysema. The latter usually indicates a fracture involving a paranasal sinus

Diagnosis

- History and clinical signs
- Careful visual inspection to compare both sides of the head
- Gentle palpation of the orbital and periorbital region
- Ophthalmic examination
- Diagnostic imaging – radiography – at least two views of the skull if fractures are a possibility. Other techniques (e.g. CT and MRI) can be very useful, but will require specialist facilities
- Ultrasonography can be of value in establishing the extent of the damage and whether there is any retained foreign material

Treatment

- Surgical intervention is not normally required unless foreign material is present, there is gross loss of alignment or the orbital contents have become entrapped; such cases are best referred to a specialist centre
- In the majority of animals, medical therapy with broad-spectrum systemic antibiotics and anti-inflammatory agents is required, as is some form of topical ocular lubricant if exposure keratopathy is a likely complication

BLUNT AND PENETRATING INJURY TO THE GLOBE

Ocular trauma is caused by a variety of moving and static objects. Referral may be an early option for accurate assessment of the damage.

The prognosis is guarded with various types of penetrating injury because infection is a possibility, especially following cat claw injury and when foreign material is implanted in the lens or vitreous. Endophthalmitis (severe intraocular inflammation which does not extend beyond the sclera) may develop.

Blunt trauma is often more damaging to the globe than penetrating injury as the globe may actually rupture under the force of the impact (Figure 2.1(a,b) and, even when rupture does not occur, the shearing forces generated within the eye may cause severe damage to the intraocular tissues (Figure 2.8). The impact may be great enough to cause the globe to collapse, but more commonly the posterior scleral coat ruptures and this damage will not be apparent on ophthalmic examination.

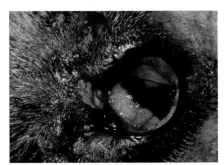

Figure 2.8 Combination of blunt and penetrating injury in a dog. The damage to the globe and eyelids of this police dog was the result of being hit by a beer bottle. Deep lacerations to the eyelids are apparent and there were also severe corneal lacerations. Extensive intraocular haemorrhage was present and the globe had ruptured. There was no possibility of restoring vision in this eye and it was removed.

Clinical signs

- The anterior segment triad associated with pain (blepharospasm, lacrimation and photophobia) is invariably present
- Blepharoedema and possible accompanying eyelid damage
- Other injuries to the head and elsewhere on the body may be present
- Corneal opacity (e.g. panstromal oedema) or obvious injury (e.g. laceration)
- Aqueous flare (protein-rich aqueous) – apparent as a subtle alteration in the transparency of the aqueous in the anterior chamber
- Aqueous leakage is likely when there is an acute penetrating injury (aqueous coagulates in air and may provide a smooth coating to an underlying prolapsed iris)
- Alteration in depth of the anterior chamber (usually shallower than normal)
- Intraocular haemorrhage (hyphaema or whole eye) can be a feature of both blunt and penetrating injuries
- Irregular or constricted pupil; if there has been full-thickness perforation the pupil margin and iris are often drawn towards the hole in the cornea.
- Thickened inflamed iris in which the fine detail is no longer apparent. Iris prolapse, ± iris incarceration, is a likely feature of penetrating injury. Blunt and whiplash injuries in animals with *granula iridica* may result in partial or complete avulsion and local haemorrhage. In animals where the drainage angle can be inspected directly, particularly horses, some tearing of pectinate fibres may also be observed following blunt trauma
- Lens luxation or signs of lens damage (e.g. capsular tears and leakage of lens material)
- Lens perforation is best appreciated by careful examination of the anterior chamber with magnification and a light source, looking from the side. Traumatic damage to the lens can result in a number of early-onset sight-threatening and painful complications, so it is sensible to refer such cases quickly for specialist assessment
- Vitreal changes (e.g. detachment of the vitreous face, subhyaloid haemorrhage [i.e. haemorrhage beneath the vitreous])
- Hyperaemia ± oedema ± haemorrhage of the optic nerve head (papilla)
- Peripapillary oedema and haemorrhage
- Retinal and choroidal oedema ± haemorrhage
- Retinal detachment

Diagnosis

- History and clinical signs
- Ophthalmic examination
- Measurement of intraocular pressure: low intraocular pressure is most commonly associated with uveitis, or globe rupture; high intraocular pressure is usually associated with glaucoma secondary to internal ocular pathology, but in trauma cases may, rarely, be a consequence of external pressure on the globe from, for example, extensive orbital haemorrhage
- Ultrasonography (or diagnostic imaging techniques such as MRI) may be useful for assessing the extent of ocular damage, especially if there are splits in the posterior ocular coats (retina, choroid and sclera), lens luxation, vitreal or retinal detachment and intraocular haemorrhage

Treatment

- Treatment of blunt injuries is symptomatic and consists of systemic and topical antibiotics and anti-inflammatory agents. The prognosis for vision is often poor, particularly in animals such as the cat, in which there is a close orbital fit of the globe within the orbit and little orbital fat
- The management of penetrating injuries is dealt with in more detail below
- Eyes that are blind and painful should be removed (Figures 2.8 and 2.1 (a,b))

THIRD EYELID INJURY

Third eyelid damage is common after cat scratch injuries. It is important to ensure that the globe is intact, as penetrating ocular injury may well have occurred at the same time.

Treatment

- Many injuries heal rapidly without surgical intervention, others require minimal debridement of damaged tissue following topical local anaesthesia (proxymetacaine hydrochloride 0.5%)
- If normal third eyelid movement has been compromised, primary repair under general anaesthesia is required. Sutures, usually in simple interrupted pattern, are placed so that they do not damage the cornea. Fine absorbable material (e.g. 6-0 polyglactin 910 or finer) is used (Figure 2.9(a,b)).

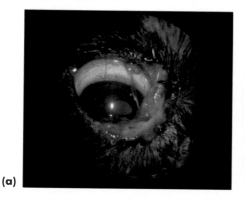 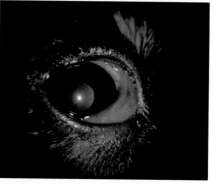

(a)   (b)

Figure 2.9(a,b) Third eyelid injury in a puppy. The third eyelid has become partially avulsed following a claw injury inflicted by a cat (a). Third eyelid function will be severely compromised if the injury is not repaired. After establishing that there was no damage to the globe, or the rest of the puppy, the third eyelid was re-attached with simple interrupted sutures of 6-0 polyglactin 910 (b) and the puppy made an uneventful recovery.

UPPER AND LOWER EYELID INJURY

Traumatic injuries to the eyelids may look dreadful but are very rewarding to treat as eyelids heal with remarkable facility because of their rich blood supply. The highly-mobile nature of the eyelids means that any wounds involving the eyelid margin require early surgical repair (Figure 2.10(a,b)).

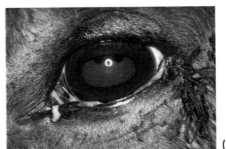

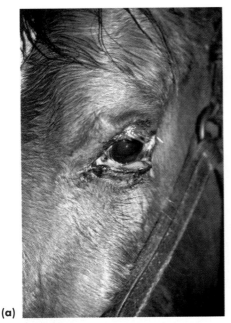

(b)

(a)

Figure 2.10(a,b) Traumatic injury to the lower eyelid of a horse (a). This was the result of becoming entangled in barbed wire. There were extensive skin lacerations that needed suturing as well as the injury to the eyelid. The eyelid was repaired with a single layer of simple interrupted sutures of 5-0 silk (b) and the horse made an uneventful recovery.

Treatment

- Eyelid lacerations should be repaired following *minimal* debridement as soon as is practicable. Primary repair is *always* the aim for this type of eyelid damage, so as to avoid later complications such as infection, cicatrisation, eyelid deformity, exposure keratopathy and epiphora.
- Most small-animal eyelid injuries requiring surgical repair are operated on under general anaesthesia. Many large-animal eyelid injuries can be repaired following sedation and local infiltration or regional anaesthesia (e.g. supraorbital nerve block for upper eyelid injuries), using a local anaesthetic such as lignocaine hydrochloride (lidocaine hydrochloride) 1% or 2%, with or without adrenaline, or mepivacaine hydrochloride 2%.
- Gross eyelid swelling can be reduced with an ice pack (e.g. a bag of frozen peas) wrapped in a towel. The wound is closed in one or two layers and, in general, one-layer closure is simpler and perfectly satisfactory. Simple interrupted sutures of 6-0 polyglactin 910 can be used to close the conjunctiva if two-layer closure is used. Skin closure is effected with a simple interrupted pattern using 4-0 to 6-0 non-absorbable suture material (e.g. silk) or absorbable suture material (e.g. polyglactin 910). A figure of eight or simple interrupted pattern can be used for the first suture, which re-apposes the tissues of the eyelid margin. Whichever pattern is used this first suture is critical as apposition must be perfect. Topical antibiotic ointment and a course of systemic antibiotic should be provided routinely for animals with

contaminated wounds. In herbivores particularly, it is also sensible to give tetanus antitòxin.

- Eyelid injuries may involve the lacrimal drainage system, causing damage to the puncta or canaliculi. If so, referral should be considered, as the repair of such injuries requires microsurgical facilities.

CONJUNCTIVAL INJURY

Blunt and penetrating ocular trauma are common causes of subconjunctival haemorrhage. Most conjunctival injuries result in extensive chemosis, which can result in conjunctival exposure and desiccation.

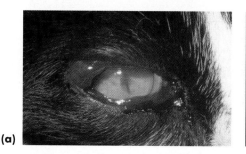
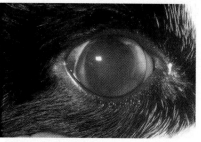

(a)   **(b)**

Figure 2.11(a,b) Subconjunctival and intraocular haemorrhage in a cat following a road traffic accident. Subconjunctival haemorrhage as the only finding is not of concern, as it will resorb naturally, usually over a period of days. In this cat, observable features of concern that indicate intraocular involvement include a tightly constricted pupil (traumatic miosis) and a small amount of haemorrhage in the pupillary aperture (a), which usually originates from the ciliary body. Pupillary dilation (traumatic mydriasis) may develop after a few hours as happened in this patient. A few days later the subconjunctival haemorrhage has almost resorbed, but the extent of intraocular haemorrhage is clear and the pupil remains dilated (b). Prognosis for retention of vision following blunt injury to the globe is invariably guarded in cats, because of the close orbital fit, and this eye remained without vision.

Treatment
- Subconjunctival haemorrhage may be left to resorb naturally over a matter of days. It is, however, important to check that the globe is intact in all cases that present with subconjunctival haemorrhage of traumatic origin (Figure 2.11(a,b)).
- Penetrating conjunctival injury may also be associated with haemorrhage and obvious conjunctival laceration. Again, it is important to check that the damage is limited to the conjunctiva alone as damage to the underlying sclera and uvea may also be present.
- Chemosis and conjunctival desiccation are not unusual after trauma. Antibiotic preparations which contain a suitable excipient (e.g. fucidic acid or chloramphenicol ointment) will lubricate the exposed conjunctiva effectively until swelling has subsided.

- Few cases require suturing, as healing is so rapid and uncomplicated, always provided that the damage is limited to the conjunctiva and does not involve deeper structures. On occasions, minimal debridement is required to remove loose flaps of tissue, sometimes combined with suturing using buried absorbable 6-0 to 7-0 sutures of polyglactin 910.

LIMBAL, EPISCLERAL AND SCLERAL INJURY

The limbus and the contiguous episclera and sclera are, in theory, susceptible to full-thickness rupture after blunt ocular injury. However, in most animals such injuries damage the posterior part of the globe rather than the anterior part of the globe. Ultrasonography and tonometry are of value in assessment. The prognosis for the eye and vision is usually very poor after severe blunt trauma (Figure 2.1(a,b)).

Penetrating injuries are often easier to diagnose, however the site of corneal penetration is not always obvious when there is blood or pus in the anterior chamber. The extent of damage to the episclera and sclera may be obscured by chemosis and an intact, or seemingly intact, conjunctiva. Careful examination of the anterior segment, paying particular attention to the depth of the anterior chamber, position of the iris and shape of the pupil, together with tonometry and ultrasonography, should help to confirm the diagnosis. The prognosis is guarded to good if the intraocular contents have not been disrupted and microsurgical repair is undertaken. The extent of corneal and scleral involvement is often best ascertained during surgical exploration (Figure 2.12(a,b)).

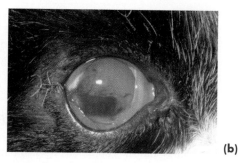

(b)

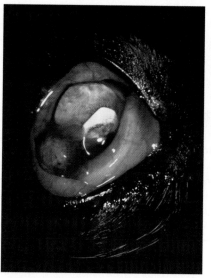

(a)

Figure 2.12(a,b) Full thickness corneal penetration, conjunctival and scleral laceration in a cat as the result of a cat claw injury (a). There is a large laterally-placed corneal wound through which the iris has prolapsed, so the pupil is deformed in consequence. A thin film of aqueous covers the prolapsed iris and the anterior chamber is partially formed; a forced Seidel test was positive. The grey area at approximately 2 o'clock to the prolapsed iris is a loose flap of badly-damaged cornea. Hyphaema is present, making it more difficult to assess potential lens damage. In this case there was none. The posterior segment was undamaged. Microsurgical repair under general anaesthesia was undertaken after reforming and deepening the anterior chamber with viscoelastic injected via a stab incision at about 90° away from the iris incarceration (in this case the dorsal cornea). Initial exploration indicated a complex wound, which extended both along and across the limbus. In such cases the conjunctiva must be opened so that the extent of any scleral injury can be ascertained and repaired. After closure of all sites other than that of iris incarceration, the uveal tissue was freed from the edges of the wound and reposited and the remainder of the cornea repaired. The appearance of the eye on the first post-operative day (b). The pupil has been dilated as part of the medical treatment (topical mydriatic cycloplegic, broad-spectrum antibiotic and non-steroidal anti-inflammatory agent). The cat made an uneventful recovery.

CORNEAL INJURY

Traumatic corneal injury is common in veterinary practice. Careful examination is required to ascertain the extent and depth of the injuries and, if it is impossible to examine the eye properly, or if there is any risk of expulsive loss of the intraocular contents, then examination under anaesthesia (EUA) may be needed. It may be sensible to obtain specialist advice before this is done, and early referral should always be considered for complex injuries if the practice lacks microsurgical facilities and expertise.

The prognosis is guarded if extensive intraocular haemorrhage is also present. In many cases it is sensible to obtain plain radiographs of the orbit, utilising two views, in case radio-opaque foreign bodies such as gunshot are the cause of the trauma. Ultrasound examination is of considerable value in assessing the extent of the damage, especially the degree of intraocular involvement, but must be performed with great caution if there is any risk of expulsion of the intraocular contents.

Clinical signs
- Acute, usually unilateral, onset of pain, blepharospasm, lacrimation and photophobia
- Corneal oedema ± third eyelid damage
- Positive Seidel test if there is aqueous leakage. This test is performed by applying fluorescein sodium to the corneal wound and examining the eye with blue light and magnification in the dark. Aqueous leakage dilutes the green fluorescein. Gentle pressure (forced Seidel test) can be applied when intermittent leakage is suspected. It is easier to assess aqueous leakage if 2% concentrations of fluorescein are used for the Seidel test (Figure 2.13(a,b)).
- Change of ocular appearance e.g. hyphaema, distorted pupil, changes in the depth or even loss of the anterior chamber, aqueous leakage or a coagulum of aqueous, iris prolapse ± incarceration of the iris, globe collapse

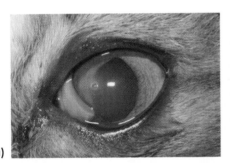
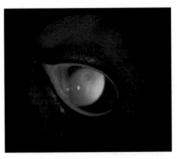

(a)
(b)

Figure 2.13(a,b) Positive Seidel test associated with a penetrating corneal injury in a Domestic Longhair. Subtle aqueous leakage was apparent with a forced Seidel test (b). Note the damage to the free border of the third eyelid from previous trauma.

Treatment
- Superficial oblique corneal lacerations, involving no more than a quarter of the corneal thickness, do not usually require surgical repair, but wound healing will often be enhanced if the loose flap of corneal epithelium is trimmed with fine scissors after applying local anaesthetic solution (proxymetacaine hydrochloride 0.5%). Protection during healing is not necessarily required, although a therapeutic soft contact lens (TSCL) can be used as a bandage lens when pain relief and protection are needed.
- For deeper non-penetrating corneal injuries support for healing may be required and choices include a therapeutic soft contact lens, collagen shield, conjunctival graft or porcine submucosal graft. A rotation conjunctival pedicle graft is an excellent means of providing support for healing. Conjunctival grafts can be used in a number of

situations where support for healing is required (e.g. corneal ulceration, descemetocoele, small corneal perforations and after keratectomies involving more than approximately one third of corneal depth). They are usually left in situ for some 2–4 weeks and then, after application of topical anaesthetic, the unattached portion of the pedicle is sectioned, between the attached graft and the limbus, using Stevens tenotomy scissors (Figure 2.14(a–g) and Box 2.2).

- When full thickness corneal damage has occurred, the wound, if small, may be self-sealing and, in this situation, a therapeutic soft contact lens, collagen shield or pedicle graft can be used. This approach can only be used if the anterior chamber is of normal depth, when there is no aqueous leakage and provided that there is no involvement of the lens or uvea (Figure 2.15). Reconstructive surgical repair is indicated when the wound is large, there is aqueous leakage or any other indication of intraocular disruption, and such cases should be referred if adequate microsurgical facilities are not available (Figure 2.16).
- A course of topical antibiotic solution, rather than ointment, is usually required (see under Ulcerative Keratitis in General and Canine Ophthalmology and as listed in Appendix 2).

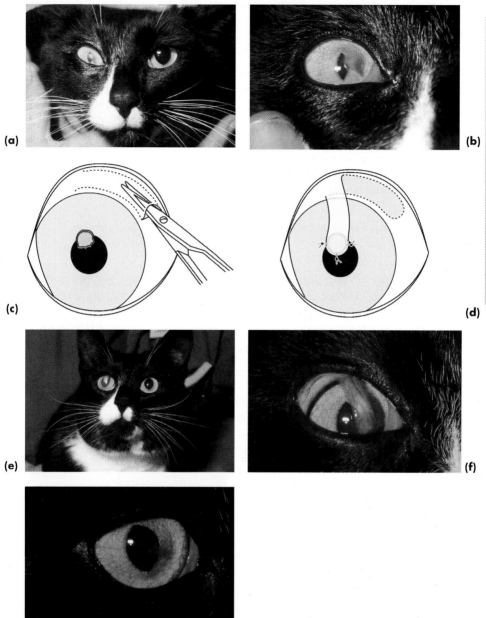

Figure 2.14(a–g) Traumatic cat scratch injury in a Domestic Shorthair. Note the faint diffuse cloudiness in the region of the injury, which is often indicative of cellular infiltration and infection. There is also constriction of the pupil on the affected side. Necrotic debris plugged a small hole in the cornea (a–b). Support for healing was provided using a rotation pedicle graft. The technique is outlined (c–d) and the graft illustrated in situ (e–f). Medical treatment consisted of ten days' topical atropine and, on the basis of culture and sensitivity, ofloxacin eye drops. The pedicle graft was sectioned after a month and the appearance, showing some residual corneal scarring is illustrated some 12 months later (g).

Box 2.2 Surgical procedure for a rotation conjunctival pedicle graft (see Figure 2.14(a–g))

1 Patient under general anaesthetic, standard aseptic skin preparation

2 A lateral canthotomy should be performed if the surgical access is poor

3 If there is any possibility of corneal perforation, it may be preferable to prepare the pedicle graft first

4 The pedicle graft is ideally harvested from the dorsal bulbar conjunctiva so that it can be orientated vertically and in line with eyelid movement

5 The extent of conjunctival dissection in relation to the position and size of the corneal ulcer should be assessed, as the graft must not be under tension when it has been placed

6 The conjunctiva is elevated with fine tissue forceps (e.g. Castroviejo or Colibri) and a small entry wound made in the conjunctiva at 90° to the limbus and some 1–2 mm from the limbus

7 Blunt dissection (e.g. Stevens tenotomy scissors) is used to undermine the conjunctiva in radial fashion, so as to create a thin transparent portion of conjunctiva that has been freed from underlying episcleral connective tissue

8 The graft is fashioned by means of two parallel radial cuts that can diverge slightly towards the base of the pedicle; the perilimbal cut should be approximately parallel to and 1 mm posterior to the limbus

9 While the recipient bed (the ulcerated area) is being prepared, the graft should be protected with a surgical swab soaked in sterile saline

10 Material for culture should be obtained from the ulcer, ensuring that swabs and scrapes include material from the edge of the ulcer

11 Instruments that are used to prepare the recipient site are discarded after use

12 Necrotic material should be cleaned from the ulcerated area by sharp dissection (e.g. Number 64 Beaver blade or corneal trephine), paying particular attention to freshening the walls of the ulcer

13 The graft is rotated into place and trimmed, if necessary, to the shape of the prepared ulcerated area (recipient site)

14 8-0 polyglactin 910 is used to suture the graft into place in the bed of the ulcer, with the first suture placed at 6 o'clock

15 The sentinel sutures (6 o'clock, 3 o'clock and 9 o'clock) should pass through the entire thickness of the conjunctiva and into the wall of the ulcer at about two thirds of corneal thickness

16 Once the sentinel sutures have been placed, other sutures are placed in similar fashion, approximately 1 mm apart, until the graft is firmly attached to the cornea

17 The bulbar conjunctiva can be left open or closed with a continuous suture of 8-0 to 9-0 polyglactin 910

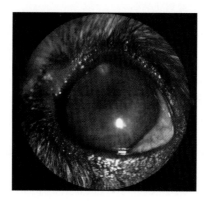

Figure 2.15 Full-thickness corneal penetration in a dog as the result of a cat claw injury. Although the eye appears quiet, careful examination with magnification indicated lens material associated with a tear in the anterior lens capsule almost underlying the site of corneal penetration. There was also a small haemorrhage from a primary retinal vessel in the damaged eye. This eye was managed medically (topical mydriatic cycloplegic, broad-spectrum antibiotic and non-steroidal anti-inflammatory agent) without surgical intervention, as the hole in the lens capsule was small enough to seal soon after the injury. The preretinal haemorrhage resorbed over two weeks.

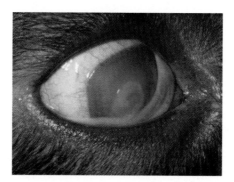

Figure 2.16 Full-thickness corneal penetration in a puppy as the result of a cat claw injury. There is marked corneal oedema and aqueous flare. The iris is swollen and its detail is no longer apparent. Careful examination indicated that lens damage had occurred and that leakage of the lens contents was continuing. There is no option other than removal of the lens contents in such cases. Small-incision surgery and use of phacoemulsification is preferable, particularly as the gross corneal thickening associated with corneal oedema makes watertight wound closure difficult.

UVEAL TRAUMA

In some injuries the uveal tract is directly traumatised. Iris prolapse is a frequent finding after ocular penetrating injury, and secondary uveitis is a common feature of many types of ocular injury. Initial damage to the uveal tract can be complicated by later secondary problems such as glaucoma (*mainly dog*), cataract formation and endophthalmitis. Penetrating injuries must be repaired as soon as they are recognised and the uveitis associated with both penetrating and blunt injuries should be treated symptomatically. Early referral should be considered for penetrating ocular injuries (Figures 2.12, 2.15 and 2.16).

Clinical signs

- Classical signs of uveitis (see below) ± indications of blunt or penetrating injury
- Hyphaema (haemorrhage in the anterior chamber) and intraocular haemorrhage may both be associated with trauma and uveitis, but they can also occur because of other problems, for example neoplasia, systemic hypertensive disease and various blood disorders, so accurate differentiation is important

LENS TRAUMA

The possibility of lens damage should always be considered when there has been penetrating ocular injury (see earlier), as a devastating *phacoclastic uveitis* can follow leakage of lens protein in *dogs* and *horses* (Figures 2.15 and 2.16). In *cats*, the initial inflammation is less intense, but in this species there is a very real risk of intraocular neoplasia developing later in life. Animals with suspected penetrating lens injuries and those with post-traumatic lens luxation should be referred to a specialist centre with the appropriate facilities and skills.

Clinical signs

- Lens luxation or subluxation is most likely after blunt injury
- Penetrating injury is most likely to be associated with capsular damage and leakage of lens material. Flocculent darkish lens material ± vitreous will be apparent on careful examination (ideally using a slit lamp at high magnification)
- Corneal oedema is often associated with lens penetration and makes accurate assessment of these cases more difficult

Treatment of penetrating lens injuries

- A small tear in the anterior capsule, without obvious loss of lens material, may self-seal swiftly, and such cases will require only symptomatic treatment for uveitis. A small capsular cataract is the only legacy of this type of injury. If there is any doubt as to the integrity of the lens capsule the animal should be referred as soon after the injury as possible.
- When there is leakage of lens material, early surgical intervention is needed, so as to avoid the likelihood of intractable and painful phacoclastic uveitis. These cases should be referred. In very young animals, the lens contents can be removed by simple irrigation and aspiration, but in most adult animals *phacoemulsification* (ultrasonic fragmentation) is used to remove the lens contents.
- It is pertinent to note that lens injuries can sometimes be associated with inoculation of infectious organisms and intralenticular infection is a potential, but rarely recognised, complication of this type of injury. Affected eyes remain painful, inflamed and, usually, opaque.

VITREAL TRAUMA

Vitreal haemorrhage may be an early complication of ocular trauma, whereas vitreal abscessation, degeneration and liquefaction are later complications. Detachment and disruption of the vitreous can often be demonstrated with ultrasonography. Vitreous prolapse into the anterior chamber may complicate ocular trauma and is usually found when traumatic lens luxation is also present.

Management

Referral will be required, as specialist equipment and expertise are both necessary for treatment. For example, prolapsed vitreous can be removed most simply from the anterior chamber using cellulose sponges and taking care to avoid traction on the vitreous base, whereas, for more complex vitreal involvement, vitrectomy may be required. Intraocular haemorrhage is left to resorb naturally and will take weeks or months to resolve, in contrast to haemorrhage in the anterior chamber, which usually takes only days to disappear.

TRAUMA INVOLVING THE OCULAR FUNDUS

Some, or all, of retinal oedema, retinal haemorrhage, retinal tears, retinal detachment, optic nerve damage and haemorrhage (subretinal, intraretinal and preretinal) may be early complications of traumatic injury to the head and eye (Figure 2.17). Examination of the eye, including the fundus, at the time of the injury may make it easier to determine the prognosis and to explain subsequent complications. The eye may be blind, or partially sighted, or appear normal immediately after the injury. In the latter case sequential examination may be necessary to detect subsequent degenerative changes in the retina, choroid and optic nerve.

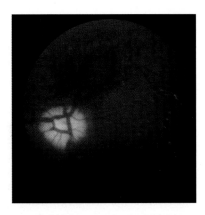

Figure 2.17 Preretinal haemorrhage from primary retinal vessels after blunt trauma to the globe. Haemorrhage in this site may take many months to resorb.

ENDOPHTHALMITIS AND PANOPHTHALMITIS AS COMPLICATING FACTORS IN OCULAR INSULT

Endophthalmitis is severe intraocular inflammation that does not extend beyond the sclera, and intraocular infections of this type, once established, become the equivalent of an intraocular abscess. The vitreous provides an ideal culture medium and toxic enzymes, low pH and low oxygen tension make treatment of established infection difficult. *Exogenous* endophthalmitis is a potential complication of penetrating ocular injury, retained intraocular foreign bodies and perforating infected corneal ulcers, although it can also be a complication of ocular surgery (Figure 2.18). Ocular infections caused by blood-borne infections are termed *endogenous* to distinguish them from those caused by the introduction of external environmental pathogens. When blunt and penetrating injuries also involve orbital tissues, panophthalmitis (severe intraocular inflammation extending into the orbit) may result.

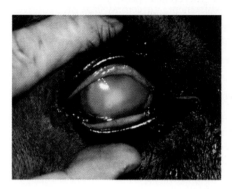

Figure 2.18 Endophthalmitis after previous penetrating injury in a horse. Intraocular implantation of foreign organic material is a relatively common cause of subsequent endophthalmitis, and the progression of intraocular infection to frank endophthalmitis can be rapid in the horse. The site of original corneal penetration is often apparent, as in this eye, even when the eye itself is pus-filled and opaque. Once endophthalmitis of this severity has developed, the only management option is to remove the eye, which is blind and painful.

Clinical signs of endophthalmitis
- Pain is often a prominent feature. Pyrexia and lethargy are common
- An ocular discharge is often present, the ocular media are cloudy or frankly opaque and the vessels of the globe are markedly congested
- Corneal vascularisation is invariably present, usually as a peripheral circumcorneal fringe of straight vessels running at 90° to the limbus
- Panuveitis with recurrent inflammation is common
- There may be corneal, conjunctival and eyelid oedema. The site of previous penetrating injury is sometimes apparent

Management of endophthalmitis
- The prognosis is very guarded, and most veterinarians would regard the management of these severe inflammations as best carried out at appropriately-equipped referral centres. For example, vitrectomy may be necessary if there is a retained foreign body and the medical management is complex whatever the cause.
- Vitreocentesis is indicated in order to obtain material for culture in a variety of media (chocolate and blood agar and Sabouraud's agar). It should be noted that culture-negative growth does not rule out bacterial infection.
- Broad-spectrum antibiotics for intravenous use are injected directly into the vitreous. Vancomycin (human dose 1 mg) or cephazolin (2.2 μg) are effective against Gram +ve organisms and amikacin (human dose 400 μg) or gentamicin (maximum dose 200 μg because of the drug's retinotoxicity) are effective against Gram −ve organisms. It is usual in human patients to use a combination of vancomycin and amikacin as the first-line treatment.
- If fungi are isolated then specialist advice should be sought.

- Systemic antibiotics, selected ideally on the results of blood culture, will also be required if the endophthalmitis is of endogenous origin.
- The prognosis for restoration of vision is poor and eyes that are irreversibly blind and painful should be removed.

Clinical signs and management of panophthalmitis

In panophthalmitis, the ocular and systemic signs are similar, but the additional involvement of the orbital tissues means that the clinical presentation can include prominence of the third eyelid and, in horses and farm animals, swelling in the region of the supraorbital fossa.

As there is potential for infection to spread along the optic nerve to the brain, it is usual to take material for culture and sensitivity and surgically remove the globe and orbital contents (*exenteration*). Based, if possible, on the results of culture, an appropriate course of systemic antibiotic treatment should also be given and antibiotic instilled directly into the operation site at the time of surgery.

COMPLICATED ULCERS AND CORNEAL INFECTION

The ancillary factors contributing to complications and the potential for infection include:
- Species: for example, ulcers in horses should always be regarded as serious
- Corneal exposure and sensitivity: for example, brachycephalic dogs are more 'at risk' than most dolicocephalic breeds
- Initiating event, extent, progression and depth of ulcer, general health of the patient and subsequent management in all species

There is a tendency to forget about ancillary factors until complications supervene. For example, it is safest to accept that any ulcer in the horse may become complicated or infected, in order to try and prevent such complications developing. The general health status of the animal should always be taken into account, both hyperadrenocorticism and diabetes mellitus can adversely influence corneal wound healing, and it could also be argued that other factors such as age and chronic disease (e.g. renal failure) might also exert an effect (Figure 2.19).

The initial history-taking must be detailed, particularly with regard to when the ulcer was first suspected, the possible aetiology and details of any treatment the animal has received. The work-up should establish if bacterial pathogens are present, as it is much easier to obtain this knowledge at the outset. Similar precautionary principles underlie assessment of the normal and protective blink response. Some idea of corneal sensitivity can be obtained by eliciting a protective blink response, using either a very fine wisp of cotton wool or, more accurately, an aesthesiometer (e.g. Cochet-Bonnet).

It is axiomatic that any treatment given should not make matters worse, so that, for example, corticosteroids are contraindicated in the majority of cases of ulcerative keratitis. The principle of 'if in doubt refer' should be followed.

OPHTHALMIC EMERGENCIES AND TRAUMA

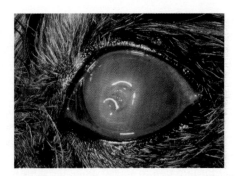

Figure 2.19 Complicated ulcer in a dog. Note the single long lash on the upper eyelid. This dog also had diabetes mellitus and reduced corneal sensitivity, which is not uncommon in diabetic patients. The tear film can provide a good culture medium in such animals, as it is usually more glucose-rich than that of normal dogs. *Pseudomonas aeruginosa* was cultured from the cornea in pure growth. Sparse numbers of Gram –ve rods (*Pseudomonas aeruginosa*) were also demonstrated from corneal scrapes, and topical treatment with tobramycin was initiated while awaiting the definitive results of culture. Subsequent sensitivity results indicated that the choice of antibiotic was appropriate.

Clinical signs
- Pain, photophobia, blepharospasm, lacrimation ± mucopurulent discharge
- Anterior uveitis in most cases, with hypopyon in some cases
- Fluorescein positive ulceration (to avoid false positives, it is important to carry out gentle irrigation with sterile saline to remove excess stain)
- Infiltration of the corneal stroma and often diffuse opacification and oedema
- Signs of liquefactive stromal necrosis (see below)
- Descemetocoele formation – exposed Descemet's membrane is fluorescein negative
- Rapid progression to corneal perforation

Management
- Identify and, if possible, remove the underlying cause and any exacerbating factors
- Corneal scraping for Gram staining and culture is essential, but undue pressure on the globe should be avoided if the cornea is compromised
- Antibiotic selection or other forms of therapy (e.g. antifungals) should, ideally, be based on the results of initial Gram stain, culture and sensitivity as well as the response to treatment
- Antibiotic selection is a critical feature of successful treatment and the available antibiotics for topical use are discussed under Ulcerative Keratitis in General and Canine Ophthalmology and listed in Appendix 2
- Support for healing may be needed, most simply as a conjunctival pedicle graft

LIQUEFACTIVE STROMAL NECROSIS ('MELTING' ULCER)

Liquefactive stromal necrosis ('melting ulcer') is a feared complication of corneal ulceration. It is a particular problem in certain species (e.g. brachycephalic animals and horses), some types of corneal insult (e.g. alkali burns) or infection (e.g. *Pseudomonas* spp ulcers) and may be a complicating factor of treatment (e.g. corticosteroid therapy) or systemic disease (e.g. hyperadrenocorticism and diabetes mellitus) (Figure 2.20(a–c)).

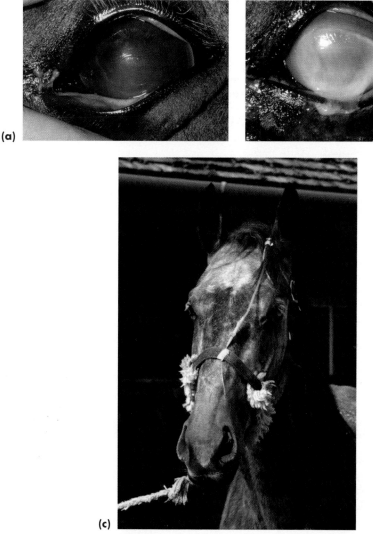

(a)

(b)

(c)

Figure 2.20(a–c) Liquefactive stromal necrosis ('melting ulcer') in a horse. This mare had inadvertently received contaminated tear-replacement solution from a multidose bottle that had been used to keep the eyes lubricated whilst she was under general anaesthesia for colic surgery. The innocuous appearance of the corneal ulcer in the left eye on the first post-operative day (a) suggests a superficial, although extensive, ulcer. The situation deteriorated rapidly over a matter of hours and the corneal liquefaction is striking (b). *Pseudomonas aeruginosa* was cultured from the tear replacement solution and both corneas. The mare responded well to intensive medical therapy delivered via a nasolacrimal lavage device (c) and was left with only minor corneal scarring.

Diagnosis

- The affected region of the cornea initially loses transparency and then progresses via oedema to frank liquefaction. Perforation is a likely and rapid complication (within hours) if the condition is not recognised. If in doubt, specialist advice should be obtained without delay.
- Scrapes and swabs should be submitted for culture and sensitivity. Gram –ve organisms such as *Pseudomonas aeruginosa* or excessive numbers of inflammatory cells confirm the likelihood of collagenolysis.

Treatment

- As a general rule, management of these cases requires specialist assistance
- Debridement of necrotic tissue should be performed and an early decision taken with regard to providing support for healing (e.g. conjunctival pedicle graft)
- Initially treatment of all types of liquefactive necrosis should be undertaken on an hourly basis, the frequency of application is only reduced when sustained improvement has been achieved
- For horses, and other large animals, it is best to insert a subpalpebral lavage device or similar at the outset, as it will make treatment easier and more accurate
- A fortified antibiotic solution or a broad-spectrum topical preparation that is effective against *Pseudomonas aeruginosa* (e.g. gentamicin or tobramycin solution) should be used and only changed if the organisms are insensitive on culture and sensitivity
- Empirical approaches include the use of topical whole fresh serum and acetylcysteine 5–10% to prevent collagenolysis
- Uveitis accompanies deep keratitis, so the pupil should be dilated with atropine 1% ± phenylephrine 10% to relieve the pain of ciliary spasm
- Non-steroidal anti-inflammatories (given orally or intravenously) are useful to relieve ocular pain and will help to stabilise the blood–aqueous barrier when uveitis is also present
- Treatment frequency can be reduced and proprietary antibiotic preparations substituted for fortified ones once the healing process is progressing satisfactorily

CHEMICAL INJURIES

Chemical injuries can occur in any species, but guard dogs, police dogs and horses are at increased risk. Referral may be required for the management of chemical injuries. Acids precipitate protein and unless they are particularly strong (i.e. pH 2.5 or less) they do not penetrate beyond the corneal epithelium. Alkalis react with fats to form soaps, which damage cell membranes. They thus have the capacity to penetrate the eye, so that their damaging effects are widespread (cornea, limbus, anterior chamber, iris, ciliary body and lens and its zonules) (Figure 2.21(a,b)). The speed of penetration of alkalis, from fastest to slowest, is ammonium hydroxide, sodium hydroxide, potassium hydroxide and calcium hydroxide. The latter, which is found in plaster and mortar, does not penetrate well, as the calcium soaps formed upon saponification are relatively insoluble and precipitate out, forming a barrier to further penetration.

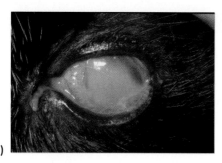
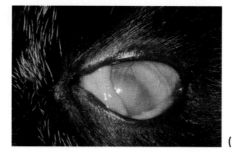

(a)   (b)

Figure 2.21(a,b) Chemical injury in a Domestic Shorthair. This was an alkali burn from sodium-hydroxide-containing cleaning fluid that was accidentally splashed into the cat's eye (a). Intensive topical medical treatment was reasonably effective given the delay between the accident and the diagnosis, although the cat was left with residual corneal scarring (b).

Clinical signs of acute chemical injury

- Conjunctival changes range from mild hyperaemia and chemosis to disastrous limbal ischaemia
- Corneal changes range from focal or diffuse corneal clouding ± punctate epithelial erosion to pancorneal opacification, ulceration and, occasionally, perforation. When alkalis or strong acids are involved, the changes are essentially similar to those of liquefactive stromal necrosis
- Other anterior-segment changes range from mild aqueous flare to frank uveitis or more generalised anterior-segment inflammation. Lens luxation can follow damage to the lens zonules
- Intraocular pressure may rise soon after the injury, probably because of an immediate shrinkage of collagen fibres

Emergency management of acute chemical injury

- As an emergency measure, the owner should be advised to irrigate the eye with copious quantities of tap water
- As part of initial veterinary assessment, the pH of the conjunctival sac should be checked and the offending chemical using standard pH paper, as well as ensuring that none of the chemical is retained within the conjunctival sac. Strong alkalis (pH 12–14) are the most damaging
- Mild chemical burns can be treated as described below for Thermal Burns

Treatment of alkali burns

- In cases of alkali burns, irrigation of the eye with tap water should be maintained until specialist help has been obtained and the animal hospitalised for treatment under close observation
- Topical treatment usually consists of citrate 10% drops every two hours, ascorbate 10% drops every two hours, chloramphenicol ointment four times daily, atropine 1% drops three times a day and fluorometholone acetate 1% drops every two hours
- Ascorbate can be used orally, for example, oral treatment for dogs with alkali burns consists of ascorbate 500 mg four times daily

OPHTHALMIC EMERGENCIES AND TRAUMA

THERMAL BURNS

Burns may be a consequence of both accidental and non-accidental injury. The eye itself is less commonly damaged than the eyelids because of the rapidity of the blink response. *Corneal* damage is usually typified by diffuse corneal haze and fluorescein uptake (the tight junctions of epithelial cells have been disrupted, thereby allowing fluorescein access to the stroma) (Figure 2.22).

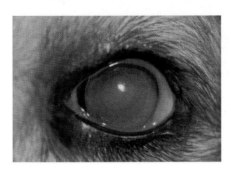

Figure 2.22 Thermal injury in a dog. Mild corneal oedema and fluorescein uptake are present as a result of superficial corneal damage caused by the intense heat generated by a chip pan that caught fire. Both corneas healed rapidly following topical treatment with antibiotic ointment and a short course of systemic analgesic was also dispensed. Respiratory problems as a result of smoke inhalation took slightly longer to resolve.

Treatment of corneal burns
- Topical antibiotic ointment and systemic analgesic are usually sufficient
- If pain is more severe because of secondary iridocyclitis, a short-acting cycloplegic should also be used

Thermal burns involving the *eyelids* are similar to those of the skin, but because the subcutaneous tissue is areolar, there may be marked swelling. Skin damage from thermal burns is classified as first degree (epidermis only), second degree (epidermis and dermis) and third degree (epidermis, dermis and subcutaneous tissue). The management of eyelid burns is based on a similar classification of the depth of involvement.

Treatment of eyelid burns
- Remove the animal from the heat source and cool the eyelid tissues as rapidly as possible (e.g. ice pack wrapped in a towel which, ideally, should be sterile)
- Administer systemic analgesics
- First-degree eyelid burns should be treated with topical antibiotic ointment, second-degree burns require antibiotic-impregnated non-occlusive dressings. Third-degree burns may require reconstructive eyelid surgery, including skin grafting, to preserve eyelid function, and such cases should be referred early
- Bacterial colonisation and eyelid infection may complicate the situation, in which case systemic antibiotic treatment will also be required
- Prophylactic tetanus treatment should be administered to horses and other herbivores

ACUTE UVEITIS

See under uveal tract for further details. If the cause is not obvious it may be sensible to seek specialist advice or refer the case at the outset (Figure 2.23).

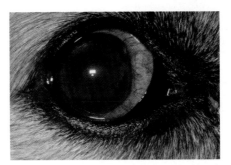

Figure 2.23 Acute uveitis in a dog. In this severe unilateral uveitis of unknown cause the eye is reddened and painful with the classical signs of blepharospasm, lacrimation and photophobia. There is a suspicious focal grey area at approximately 2 o'clock in the limbal cornea that may be indicative of a previous penetrating injury and it is important to rule out a retained foreign body in this area. The whole cornea is mildly oedematous, hyphaema is present, iris detail is lost and the pupil is constricted. When viewed from the side it was possible to see that the anterior chamber was shallow as a result of profound iris inflammation.

Salient clinical signs of acute anterior uveitis
- Pain, photophobia, blepharospasm and lacrimation
- Ocular redness, often most marked in the perilimbal area above the ciliary body (*perilimbal hyperaemia*)
- Mild corneal opacity
- Aqueous flare
- Loss of iris detail; iris will be swollen because of inflammation
- Anterior chamber is shallower than normal because of iris inflammation
- Constricted (*miotic*) pupil, which does not change shape under different lighting conditions
- Although the direct pupillary light response is absent, the consensual pupillary light response is usually present in unilateral cases
- Low intraocular pressure
- Variable effect on vision, but can be a cause of sudden blindness in severe cases

ACUTE GLAUCOMA

If the practice lacks facilities for accurate measurement and monitoring of intraocular pressure and examination of the drainage angle, of both eyes, with a goniolens, suspected cases should be referred as a matter of urgency (Figure 2.24).

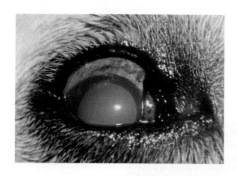

Figure 2.24 Acute glaucoma in a dog. The eye is painful, there are conjunctival and episcleral congestion, panstromal corneal oedema, a clear anterior chamber of normal depth, apparently normal iris detail and a widely dilated pupil. The intraocular pressure measured with an applanation tonometer (Mackay Marg) was 55 mm of mercury.

Salient clinical signs of acute glaucoma in the dog

- Pain, photophobia, blepharospasm and lacrimation
- The patient may be head shy and reluctant to move because the pain is so severe. Affected animals may also lose their appetite and, occasionally, they vomit
- Ocular redness due to ciliary injection and conjunctival and episcleral congestion. A circumcorneal brush border of blood vessels may be apparent within a few days of onset, especially if there is marked corneal oedema
- Corneal oedema (if the intraocular pressure is greater than 40–50 mm Hg)
- Dilated (*mydriatic*), non-responsive pupil, *but* note that when a previous uveitis has caused extensive posterior synechiae (adhesions), the pupil will be immobile and constricted (*miotic*)
- There is no direct or consensual pupillary light response
- High intraocular pressure (in excess of 30 mm Hg)
- Abnormal anterior chamber depth – e.g. iris inflammation and iris bombé will cause the anterior chamber to be shallower than normal, posterior lens luxation will cause the anterior chamber to be deeper than normal. There may, however, be no change in the depth of the anterior chamber
- Reduced vision or blind: affected animals can become acutely blind within hours of the onset of glaucoma. Owners are unlikely to notice a partial unilateral reduction in vision, but may, if observant, pick up unilateral blindness

PRIMARY LENS LUXATION

Primary lens luxation is the commonest cause of acute glaucoma in terrier breeds and cases should be referred as a matter of urgency if the expertise and facilities for intraocular surgery are not available (see Section 3, pp 148–149) (Figure 2.25).

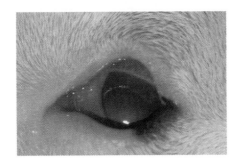

Figure 2.25 Primary lens luxation with secondary glaucoma in a Miniature Bull Terrier. The classical pain triad of lacrimation, blepharospasm and photophobia was present. The eye is reddened, the lens is lying in front of the iris and the dorsal lens equator is highlighted by the light source. Contact of the anteriorly luxated lens with the posterior cornea has caused localised corneal oedema. The intraocular pressure (Mackay Marg tonometer) was 65 mm Hg. Lens luxation occurred in the fellow eye some weeks later.

Clinical features of acute lens luxation (in addition to those of glaucoma outlined above)

- Local corneal oedema if the lens is, or has been, anterior. The anteriorly-luxated lens can cause mechanical damage to the endothelial cells of the posterior cornea
- The lens can be visualised in an abnormal position – in the anterior chamber, pupillary aperture, immediately posterior to the iris or within the vitreous. Part, or all, of the edge of the lens (equator) can be highlighted as a bright reflective rim with penlight illumination. If the lens has moved from an axial position, an *aphakic crescent* may be apparent. The lens moves with ocular movement (phacodenesis) and can change position within the eye, although an anterior position is commonest when intraocular pressure is high
- Anterior-chamber depth may be abnormal, e.g. deep, if the lens is in the anterior chamber, or has dropped back into a liquefied vitreous, shallow if the lens and vitreous are causing pupil block
- Trembling of the iris (*iridodenesis*) when the dog moves its head, as the iris has lost the support of the lens
- Vitreous may be apparent in the anterior chamber, visible as faint, cloudy opacities at the pupillary margin

SUDDEN LOSS OF VISION

If the cause is not obvious, it is sensible to seek early specialist help: some types of acute visual loss benefit from early intervention if sight is to be restored, and electroretinography (ERG) is a critical tool in the evaluation of vision loss. The causes can be empirically grouped into those that affect the normal transparency of the ocular media, those that affect retinal function and those that affect the central nervous system (optic nerve to visual cortex). In addition to local ocular insults as a cause of vision loss, many generalised diseases are associated with acute blindness.

Causes of sudden blindness

- Acute-onset pancorneal opacity (e.g. panstromal oedema)
- Lipaemic aqueous because of chylomicronaemia
- Uveitis (anterior, posterior and panuveitis)
- Acute glaucoma (mainly dog)
- Globe rupture
- Haemorrhage (intraocular haemorrhage, local intracranial and extracranial haemorrhage and generalised severe haemorrhage) can all be causes of sudden blindness
- Retinal detachment (e.g. systemic hypertensive disease – intraocular haemorrhage may also be present)
- Sudden acquired retinal degeneration (SARD) in the dog
- When the blood supply to the optic-nerve head is severely disrupted, ischaemic optic neuropathy can result. Acute blindness associated with ischaemic optic neuropathy is an occasional complication of both primary and secondary haemorrhage, septic emboli and the surgical ligation of arteries. In horses, arterial ligation (e.g. maxillary, greater palatine, internal, external carotid) is a treatment for epistaxis associated with guttural-pouch mycosis and an occasional cause of acute vision loss on the ipsilateral side
- Optic neuritis and retrobulbar neuritis (e.g. associated with distemper virus)
- Toxic damage (e.g. toxic hepatic encephalopathy, quinolone antibiotics, anthelmintics like ivermectin, salt poisoning and lead poisoning) (Figure 2.26)
- Severe ocular trauma (e.g. intraocular haemorrhage, globe prolapse) and head trauma (e.g. poll injuries in horses, as a result of rearing and falling over backwards, can cause partial or complete shearing of the optic nerve as it leaves the brain through the optic canal)
- Metabolic disease e.g. hypoglycaemia in all species
- Intracranial lesions such as brain tumours (e.g. optic chiasma compression by neoplasm), haemorrhage, hydrocephalus, tentorial herniation
- Consequence of hypoxia/anoxia (e.g. anaesthesia-associated and following cardiac arrest in all species)
- Feline ischaemic encephalopathy (cerebral vascular infarction)
- Post-ictal (epilepsy)

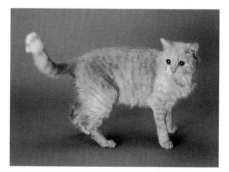

Figure 2.26 Sudden blindness in a cat within 18 hours of oral administration of the quinolone antibiotic enrofloxacin. Note the widely-dilated pupils, which were unresponsive to light. Retinal changes in this cat are illustrated in the feline section.

Clinical findings
- The history can be of crucial importance, but on occasions is misleading, particularly when the loss of vision is the result of non-accidental injury
- External signs of damage to the head or eye may be apparent
- Partial or complete unilateral or bilateral blindness
- Sudden bilateral loss of vision usually renders animals nervous, easily startled and unable to function normally, even in a familiar environment. Unilateral blindness may not be recognised as quickly, although affected animals may show a similar behaviour pattern when approached on the affected side
- Normal or abnormal pupillary light reflexes (usually abnormal)
- Intraocular haemorrhage, or other signs of intraocular damage
- Retinal detachment, or more subtle retinal changes
- Optic nerve head (ONH) oedema (papilloedema) ± peripapillary and retinal haemorrhage
- When the cause of blindness is central only, there will be no indication of intra-ocular abnormality

Management
- Accurate case assessment is crucial, as it helps to determine if the damage is reversible or irreversible
- Treatment regimes for common causes of vision loss are listed in the relevant sections under specific conditions

SUDDEN OCULAR PAIN

If the cause is not obvious after careful examination, and particularly if the pain is intractable, it is important to seek early specialist advice. Reduction of ocular pain after the application of topical local anaesthetic (e.g. proxymetacaine hydrochloride 0.5%) implies external eye disease (e.g. ocular surface disease, ulcerative keratitis) rather than an intraocular problem (e.g. uveitis, glaucoma). Successful treatment depends upon establishing and eliminating the cause and the treatment of common causes of ocular pain are listed in the relevant sections under specific conditions (Figure 2.27(a–c)).
- Traumatic damage to eye, adnexa, orbit (including foreign bodies)
- Retrobulbar (orbital) abscess and orbital cellulitis
- Endophthalmitis and panophthalmitis
- Allergic blepharoconjunctivitis (mainly horse): acute conjunctivitis in all species is usually uncomfortable, rather than frankly painful
- Ectopic cilia and, less commonly, distichiasis and other lash and hair problems (mainly dog) producing corneal irritation or frank ulceration
- Acute dry eye, particularly if there is accompanying corneal ulceration
- Ulcerative keratitis (superficial ulcers are often more painful than deeper ulcers)
- Acute uveitis
- Acute glaucoma (mainly dog)

OPHTHALMIC EMERGENCIES AND TRAUMA

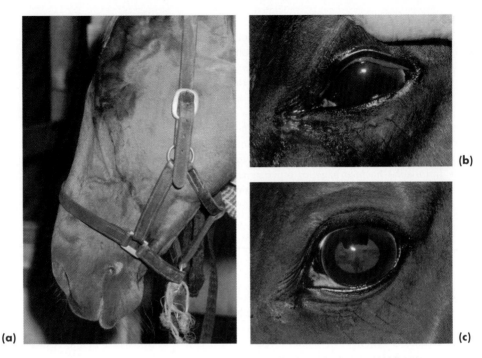

(a)

(b)

(c)

Figure 2.27(a–c) Sudden ocular pain in a horse (a). This horse had sustained blunt trauma to the globe hours earlier. Sedation and an auriculopalpebral nerve block were administered and subsequent examination revealed intense miosis and hyphaema (b). Medical treatment with atropine 1% and prednisolone acetate 1% was instituted. The pain diminished within an hour of treatment commencing and recovery was uneventful. The haemorrhage had almost resorbed two days after initial presentation (c) and the horse went on to make a complete recovery.

REFERRALS

The list given in Box 2.3 should not be regarded as exhaustive. Referral should always be considered as one of the management options for difficult cases and the art of referral lies in recognising not only which cases to refer, but how and when to refer them. A letter of referral should set out the reason for referral, any information of relevance, the results of investigations and any treatment that has been given. It is discourteous, and usually unhelpful, to send computer print-outs of the patient's life history, and even worse to send no information whatsoever. Problems requiring urgent or emergency referral are signified by an asterisk (*) and for these cases brief details (including treatment) can be passed to the receptionist at the time of making the appointment, emailed or faxed through or sent with the client.

Box 2.3 Ocular conditions for possible referral

- Acute proptosis and prolapse when the aetiology is not obvious*
- Orbital neoplasia (and other orbital problems for which surgery may be required)
- Complex adnexal and intraocular neoplasia
- Endophthalmitis and panophthalmitis*
- Complicated blunt and penetrating trauma, including complex foreign bodies*
- Complex eyelid problems, including cases which require revision because of previous failed eyelid surgery
- Parotid duct transposition, unless proficient and practised in the technique
- Deep corneal ulcers and penetrating corneal injuries*
- Liquefactive stromal necrosis including alkali burns*
- Corneal problems requiring keratectomy or keratoplasty
- Acute glaucoma*
- Lens luxation in the dog* and other species
- Cataract surgery (dogs with diabetic cataracts should be referred as soon as possible for assessment)
- Acute canine* and equine* uveitis and uveitis where the aetiology is complex or not obvious
- Sudden blindness*
- Unexplained ocular pain or redness (urgency of referral depends upon the degree of pain)

* Denotes urgent or emergency referral

OPHTHALMIC EMERGENCIES
AND TRAUMA

SECTION 3
GENERAL AND CANINE OPHTHALMOLOGY

INTRODUCTION

In this section, the basic principles of veterinary ophthalmology are described using the dog as the type species. Knowledge of normal ocular anatomy underpins the recognition of ocular abnormality (Figure 3.1(a–c)). Subsequent sections will highlight species differences, so as not to repeat much of the material outlined in this section. The common canine ocular and adnexal conditions and those that are important to recognise because of the serious implications of misdiagnosis are summarised in Box 3.1.

In many countries, dogs that are to be used for breeding are examined for inherited eye disease, and in some countries there is also a DNA testing scheme. In the USA, canine hereditary eye disease certification is run by the Canine Eye Registration Foundation (CERF) and for much of Europe the European College of Veterinary Ophthalmologists (ECVO) fulfils this function. In the UK, the ECVO plays a lesser role, and examination for hereditary eye disease comes under the auspices of the British Veterinary Association/Kennel Club/International Sheep Dog Society (BVA/KC/ISDS) Eye Scheme. An up-to-date list of the conditions and breeds covered by this scheme is published annually by the British Veterinary Association (*In Practice* Supplement on Hereditary Eye Disease) and the pamphlet is available free from the British Veterinary Association.

GENERAL AND CANINE OPHTHALMOLOGY

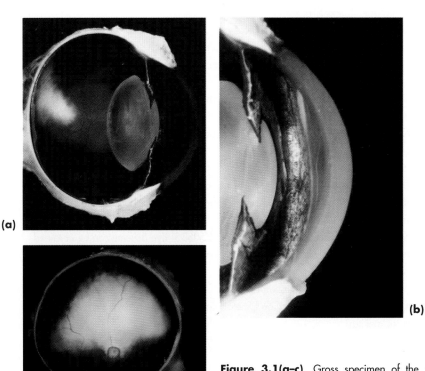

(a)

(b)

(c)

Figure 3.1(a–c) Gross specimen of the normal canine globe (a); higher power view of the anterior segment (b); fundus (c) (with acknowledgements to J. R. B. Mould).

Box 3.1   Common and important canine ocular and adnexal conditions

- Trauma
- Primary and secondary neoplasia (e.g. benign eyelid neoplasia and multicentric lymphoma)
- Periocular abnormalities associated with abnormal skull shape (e.g. brachycephalic dogs) and poor facial anatomy (e.g. nasal folds)
- Upper and lower eyelid imperfections (e.g. entropion)
- Third eyelid imperfections (e.g. kinked cartilage and prolapse of the nictitans gland)
- Horner's syndrome (e.g. idiopathic type in Golden Retriever)
- Distichiasis in many breeds of dog
- Ectopic cilia (much less common than distichiasis, but important to recognise as a cause of acute ocular pain)
- Dry-eye syndromes (particularly immune-mediated keratoconjunctivitis sica in breeds like the West Highland White Terrier)
- Conjunctivitis and its differential diagnosis
- Epithelial basement membrane dystrophy (important in the differential diagnosis of ulcerative keratitis)
- Other causes of ulcerative keratitis
- Corneal lipid deposition (may be indicative of systemic disease)
- Chronic superficial keratoconjunctivitis (pannus)
- Uveitis (uncommon, but important to recognise and differentiate from other causes of 'red eye')
- Primary and secondary glaucoma (uncommon, but important to recognise and differentiate from other causes of 'red eye')
- Primary lens luxation and secondary glaucoma (mainly terriers)
- Cataract
- Sudden blindness and its differential diagnosis
- Inherited diseases of the eye (e.g. cataract and fundus conditions) and adnexa (e.g. eyelid defects) are relatively common in pedigree dogs. Further information about those eye conditions currently included in the British Veterinary Association/Kennel Club/International Sheep Dog Society (BVA/KC/ISDS) Eye Scheme can be obtained from the annually-updated *In Practice* article on Hereditary Eye Disease published by the *Veterinary Record*
- Common generalised problems with ocular manifestations include a variety of infectious diseases (e.g. distemper) and metabolic diseases (e.g. hypothyroidism and diabetes mellitus)

GLOBE AND ORBIT

Anatomy
- In the dog, as in other domestic animals, the orbital floor is incomplete and the medial wall of the orbit relatively thin
- Incomplete bony orbital rim with the dorsolateral portion completed by dense collagenous orbital ligament
- The extraocular muscles encircle the optic nerve and form a cone that is directed caudally, ventrally and medially towards the optic foramen; the apex of the cone is caudal and the base rostral
- Orbital contents – globe, extraocular muscles, blood vessels, nerves and intraorbital fat
- The lacrimal gland lies deep to the orbital ligament and the zygomatic salivary gland is present in the ventral orbit in a recess of the maxilla ventral to the globe
- Disease processes in the frontal and maxillary sinuses, caudal nasal chamber, caudal molar tooth roots, pharynx and muscles of mastication, the lacrimal and the zygomatic salivary glands may impinge on the orbit

CONDITIONS OF THE CANINE GLOBE AND ORBIT

Causes of enophthalmos (backward displacement of the globe)
- Small eye – may be congenital (e.g. cystic eye and microphthalmos) or acquired (e.g. ruptured globe and phthisis bulbi)
- Dehydration and debility
- Horner's syndrome
- Anterior-segment pain with active retraction of the globe by action of the retractor bulbi muscles
- Tetanus
- Chronic stage of masticatory myositis

Causes of exophthalmos (forward displacement of the globe)
- Traumatic prolapse/proptosis of the globe
- Inflammation of periorbital tissues: retrobulbar foreign body, orbital cellulitis, retrobulbar abscess
- Retrobulbar neoplasia and neoplasia that has invaded from adjacent regions (e.g. nasal chamber)
- Acute stage of masticatory myositis (third eyelid is prominent as the swelling is extraconal, see below) and extraocular polymyositis (third eyelid is not prominent as the swelling is intraconal, see below)
- Zygomatic inflammation, mucocoele formation and other cystic swellings are uncommon causes
- Orbital vascular abnormalities, both congenital and acquired, are rare causes (e.g. arteriovenous shunts)
- Temporomandibular osteopathy in the West Highland White Terrier (very rare cause of exophthalmos, as the periosteal proliferation is usually sufficiently ventral to have no effect on globe position)

INVESTIGATION OF ORBITAL DISEASE

History
- Acute onset with pain suggests inflammation, which is a reasonably common cause, gradual onset without pain is more likely to be neoplasia, a cyst or a zygomatic mucocoele (of these three, neoplasia is the most common).
- History of trauma preceding the onset of clinical signs can be helpful, but note that there may be a gap of days or weeks between the original injury and the observed problem and often the cause is unknown.

Examination
- A full examination of the animal, the eyes and adnexa should be undertaken.
- It is essential to examine the eyes both from in front and from above; exophthalmos is more obvious than globe enlargement when the eyes are examined from above.
- Check the position of the third eyelid; it may be more prominent than usual if there is an orbital lesion, especially if the orbital lesion lies outside the endorbital muscle cone (*extraconal*). *Intraconal* lesions (those within the endorbital muscle cone) do not usually result in third-eyelid protrusion, the proptosis is usually axial and strabismus (squint) is subtle or absent.
- Note whether strabismus is present. Strabismus may reflect the position and size of an orbital (usually extraconal) or paraorbital lesion, but can also be the result of muscle or nerve damage, or indicative of CNS involvement. Occasionally it will be necessary to perform a forced-duction test to ascertain if strabismus is the result of fibrosis (e.g. associated with the chronic stage of myositis) or entrapment (e.g. following orbital trauma) or is of neurological origin. Under general anaesthesia, the conjunctiva and underlying Tenon's capsule is grasped close to the limbus and the globe is manipulated to ascertain the degree of free movement. Mobility will be normal if the origin of the strabismus is neurological.
- Attempt to repulse both globes back within the orbit by gentle pressure through the closed upper lid; a unilateral space-occupying lesion (SOL) will produce an obvious disparity between the two eyes, with increased resistance being felt on the affected side.
- Check the blink response and mobility of all three eyelids and ensure that there is no exposure keratopathy.
- Check that there is no pain or difficulty in opening the mouth.
- Check whether a nasal discharge is present and ensure that there is free passage of air from the nostrils using a wisp of cotton wool.
- Check the local lymph nodes to ascertain if they are of normal size.
- Diagnostic imaging of the orbit can be helpful in the investigation of orbital disease. In general, radiography is the least useful unless there is bony involvement or a radio-opaque foreign body. Ultrasonography may be of value and CT and MRI provide superb soft-tissue detail.

Possible ocular and oral signs of orbital space occupying lesions
• Exophthalmos
• Third eyelid prominence
• Strabismus
• Increased resistance to globe retropulsion, especially obvious in unilateral cases
• Corneal profile will be more obvious on the affected side when viewed from above
• Lagophthalmos (inability to close the lids) ± exposure keratopathy
• Conjunctival hyperaemia/congestion/chemosis
• Periorbital swelling
• Pain or difficulty in opening the mouth
• Swelling or other abnormality caudal to last upper molar tooth

ORBITAL NEOPLASIA

History, aetiology and clinical signs
• Tumours may arise from any of the orbital tissues, or by extension from neighbouring tissues (e.g. nasal), or because of secondary spread (e.g. multicentric lymphoma).
• The history is usually that of a slowly-developing exophthalmos with third eyelid prominence and globe deviation: findings that enable space occupying orbital lesions to be differentiated from globe enlargement (Figure 3.2(a–b)). Pain is not usually a feature in these slowly progressive cases with orbital neoplasia.
• The patient is usually middle aged or old.
• There are exceptions: beware the situation in which a rapid-onset with pain tempt a diagnosis of retrobulbar abscess, for there are occasions in dogs of any age when a highly-aggressive tumour can mimic inflammatory disease.
• Always check the nasal airflow (using a fine wisp of cotton wool) and the local lymph nodes (by palpation) when neoplasia is suspected.
• The ocular signs can be very helpful. For example, a nasal tumour that has infiltrated the orbit may produce lateral globe deviation as well as the expected exophthalmos and third eyelid prominence. In addition to ocular signs, there may also be reduced airflow, a nasal discharge or haemorrhage from the nostril on the affected side.

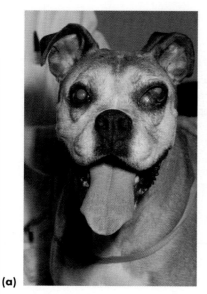 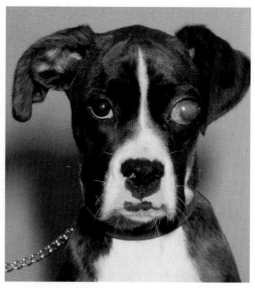

(a)   (b)

Figure 3.2 **(a)** Orbital neoplasia in an old Boxer. Prominence of the third eyelid is the most obvious feature and there is also an upward and outwards squint, both of which are helpful in establishing the ventromedial position of the space-occupying mass. The dog's open mouth and absence of any signs of pain indicate that the cause is more likely to be neoplastic than inflammatory, as was indeed the case. This dog should be compared with that in (b). **(b)** A young Boxer with an enlarged globe because of glaucoma secondary to previous trauma (penetrating cat claw injury) in which there is no third-eyelid prominence. In (a) the corneal profile was more obvious on the affected side when viewed from above.

Diagnosis and management

- Most cases are best referred if there is a prospect of retaining a functional eye, or if the extent and nature of the tumour are unclear, especially as the prognosis is guarded.
- Ultrasound-guided fine needle aspiration/biopsy of the lesion, or sampling from a local lymph node, may provide diagnostic material, but many orbital lesions are not easily accessible.
- The use of computed tomography (CT) and magnetic resonance imaging (MRI) have greatly improved the investigation of neoplasia in and near the orbit. The two techniques are complementary rather than exclusive, although MRI is the more generally useful, especially if there is intracranial involvement.
- Skull radiography is useful if there is bony involvement, intraoral views are helpful if dental involvement is suspected and chest radiography should be performed if there is any suspicion of distant metastasis.
- **Under no circumstances** should orbital exploration be attempted without a precise knowledge of orbital anatomy, the requisite skills in orbital surgery and an accurate diagnosis for which refined imaging techniques are *mandatory*.

ENUCLEATION OF THE GLOBE AND EXENTERATION OF THE ORBIT

Removal of the globe is indicated for blind, painful eyes (e.g. unresponsive glaucoma), for eyes with inoperable intraocular tumours, for irreparably damaged eyes and for serious infections of the eye that have not responded to treatment (e.g. endophthalmitis). Orbital exenteration may be needed if there is inflammatory or neoplastic orbital involvement. Samples for culture and sensitivity should be taken prior to surgery if infection is present.

The commonest methods of globe removal are trans-palpebral and transconjunctival enucleation. Prostheses (e.g. silicone implants) are sometimes used following globe removal and are of potential value in young growing animals to minimise skull deformity. In other situations their use is more equivocal, as the animal is unconcerned about the cosmetic result. Evisceration (removal of the ocular contents via a perilimbal incision) and implantation of a prosthesis into the remaining corneoscleral shell is performed with much greater frequency in the USA than in Europe and this may reflect, in part, owner attitude and expectations.

Trans-palpebral (en-bloc) enucleation
- General anaesthesia
- Usual preparations for aseptic surgery
- Infiltration of the orbit with local anaesthetic provides good peri-operative and post-operative analgesia. Use bupivacaine and lignocaine (4:1 ratio) and a total dose of 3–5 ml
  - Palpate orbital rim and globe to affirm landmarks
  - Use 1″ needle for small dogs and 1½″ needle for large ones
  - Enter orbit medially at 2 o'clock following the orbital wall caudally, draw back before injecting anaesthetic in the posterior orbital region
  - Repeat laterally at 8 o'clock, again drawing back before injecting anaesthetic behind the globe
  - Massage the eye gently, unless it is likely to rupture, to spread the local anaesthetic within the orbit
- The eyelids are held closed with Allis tissue forceps, or sutured together so as to provide a bridle suture for handling. Make an encircling skin incision that will permit the skin edges to be apposed without tension later
- The underlying tissues are dissected as far as the orbital margin taking care not to penetrate the conjunctival sac
- Heavy scissors are used to section first the lateral canthal ligament and then the shorter medial canthal ligament
- Gentle traction is applied to the lids to elevate them so that their connection with the orbital margin can be sectioned. The globe and extraocular muscles should be handled gently so as to avoid potential vagal effects (bradycardia via the oculocardiac reflex)
- The attachments of the globe to the orbit are sectioned, if possible identifying each individual extraocular muscle then sectioning it as close to the globe as possible
- The optic nerve is clamped with curved forceps, taking care to avoid excessive traction. A scalpel blade or curved scissors are used to section the nerve between the

globe and the forceps. It is not essential to ligate the optic nerve if it has been clamped, but the forceps should be left on for at least 5 minutes

- Before closing it is important to check that all haemorrhage is under control. The orbit should *not* be packed as this increases the risk of infection, may be uncomfortable for the patient and gives a poorer long-term cosmetic result
- Absorbable sutures (e.g. 5-0 to 6-0 polyglactin 910) are placed through connective tissue/muscles to close the dead space. Usually two or so interrupted sutures may be placed deeply and continuous sutures subcutaneously in order to achieve tight closure. The skin is closed with simple interrupted sutures (e.g. 3-0 to 4-0 nylon or polyglactin 910)
- If wound seepage is a problem, pressure can be applied by suturing a tightly rolled up large swab over the wound and removing it after two days
- Immediate systemic postoperative analgesia should be provided
- If the globe or orbit is infected, topical antibiotic can be instilled into the orbit when the globe has been removed and a course of systemic broad-spectrum antibiotic provided. The selection of antibiotic should be based on previous culture and sensitivity results
- Non-absorbable sutures are removed after 7–10 days

Trans-conjunctival (sub-conjunctival) enucleation
- This technique should not be used when there is orbital neoplasia or infection
- The eyelids remain open during the procedure and the conjunctival space is opened by an initial incision close to the limbus
- Pathogens may be inadvertently introduced into the orbit once the conjunctival space is entered
- Less extraocular tissue is removed and there is usually less haemorrhage
- Once the globe has been removed, the conjunctival sac, nictitating membrane and eyelid margins are excised
- Retained conjunctival tissue may become cystic and lead to sinus formation

Exenteration
- Exenteration involves removal of the globe and all other orbital tissues. The indications for this technique include orbital neoplasia (primary tumours and those that have extended from the globe) and non-responsive orbital infections (usually panophthalmitis).
- The surgical technique involves dissection close to the wall of the orbit and is invariably associated with more haemorrhage than the others described.

EYELIDS

ANATOMY AND PHYSIOLOGY

The eyelids function to protect and lubricate the eye and the *integrity of all three eyelids* is important in terms of these functions.

Upper and lower eyelids
The upper and lower eyelids consist of three layers. The outer layer of skin contains hair follicles, eyelashes (upper eyelid only) and their respective sebaceous glands. The

middle layer consists of muscle, tarsal (*meibomian*) glands and the collagenous connective tissue known as the *tarsal plate*. The inner layer is palpebral conjunctiva. Skin
and conjunctiva meet at a mucocutaneous junction known as the *eyelid margin*. The
eyelids are richly supplied with nerves, blood vessels and lymphatic tissue.

Third eyelid

The third eyelid (nictitating membrane, *membrana nictitans*) arises as a fold from the
ventromedial aspect of the conjunctiva. The free border is usually darkly pigmented.
The amount of third eyelid which is visible in the normal dog largely depends on the
relationship between the globe and orbit; thus in brachycephalic breeds with a shallow
orbit the third eyelid is unobtrusive, whereas third eyelid prominence is a conspicuous
feature of those dolicocephalic breeds with small eyes. Retraction of the globe into the
orbit results in passive protrusion of the third eyelid.

The third eyelid consists of inner (*bulbar*) and outer (*palpebral*) conjunctiva (*nictitating conjunctiva*) and both surfaces are covered by nonkeratinised stratified squamous epithelium. The stroma is fibrous connective tissue and a T-shaped hyaline
cartilage plate reinforces the structure of the third eyelid. There is substantial glandular and lymphoid tissue. A superficial seromucous gland, the *nictitans gland*, is located
at the base of the T-shaped cartilage, and this gland contributes significantly to the
preocular tear film (PTF).

EXAMINATION OF THE EYELIDS

Examination of the upper and lower eyelids

- Careful examination of the eyelids should be performed in good light and with magnification. The outer and inner surfaces should be inspected as well as the fornices
  and lid margins. It is easy to miss penetrating injuries, sparse distichia, ectopic cilia
  and foreign bodies
- Swabs and impression smears should be taken when relevant. Local anaesthesia is
  not usually necessary for this, but will be required for eyelid biopsies

Examination of the third eyelid (nictitating membrane)

- Examination of the outer (palpebral) surface is achieved by applying gentle pressure
  to the globe through the upper eyelid in order to repulse the globe and mechanically
  protrude the third eyelid
- The inner (bulbar) surface can be examined following topical application of local
  anaesthetic drops (e.g. proxymetacaine hydrochloride 0.5%)
  - The slightly-raised ridge close to the free border of the third eyelid is grasped with
    thumb forceps (taking care to avoid inadvertent damage to either the cornea or
    the free border of the third eyelid)
  - The inner surface is inspected by gently pulling the leading edge away from the
    eye
- Whilst examination of the inner aspect of the third eyelid is not performed routinely,
  it is an *essential* part of ophthalmic examination if there is any possibility of a *foreign
  body* (e.g. grass seed)
- Direct inspection of the lymphoid tissue on the inner surface of the eyelid is also of
  importance in chronic conjunctivitis cases, as follicular hyperplasia can cause direct
  low-grade physical trauma to the cornea

CONDITIONS OF THE CANINE THIRD EYELID

Causes of prominence – and apparent prominence – of the third eyelid

- *Anatomical* e.g. small eyes
- *Reduced volume of orbital contents* e.g. because of debility and severe dehydration, loss of retrobulbar fat, atrophy of the pterygoid muscles
- *Lack of pigment*, particularly if unilateral, can give a spurious impression of prominence
- *Horner's syndrome*
- *Dysautonomia* (much less common in the dog than the cat – see Section 4, pp 182–183
- *Scrolling of third eyelid cartilage*
- *Hypertrophy and prolapse of the nictitans gland*
- *Cystic swelling* of the nictitans gland is a rare cause of prominence
- *Pain* produces globe retraction and consequent protrusion of the third eyelid (Figure 3.3)
- *Inflammation* e.g. plasmacytic conjunctivitis (see Pannus this section, pp 120–122) and chronic lymphoid hyperplasia
- *Trauma, injury and infection*
- *Systemic and generalised problems* e.g. tetanus
- *Neoplasia* primary (rare) and secondary (most commonly lymphoma)
- *Retrobulbar space-occupying lesions* e.g. inflammation or neoplasia
- *Drug-induced* e.g. phenothiazine tranquillisers

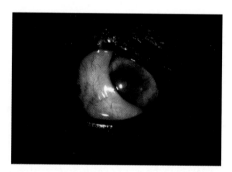

Figure 3.3 Prominence of the third eyelid. This Border Collie lacks pigment in the third eyelid as a normal variant. The eye is painful because of ciliary spasm (note the pupil constriction) as a result of a penetrating corneal injury (the circular white dot) of unknown cause an hour previously. It is important to ensure that there are no additional complications such as aqueous leakage, retained foreign material or intraocular damage in such cases. No such complications were present, and the dog made a complete recovery after symptomatic treatment with a mydriatic cycloplegic (atropine) and antibiotic drops (chloramphenicol).

Pigment variations

The free border of one or both third eyelids is usually pigmented. Non-pigmented third eyelids are common and part of normal variation, their pink colour and lack of pigment should be differentiated from colour variations due to inflammation and from the pigment loss associated with plasmacytic conjunctivitis (see this section, pp 120–121).

Horner's syndrome

Horner's syndrome indicates damage to the efferent sympathetic nerve supply to the eye at any point along its three-neurone pathway between the brain and eye. The first-order neurones pass from the hypothalamic region of the brain via the lateral tectotegmental spinal pathway to emerge in the chest at T1–T3. The second-order preganglionic neurones join the vagus nerve to form the vagosympathetic trunk and synapse in the cranial cervical ganglion caudoventral to the ear. Third-order postganglionic neurones run through the tympanic bulla and middle ear, enter the skull and transit the cavernous sinus, then leave the skull via the orbital fissure to supply the eye and orbit.

Ophthalmic features

- *Miosis* (pupil construction) with the affected pupil being smaller than the normal one under all conditions of illumination – inequality of pupil size is termed *anisocoria*. Miosis may be the only ophthalmic feature in lesions affecting the brachial plexus when damage is limited to the T1 nerve root of the T1–T3 sympathetic outflow
- *Ptosis* (drooping) of the upper eyelid. There may also be a mild lower eyelid ectropion. Both are the result of loss of smooth-muscle tone in the eyelids (Müller's muscle)
- *Enophthalmos*, because of loss of muscle tone in the smooth muscle of the orbit
- *Prominence* of the third eyelid occurs secondarily to the enophthalmos
- *Conjunctival hyperaemia* occurs because of loss of peripheral vascular tone. This feature is usually more obvious in the early stages

Aetiology

As the cranial cervical ganglion is anatomically close to the tympanic bulla, ear problems are probably one of the commonest causes of Horner's syndrome, but other possible causes include central nervous system disease, thoracic disease and lesions involving the neck and head, including the cavernous sinus. Neoplasia, inflammation or trauma affecting any of these regions may be relevant.

A form of idiopathic Horner's syndrome, usually third order, is relatively common in the Golden Retriever. No treatment is required for these cases and the appearance will gradually return to normal over a period of weeks or months.

Pharmacological testing to localise the lesion

Although a number of pharmacological agents can be used to help localise the site of the lesion, topical phenylephrine 10% is the agent most commonly used. One drop of the drug is applied to each eye and the time taken to achieve pupillary dilation is noted as an indication of denervation hypersensitivity (Box 3.2). It should be noted that the results can be equivocal and that it is often only possible to differentiate preganglionic lesions from postganglionic lesions.

GENERAL AND CANINE OPHTHALMOLOGY

Box 3.2   Time to pupillary dilation as indication of denervation hypersensitivity

- 60–90 minutes suggests a normal eye, or first-order Horner's syndrome
- 20–45 minutes suggests second-order Horner's syndrome
- Less than 30 minutes suggests third-order Horner's syndrome

---

Scrolling of the third eyelid cartilage

The cartilage may be abnormally kinked, usually in the vicinity of the upper part of the T. The kinking results in eversion or, less commonly, inversion of the third eyelid. The appearance is unsightly and the functional mobility of the third eyelid may be impaired. The problem is often developmental and is quite common in some of the larger breeds of dog (e.g. Great Dane, St Bernard, Mastiff and Weimaraner) (Figure 3.4(a)). The deformity may be a consequence of unequal growth between the cartilage and the conjunctiva during development.

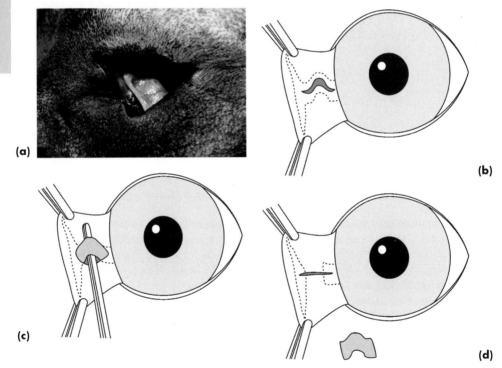

(a)

(b)

(c)

(d)

Figure 3.4   (a) Scrolling of the third-eyelid cartilage in a Great Dane. **(b–d)** The kinked portion of the cartilage in (a) was surgically removed to restore normal anatomical relations between the third eyelid and the globe (b–d).

Clinical signs

- The appearance is characteristic, as the kink can be appreciated by simple visual inspection

- Although the majority of cases have a kink in the long arm of the T, others may have deformity of the short arms
- In some dogs, prolapse of the nictitans gland is also present

Treatment
- If the scrolling is causing no problems, then treatment is not required
- If tear film distribution is affected, with or without accompanying prolapse of the nictitans gland, then surgery is usually the treatment of choice

   Surgery involves removal of the kinked section of cartilage only, normally utilising an approach via the inner aspect of the third eyelid. Following general anaesthesia, the third eyelid is everted and stabilised with stay sutures, or a pair of Allis tissue forceps, placed so as to avoid inadvertent damage to the free border. The overlying conjunctiva is incised, most commonly at 90 degrees to the free margin over the long arm of the 'T' and the affected portion of cartilage is filleted out and excised. It is important to ensure that no sharp edges of cartilage protrude. No suturing is required. If there is also a prolapse of the nictitans gland, it can be relocated as described below (Figure 3.4(b–d)).

Hypertrophy and prolapse of the nictitans gland
Protrusion of the nictitans gland over the free border of the third eyelid is of characteristic appearance (popularly known as 'cherry eye') and is relatively common (Figure 3.5(a)). It should be distinguished from neoplasia, which is uncommon. There appears to be a breed predisposition in, for example, the Beagle, Bulldog and Boston Terrier, but it is an occasional finding in many breeds of dog. The condition may be caused by inherent instability of the connective tissue which anchors the gland at the base of the third eyelid, it may also be a direct consequence of chronic glandular hypertrophy. Whatever the initiating cause, the prolapsed gland becomes reddened in its abnormal location and most owners find it unsightly.

GENERAL AND CANINE OPHTHALMOLOGY

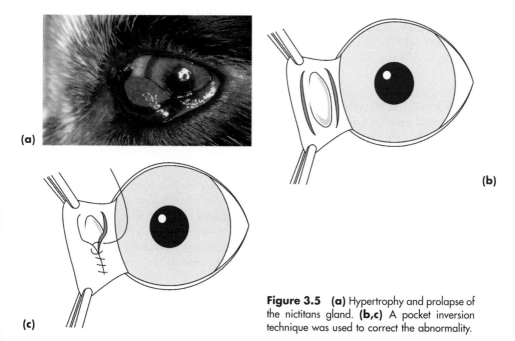

(a)

(b)

(c)

Figure 3.5 (a) Hypertrophy and prolapse of the nictitans gland. **(b,c)** A pocket inversion technique was used to correct the abnormality.

Clinical signs
- The glandular tissue protrudes beyond the free border of the third eyelid. In obese animals the appearance may be particularly florid
- Kinking of the cartilage of the third eyelid may also be present

Differential diagnosis
- Primary and secondary neoplasia
- Chronic inflammatory disease
- Cysts

Treatment
Excision of the prolapsed gland should *not* be carried out, because of the deleterious effects on tear production. Instead it should be relocated. There are a number of published techniques of which the pocket inversion technique (Figures 3.5(b,c)) is the easiest to perform.

Pocket inversion technique
Following general anaesthesia, the third eyelid is everted and stabilised with stay sutures or a pair of Allis tissue forceps, placed so as to avoid inadvertent damage to the free border. A curved incision is made parallel to the free border of the third eyelid, proximal to the prolapsed gland. A second curved incision is made distal to the pro-lapsed gland. The gland is covered by suturing the proximal edge of the first incision and the distal edge of the second incision together, effectively burying the prolapsed gland in a pocket.

The continuous buried sutures of 6-0 polyglactin 910 commence with a buried knot externally on the outer aspect of the third eyelid and also finishes externally with a second buried knot, so as to avoid any possibility of corneal abrasion. It is usual to leave small gaps at each end of the suture line so that the nictitans gland secretions can reach the conjunctival sac.

Surgery may be frustrating because the gland can reprolapse in giant breeds of dog and those with prominent eyes. In the event of reprolapse it may be better to seek specialist advice.

Third eyelid inflammation
As the third eyelid is covered by conjunctiva it can be involved in acute and chronic conjunctivitis (see this section, pp 102–103).

Third eyelid neoplasia
Primary neoplasia is rare. Examples reported in the dog include papilloma, melanoma, adenocarcinoma, adenoma, squamous cell carcinoma, haemangioma, angiokeratoma and mastocytoma. Secondary involvement is most commonly a consequence of multi-centric lymphoma and systemic histiocytosis. It is important that primary tumours of the third eyelid are differentiated from primary tumours that have infiltrated from elsewhere (e.g. nasal tumours) and from secondary tumours.

Treatment
- Primary localised tumours can be excised with the patient under general anaesthesia

and this is one of the few situations in which it is permissible to sacrifice part or all of the third eyelid
- All third eyelid tumours should be submitted for histopathological examination
- Lifelong tear replacement therapy will be required in those animals in which corneal health is compromised by third eyelid loss

CONDITIONS OF THE CANINE UPPER AND LOWER EYELIDS

Ophthalmia neonatorum
The eyelids of neonatal puppies remain naturally fused (*ankyloblepharon*) for some 7–15 days postnatally. Occasionally infection behind the fused eyelids results in *ophthalmia neonatorum* (neonatal conjunctivitis) and the situation must be recognised if complications such as globe rupture and endophthalmitis are to be avoided. Canine herpes virus and bacteria such as coagulase-positive Staphylococci are the usual cause. *Ophthalmia neonatorum* is commoner in kittens than puppies and is illustrated in Section 4, pp 183–185.

Clinical signs
Swelling is apparent behind the fused eyelids and there is usually an ocular discharge or beads of pus in the medial canthal region.

Treatment
- Premature opening of the eyelids is required if vision-threatening complications (ulceration, perforation, endophthalmitis) are to be avoided
- It is usually possible to separate the eyelids in the conscious puppy. A topical local anaesthetic can be applied to the medial canthus beforehand
- One tip of blunt-tipped tenotomy scissors is inserted medially and slid gently and with considerable care along the presumptive opening, in the same way as a paper knife is used to open an envelope. Avoid applying pressure to the globe while separating the eyelids
- Once the eyelids have been separated, all ocular discharge should be gently cleaned away and appropriate topical medical treatment using an antibiotic in an oily excipient (chloramphenicol ointment or fusidic acid gel) should be applied to ensure that the eyelids remain open. Note that the ocular media may not be transparent if the puppy is less than five weeks of age. This is a normal feature of carnivore eyes, as postnatal development continues for some 12 weeks after birth
- General nursing care, as appropriate, should accompany local ocular treatment

Entropion
Entropion is the in-turning (inversion) of the whole eyelid or part of the eyelid and is a common problem in dogs. The types include spastic entropion (a result of anterior-segment pain), anatomical entropion (breed related), cicatricial entropion (a result of fibrosis and scarring) and atonic entropion (a consequence of laxity and often associated with senility).

Entropion is common in certain breeds and is probably inherited in many dogs with anatomical entropion. When examining affected animals it is important to make the assessment without distorting the eyelid appearance by handling the head. Sedation or general anaesthesia should also be avoided when calculating the extent of the entropion, particularly if surgery is contemplated. If surgery is required it is performed with the patient under general anaesthesia.

Spastic entropion
If a spastic component is suspected, topical local anaesthesia is an essential part of the investigative procedure. If the blepharospasm and accompanying entropion resolve following the application of local anaesthetic, it is obvious that entropion surgery is not required as the entropion is of pain-related (spastic) origin. It is important to establish and eliminate the reason for the anterior-segment pain.

Anatomical entropion
Anatomical entropion is a unilateral or bilateral condition that may affect part of the eyelid or the whole length of the eyelid. Although the lower eyelid is most commonly affected, both upper and lower can be involved. The situation can be further complicated by the lateral canthal ligament providing poor support (as in breeds with a diamond-shaped eye) or the ligament being too taut. The age of onset is variable: in breeds such as the Shar Pei, the condition may develop almost as soon as the eyelids first open (Figure 3.6(a)), whereas in other breeds the entropion develops at a few months of age.

Many breeds of dog can be affected by entropion and a dominant mode of inheritance may operate in some of them. The possible genetic implications should be discussed with the owner for *any* eyelid disorder that demonstrates a familial trait. The aim of such counselling being the prevention of heritable malformations, rather than their perpetuation by continued breeding.

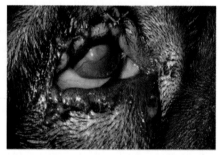

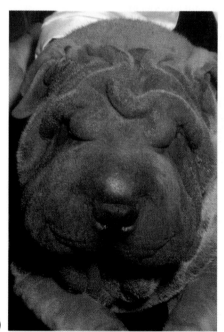

(a)

(b)

Figure 3.6 (a) Anatomical entropion in a young Shar Pei. **(b)** A temporary tacking procedure is used to evert the eyelid margins in entropion. For mild cases, only the lower eyelid requires suturing, but in the majority of cases both upper and lower eyelids are sutured (with acknowledgements to D. J. Gould).

In young animals with mild entropion it is sometimes possible to delay corrective excisional surgery until maturity. If, however, there is any pain and discomfort, or if corneal damage is occurring, then treatment must be undertaken. Temporary sutures without incision (see below) provide the easiest solution in young animals and temporary tacking procedures often break the cycle of irritation and blepharospasm that exacerbates the existing entropion; so producing a satisfactory long term solution (Figure 3.6(b)).

Cicatricial entropion

Cicatricial entropion is not particularly common in small animals. Causes include previous surgery, trauma, chronic inflammation and injuries from caustic chemicals.

Atonic (senile) entropion

Atonic entropion is seen most commonly in the aged Cocker Spaniel and the accompanying trichiasis (normal eyelashes in contact with the cornea) can produce corneal damage. The discomfort produced by the condition may result in self-inflicted trauma, and it is not unusual for affected patients to develop further problems such as blepharitis and periorbital dermatitis.

Correction of the entropion is all that is required for mild cases, whilst more radical procedures are needed for severe cases. A course of systemic antibiotic is needed prior to surgery in those animals with established blepharitis or dermatitis. Staphylococci and streptococci are the commonest causative organisms, and oral penicillin, or similar, given for three weeks, is indicated.

Entropion surgery

There are many surgical techniques for entropion correction, but in general the simplest effective method of repair for the type of entropion present is the one which should be selected. It is worth emphasising, however, that techniques such as the injection of materials like liquid paraffin into the eyelid *have no place* in the treatment of entropion in any species; chronic complications of this approach include cellulitis, lipogranuloma formation and severe eyelid distortion.

More difficult cases, especially in dogs with large skulls, may require a combination of blepharoplastic techniques, including section of the lateral canthal ligament (lateral canthal tendonotomy) and are probably best referred.

Temporary suturing

Temporary suturing without incision may be used in young animals (e.g. Shar Pei). Vertical mattress sutures are usually employed, using 5-0 silk, braided nylon or polyglactin 910 on a reverse cutting needle (Figure 3.6(b)). Sufficient skin is pinched between forefinger and thumb just below the eyelid margin to restore normal anatomical relations and some 3–4 vertical mattress sutures are inserted. This temporary tacking procedure is an effective means of everting the eyelid in dogs, lambs and foals with neonatal entropion.

Hotz-Celsus procedure

The Hotz-Celsus procedure of skin–muscle resection is the commonest excisional technique used for uncomplicated entropion. At the time of examination of the conscious, unsedated dog a simple diagram of the proposed surgery should be drawn and *not*

GENERAL AND CANINE
OPHTHALMOLOGY

revised once the animal is more relaxed because it is sedated and/or anaesthetised. A finger, lid plate, tongue depressor or scalpel handle is placed within the conjunctival sac to tense the lid and protect the cornea and, of these, a finger is the most effective.

An incision is made parallel to the affected portion of eyelid, and it is important that the first incision is placed sufficiently close to the lid margin (approximately 2 mm). The second incision is elliptical, made at a distance far enough away from the first to correct the entropion. The incised skin and muscle is usually removed with Stevens tenotomy scissors or by sharp dissection with a scalpel, using a 15-gauge Bard-Parker blade.

The defect is closed with simple interrupted 5-0 or 6-0 silk sutures which are removed 5–7 days later. Alternatively, absorbable material such as 5-0 to 6-0 polyglactin 910 may be used. The suture knots are placed as far from the eyelid margin as possible (Figure 3.7(a,b,c) and 3.8(a,b,c,d)).

When the Hotz-Celsus procedure is used to correct medial canthal lower eyelid entropion, the incision made is triangular in shape, with its base closest to the eyelid margin (Figure 3.12(b,c)).

Y- to V-plasty

Y-to-V plasty is a procedure that is used for simple cases of cicatricial entropion.

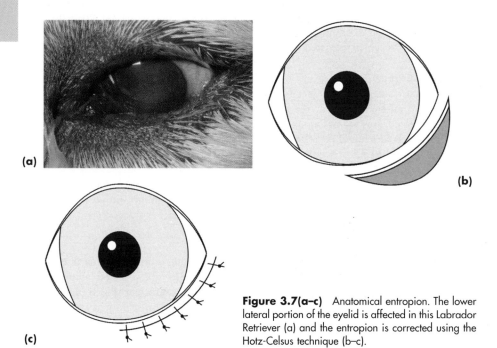

Figure 3.7(a–c) Anatomical entropion. The lower lateral portion of the eyelid is affected in this Labrador Retriever (a) and the entropion is corrected using the Hotz-Celsus technique (b–c).

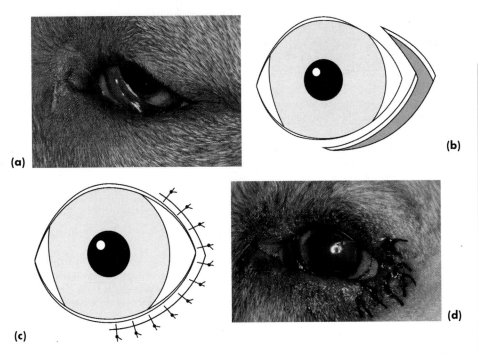

Figure 3.8(a–d) Anatomical entropion. If there is also a tendency for the eyelid to 'kink' at the lateral canthus (a), the Hotz-Celsus technique is modified by extending the tissue excision to incorporate a portion of the upper eyelid as illustrated (b–d).

Ectropion

Ectropion is an outward turning of the eyelid (Figure 3.9(a)). In mild form some breeders would consider it a 'desirable' breed feature. As such it is reproducible and presumed to be inherited in many of the affected breeds. There is a gap between the eyelid and the cornea so that the conjunctiva and cornea are relatively exposed, the tear film is poorly distributed and there is an increased propensity for foreign material to gain access to the lower conjunctival sac. However, ectropion rarely produces any major discomfort for the animal and in many cases it is better to leave it alone, providing that recurrent conjunctivitis and/or keratitis are not causing problems.

In some dogs the degree of ectropion varies considerably according to whether the animal is relaxed and tired or alert. If normal conformation is present in the alert state, surgery is not usually required.

Ectropion may be anatomical (usually a consequence of selective breeding), cicatricial, atonic and paralytic.

Anatomical ectropion

Anatomical ectropion usually involves the lower eyelid (Figure 3.9(a)), except when more complicated deformity results in a 'diamond eye'. Lower eyelid ectropion is a typical feature of breeds such as the Bassett Hound, St Bernard and Clumber Spaniel.

Cicatricial ectropion

Cicatricial ectropion has the same possible origins as cicatricial entropion.

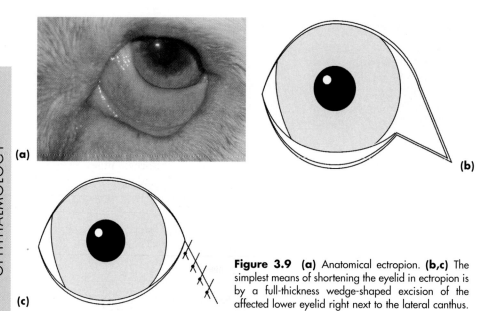

(a)

(b)

(c)

Figure 3.9 **(a)** Anatomical ectropion. **(b,c)** The simplest means of shortening the eyelid in ectropion is by a full-thickness wedge-shaped excision of the affected lower eyelid right next to the lateral canthus.

Atonic ectropion
Atonic ectropion is usually a consequence of senility and predominantly affects the lower eyelid, just as senile atonic entropion affects predominantly the upper eyelid.

Paralytic ectropion
Paralytic ectropion is usually a consequence of facial (VIIth) nerve paresis or paralysis, but is also occasionally seen in mild form in dogs with Horner's syndrome.

Ectropion surgery
There are many possible techniques for the correction of ectropion, some of which are unnecessarily complicated unless there is a real problem with defective eyelid tone. Wedge excision (Figure 3.9(b,c)) is the commonest technique and is used for the treatment of both ectropion and eyelid neoplasia.

Wedge excision
The assessment of these cases is made exactly as already outlined for entropion surgery. The appropriately-sized wedge of tissue is excised right next to the lateral canthus and the lid is closed using a single layer of 5-0 to 6-0 simple interrupted silk or polyglactin 910 sutures. The first suture re-apposes the eyelid margin and may be inserted as a figure of eight suture or a simple interrupted suture, but, whichever is selected, apposition must be perfect.

V-to-Y plasty
V-to-Y Plasty is very useful for simple cases of cicatricial ectropion.

Macropalpebral fissure – 'diamond' eye
The 'diamond-shaped' eye is achieved through selective breeding. Breeds affected

include the Bloodhound, Clumber Spaniel and St Bernard (Figure 3.10). The conformation of the skull and the amount of redundant skin, together with overlong eyelids and weak support from the lateral canthal ligament, combine so that there is a tendency for the central portion of the eyelid margin to evert and the medial and lateral eyelid margins to involute. There is thus combined ectropion and entropion and, often, a degree of exposure keratopathy. Permanent spastic entropion and secondary keratitis eventually supervene.

Treatment
Surgery is complex and can include some, or all, of eyelid shortening by wedge excision, Hotz-Celsus resection and re-alignment of the lateral canthal tendon, so such cases are better referred.

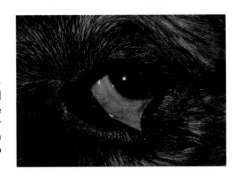

Figure 3.10 Macropalpebral fissure ('diamond eye') in a St Bernard. This was corrected by removing full-thickness wedges from the lateral aspects of both the upper and lower eyelids to shorten the eyelids, together with tensioning the lateral canthus by direct suture to the periosteum of the zygomatic arch.

Micropalpebral fissure – blepharophimosis
This is seen as an isolated feature in breeds such as the Shetland Sheepdog or combined with other eyelid problems such as entropion and excessive skin folds in breeds such as the Chow Chow (Figure 3.11).

Treatment
- Treatment is not always required, but may be complex when it is needed because of the other accompanying abnormalities
- The simplest way of increasing the palpebral fissure is by modified lateral canthotomy

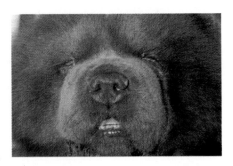

Figure 3.11 Micropalpebral fissure (blepharophimosis) in a Chow Chow. This dog also had small eyes, and animals with this degree of anatomical abnormality require referral.

Pekingese and pug adnexal disease

Possible problems (Figure 3.12(a))

- Prominent globe/shallow orbit (excessive palpebral aperture)
- Anaesthetic cornea (insensitive)
- Inadequate blink (lagophthalmos)
- Distichiasis (see this section, pp 90–91)
- Medial canthal hairs and/or hairy caruncle
- Medial lower eyelid entropion
- Nasal folds

Solutions

- Shorten eyelid opening (permanent medial or lateral canthorrhaphy – usually best referred for this technique)
- Medial lower eyelid entropion can be treated using the modified Hotz-Celsus technique outlined earlier (Figure 3.12(b,c))
- Medial canthoplasty is the simplest means of shortening the eyelids, negating the effects of lower medial entropion, medial canthal hairs and a hairy caruncle (usually best to refer cases for this technique)
- Catholysis for distichia if the extra eyelashes are causing a problem (animals with troublesome distichiasis may require referral)
- Nasal folds can be excised with strong sharp scissors and the skin defect closed with simple interrupted sutures or a continuous running suture, using 5-0 silk or polyglactin 910
- Tear replacement therapy may also be required

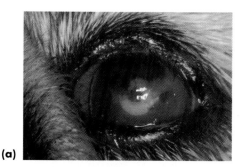

(a)

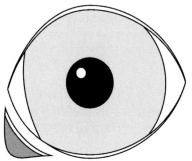

(b)

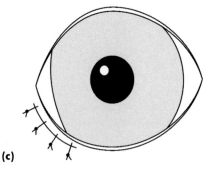

(c)

Figure 3.12 **(a)** Multiple adnexal abnormalities in a Pekingese. Previous partial tarsal plate excision had exacerbated the situation as distichia were still present, but many of the hairs had become misdirected and corneal ulceration was present in the left eye, illustrated here. **(b,c)** Quality of life for the dog in (a) was improved considerably by a modified Hotz-Celsus technique to correct the medial lower eyelid entropion, excision of the nasal folds, catholysis for the distichiasis and a short course of tear replacement therapy.

Cocker spaniel adnexal disease
Possible problems (Figure 3.13(a,b))
- Upper eyelid entropion, usually age-related (atonic) and trichiasis (see this section, p. 90)
- Lower eyelid ectropion, usually age-related (atonic)
- Distichiasis
- Inadequate tear production (KCS)
- Inadequate tear distribution
- Secondary blepharoconjunctivitis

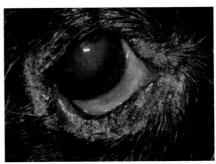

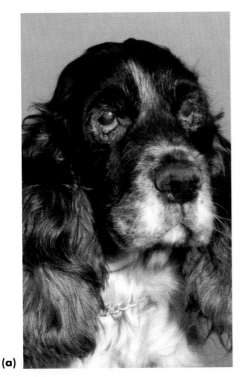

(b)

(a)

GENERAL AND CANINE OPHTHALMOLOGY

Figure 3.13(a,b) Multiple adnexal abnormalities in a Cocker Spaniel. Anatomical imperfection was associated with lower eyelid ectropion and upper eyelid entropion with trichiasis (the normal upper eyelashes are in contact with the cornea). Sparse distichia were present in the upper and lower eyelids of both eyes. Tear production was low in both eyes (Schirmer I tear test of 5 mm/minute in each eye). Secondary blepharitis (*Staphylococcal* spp on culture) and corneal pathology were apparent. The dog was given systemic and local antibiotic treatment over a four-week period for the staphylococcal infection. Tear replacement therapy was also instituted for the dry eye after ascertaining that there was no underlying treatable cause, such as hypothyroidism. Rhytidectomy was the surgical procedure chosen to restore normal anatomical relations in this dog.

Solutions
- Antibiotic therapy for the blepharoconjunctivitis (may require local application as well as systemic treatment) for at least three weeks

- Medical treatment for KCS (rarely surgical)
- Catholysis for distichia if the extra lashes are causing a problem (cases may require referral)
- Surgical treatment for anatomical problems. Minor problems can be corrected by eyelid surgery (many techniques), whereas major problems (so called 'slipped facial mask') require more complex surgery (e.g. face lift or rhytidectomy). Many of these cases are best referred

Trichiasis

Trichiasis denotes normal eyelashes in contact with the cornea. It is seen in conjunction with entropion or as a consequence of laxity or deformity of the upper eyelid. Untreated trichiasis will cause keratitis and, in chronic cases, pigmentation of the area of cornea subjected to low-grade trauma is the most prominent feature. Medial-canthal hair (caruncular region) and facial hair (e.g. associated with medial lower eyelid entropion and nasal folds) in contact with the cornea will also cause similar problems. Medial canthal hair is seen most commonly in breeds such as the Lhasa Apso, Shih Tsu and Tibetan Spaniel and is invariably a cause of chronic epiphora.

Treatment

- Minor cases of trichiasis are most readily treated by the most appropriate type of entropion surgery. When the trichiasis is part of a more complex presentation, as in some aged Cocker Spaniels, a more radical approach (e.g. Stades procedure or rhytidectomy) may be needed and referral is necessary
- Medial canthal hairs may be treated by medial canthoplasty, by excision of the caruncle, or hair follicles can be destroyed using catholysis. When there is also subtle medial lower eyelid entropion a medial canthoplasty or Hotz-Celsus resection of the affected region of eyelid can be performed
- Nasal folds can be excised with strong sharp scissors and the skin defect closed with simple interrupted or continuous sutures as outlined previously

Distichiasis

Extra eyelashes are common in a number of purebred and crossbred dogs. The extra lashes usually arise from the tarsal (meibomian) gland orifice and there may be one or several cilia emerging from each opening. In affected animals, the meibomian gland openings are often more haphazardly arranged than in normal animals. The problems caused by the extra lashes depend on the relationship between the eyelids and the cornea, particularly the degree of globe prominence, and the stiffness and length of the cilia (Figure 3.14).

Breeds affected include the Boxer, Bulldog, Flatcoated Retriever, Miniature Long-haired Dachshund, Miniature and Toy Poodle, Pekingese, Rough Collie, Shetland sheepdog and some spaniels (American and English Cocker, Welsh Springer). It is worth advising owners as to the possible inherited nature of distichiasis in most of the breeds in which it is seen.

Treatment

If the extra lashes are causing the dog no problem other than premature disruption of the tear film then they should be left alone, especially as some procedures (e.g. partial tarsal-plate excision) destroy meibomian-gland function.

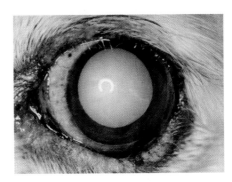

Figure 3.14 Distichiasis. This American Cocker Spaniel had been referred for cataract surgery and the distichia were an incidental finding, as the dog had lived with distichiasis without apparent untoward effect for most of its life. Note that the cataract is total and tending to hypermaturity with concomitant darkening of the iris.

Catholysis

Catholysis is an excellent method of treatment for those dogs which have problems, but general anaesthesia, good magnification and a commercial electroepilation unit are required and the procedure is moderately time consuming, so cases are often referred. Only those extra lashes that are visible can be destroyed, although if the eyelids are squeezed gently at the time of the procedure other lashes may be partially extruded.

The catholysis needle is placed directly into the affected meibomian gland opening and the hair follicles are destroyed using a setting of 3–5 milliamps for approximately ten seconds for each distichium. Because of the cyclical growth pattern of hairs, a second treatment is occasionally necessary, to deal with distichia that have subsequently emerged from untreated openings.

Cryosurgery

Cryosurgery with either nitrous oxide or liquid nitrogen, using a small cryoprobe and a double freeze-thaw cycle, is also an effective and selective means of treatment, as the hair follicles are more susceptible to cold than the meibomian glands. Owners should be warned of the temporary, rarely permanent, loss of eyelid pigment that will follow. The procedure is carried out under general anaesthesia. There is more eyelid swelling in the immediate postoperative period than is encountered after catholysis, but this can be reduced by the judicious use of non-steroidal anti-inflammatory agents. It is usually better to consider referral unless familiar with the use of cryosurgery at this site.

Ectopic cilia

The cilia (multiple), or cilium (single), emerge through the palpebral conjunctiva and impinge directly on the cornea. The condition is therefore painful and may present acutely with the typical signs of anterior-segment discomfort (pain, blepharospasm and excessive lacrimation). The usual location for these lashes is underneath the middle part of the upper eyelid a few millimetres from the eyelid margin (Figure 3.15(a)), but a careful search may be required as the cilia can arise in other sites. As with distichia the extra lashes usually arise from hair follicles within the meibomian glands.

Breeds of dog affected include the Bulldog, Flatcoated Retriever, Pekingese, Cocker Spaniel, Rough Collie, Shetland Sheepdog and Yorkshire Terrier.

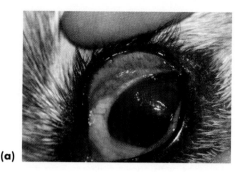

(a)

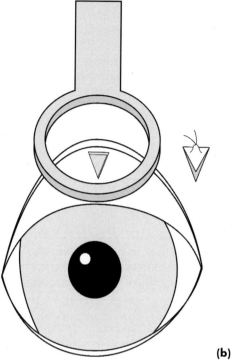

Figure 3.15 **(a)** Ectopic cilium. The ectopic cilium in this Shetland Sheepdog has caused a superficial corneal ulcer and the position and shape of the ulcer mirrors accurately the excursion of the upper eyelid. **(b)** Sharp excision from the palpebral surface of the eyelid was used to remove the hair-producing follicle in (a). The ulcer healed uneventfully without any additional treatment after the underlying cause was removed.

(b)

Treatment
- The most effective technique is simple resection of the hair-producing follicle(s) from the palpebral aspect of the eyelid under general anaesthesia (Figure 3.15(b))
- Tarsal cyst forceps are useful for stabilising the eyelid and reducing haemorrhage. A sharp triangular-shaped incision is made around the extra lash, making sure that it is deep enough to remove the follicle from which the cilium or cilia arise. No sutures are required

Dermatoses
Other eyelid diseases are reasonably common in the dog. There are a number of possible causes, which include parasitic (e.g. demodectic and sarcoptic mange), mycotic (e.g. *Microsporum* spp and *Trichophyton* spp) and bacterial infection (e.g. *Staphylococcus* spp). Non-infectious causes include hypersensitivity reactions (e.g. atopy, contact hypersensitivity reactions, food intolerance), immune-mediated diseases (e.g. pemphigus complex, uveodermatological syndrome, discoid and systemic lupus erythematosus), zinc-responsive dermatoses and mucocutaneous pyoderma. In non-temperate climates, eyelid involvement may be a feature of generalised fungal disease.

Accurate diagnosis is based on the history and clinical appearance with additional help from other methods such as impression smears, culture (in a range of growth media) and, most importantly, biopsy. Routine histopathology may need to be supplemented by special techniques such as immunofluorescence, especially for putative immune-mediated problems. Intradermal skin tests and skin biopsy may also be appropriate and details should be obtained from standard veterinary dermatology texts.

Acute eyelid inflammation

- Hypersensitivity reactions, of which atopy is the commonest, are not uncommon. Atopic dermatitis can also present as a chronic problem, with breeds such as the English Setter, Labrador Retriever and West Highland White Terrier being over-represented. Eyelid involvement includes conjunctivitis and there may also be changes elsewhere (e.g. skin)
- Juvenile pyoderma may be a type of bacterial hypersensitivity. It typically affects the head region only, affects puppies less than three months of age and responds to systemic treatment with broad-spectrum antibiotics and immunosuppressive doses of corticosteroids
- Reactions to insect bites and stings should also be considered when there is an acute presentation – usually swollen eyelids ± facial swelling

Chronic eyelid inflammation

- Meibomianitis is the commonest chronic eyelid infection reported in the dog. Although it may have acute origins it is most likely to be diagnosed when chronic, particularly if granuloma formation (chalazion) supervenes
- Management of meibomianitis can be difficult. Warm compresses can be helpful and meibomian secretion should be expressed and cultured before an appropriate topical and systemic broad-spectrum antibiotic is selected for long-term treatment
- When chalazia have formed, excision and curettage of the inspissated material utilising an approach via the palpebral conjunctiva may be required

Neoplasia

Primary eyelid neoplasia is common in dogs, and such tumours are usually benign (Figure 3.16(a)). Sebaceous adenoma and adenocarcinoma, melanoma and papilloma account for approximately 80% of eyelid neoplasms. Others reported include squamous cell carcinoma, basal cell carcinoma, sebaceous gland epithelioma, histiocytoma and mast cell tumour. Most canine eyelid tumours are removed surgically under general anaesthesia.

Treatment

The majority of canine primary eyelid tumours can be excised by a deep full-thickness modified wedge excision (deep and house-shaped or V-shaped), taking care to check the full extent of the tumour before surgery (look beneath the eyelid) (Figure 3.16(b)). A 2 mm rim of normal tissue should be included. The eyelid can be closed in one layer using 5-0 to 6-0 non-absorbable (silk) or absorbable (polyglactin 910) suture material on a cutting needle. The eyelid margin is closed first, with either a figure of eight suture or a simple interrupted suture, the remainder of the incision is closed with simple interrupted sutures (Figure 3.16(c)). In most dogs direct closure is possible with loss of up to a third of the eyelid length. When this amount is exceeded it is simplest to use a sliding lateral canthoplasty to relieve tension and prevent eyelid distortion as an adjunct to primary closure (Figure 3.16(d,e)).

Referral should be considered for more complex problems, as there are a considerable number of possible blepharoplastic techniques. As a general principle, eyelid surgery should be kept simple, and the aim is to ensure normal congruity (accuracy of apposition between the eyelid and the globe) and mobility. A surgically-created eyelid should have a conjunctival- or mucous-membrane-lined inner surface and some form of hairless eyelid margin (e.g. transposed eyelid margin as with the Mustardé technique, or transposed buccal mucosa as with lip-to-lid procedures) so that there is no possibility of skin hairs coming into contact with the cornea.

- Rarely, surgery may need to be combined with other treatments such as cryotherapy or radiotherapy.
- Any atypical or unusual tumours must be submitted for histopathology.

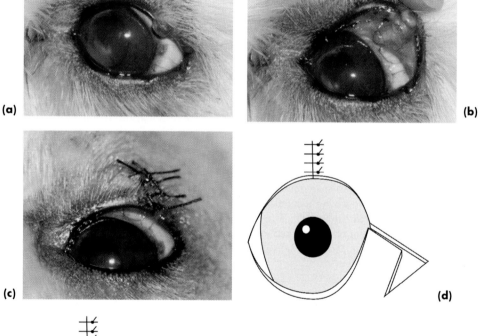

Figure 3.16 **(a)** Eyelid neoplasia (sebaceous adenoma) in a West Highland White Terrier. **(b)** When the eyelid in (a) is everted, the extent of the tumour is apparent. **(c)** A full thickness V-shaped incision was used to excise the mass and the wound closed in one layer with simple interrupted sutures of 5–0 silk. **(d,e)** When eyelid tumours are large enough to distort the eyelid contour after primary closure a simple releasing technique (sliding lateral canthoplasty) can be used at the lateral canthus.

GENERAL AND CANINE
OPHTHALMOLOGY

LACRIMAL SYSTEM

INTRODUCTION

The lacrimal system consists of the lacrimal and nictitans glands; the accessory glands (e.g. the meibomian or tarsal glands and the glands of Zeiss and Moll); the *preocular tear film* (PTF); the lacrimal lake; the upper and lower lacrimal puncta and canaliculi; the lacrimal sac (which is a defined structure in humans, but not in domestic animals); the nasolacrimal duct and the nasal ostium or punctum. The tears usually drain into the vestibulum of the nasal cavity. In brachycephalic dogs (and most cats) the nasolacrimal duct is short and wide and often opens more caudally, so that the tears drain into the nasopharynx (Figure 3.17).

The PTF is complex, and consists of an external oily (lipid) layer (mainly from meibomian glands), aqueous (lacrimal and nictitans glands) and mucin (conjunctival goblet cells and surface epithelial cells). The normal canine tear film has a pH of 6.8–8.0 with a mean of around 7.5.

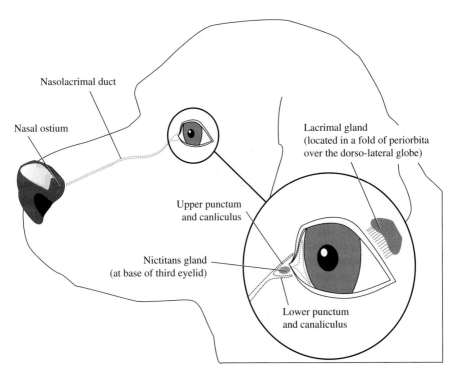

Figure 3.17 The canine lacrimal system. The main secretory components comprise the nictitans and lacrimal glands (shown in light grey at the medial and dorsolateral canthus respectively), the conjunctival goblet cells and the meibomian glands in the eyelid margins. The excretory components consist of the upper and lower puncta and their respective canaliculi. These conjoin at the vestigial lacrimal sac to form the nasolacrimal duct, which terminates rostrally as the nasal ostium.

GENERAL AND CANINE
OPHTHALMOLOGY

The preocular tear film covers the ocular surface and quantitative, qualitative or tear-film distribution problems should always be considered when the ocular surface appears abnormal. Note that the ocular surface is a term used to describe the continuous epithelium which covers the third eyelid, extends from the eyelid margins onto the back of the eyelids, into the fornices and onto the globe. It includes the conjunctival, limbal and corneal epithelium.

INVESTIGATION OF LACRIMAL DYSFUNCTION IN SMALL ANIMALS

- Investigation of lacrimal dysfunction requires careful inspection of the external eye and adnexa, paying particular attention to conformation, eyelid congruity, the frequency and adequacy of blinking, the presence, position and size of the lacrimal puncta and the position of normal and extraneous hairs. The nature and position of any ocular discharge and the site and extent of any inflammation must also be assessed.

- The aqueous portion of the tear film is most commonly assessed using the Schirmer I Tear Test (Figure 3.18) and the test should be performed before any solutions are applied to the eye. The test strip is bent at the notch and the short portion is placed in the ventral conjunctival sac. In normal dogs a reading of 15 mm ± 5 mm is obtained for reflex tear production over one minute. Readings of less than 5 mm per minute are significant. Fear, sedation and general anaesthesia all reduce the values.

- Scrapes, impression smears and swabs should, if relevant, be taken before the tissues are handled to any extent to avoid inadvertent contamination.

- Fluorescein dye can be used to assess the patency of the nasolacrimal drainage system. Fluorescein usually appears at the nostrils within five minutes of installation into the lower conjunctival sac. However, in brachycephalic dogs, the back of the tongue and throat region should also be examined if fluorescein does not appear at the nostrils. The dye is most readily detected in the dark using a light source fitted with a cobalt blue filter. If there is doubt as to patency, further investigation is warranted.

- The system can be irrigated (under local or general anaesthesia) via a lacrimal cannula placed in the upper punctum. Patency of the lower punctum and canaliculus is established first (digital pressure should be applied to the lacrimal sac region), then the lower punctum is occluded so that patency of the nasolacrimal duct can be demonstrated. Fluid for culture is usually collected from the nostrils if culture is required and the samples should be cultured both aerobically and anaerobically. When the whole system is to be catheterised, general anaesthesia is required. The nasal ostium is not visible in the dog without special equipment.

- Dacryocystorhinography is useful on occasions; plain films should be taken before the injection of iodine-based contrast medium via the upper punctum and canaliculus. The lower punctum is usually occluded with fine mosquito forceps. Lateral and dorsoventral radiographic views should be taken within a few seconds of injection. Slightly oblique views may also be useful to avoid superimposition of, for example, the tooth roots.

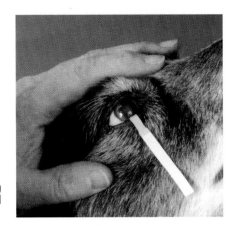

Figure 3.18 Schirmer I tear test being carried out. In this dog production was normal (15 mm/minute).

CANINE LACRIMAL SYSTEM PROBLEMS – THE DRY EYE

Whilst aqueous deficiency (keratoconjunctivitis sicca or 'dry eye') is the commonest clinical condition, lipid abnormalities (e.g. after partial tarsal plate excision) and mucin abnormalities (e.g. associated with chronic conjunctivitis) can also occur as independent problems.

Defective spreading of tear film is usually associated either with eyelid problems (absence, defects, masses, abnormal lashes), prominent or enlarged eyes or abnormal blinking (e.g. of neurological origin).

If complex ocular surface disorders are suspected, or if there is inadequate response to tear replacement therapy, it is sensible to seek specialist advice.

Keratoconjunctivitis sicca
Incidence
Keratoconjunctivitis sicca (KCS) is a common and frequently misdiagnosed problem, most likely to be mistaken for a simple 'conjunctivitis'.

Aetiology
- *Congenital* causes include aplasia or hypoplasia of the lacrimal gland ± nictitans gland. In affected animals (e.g. Yorkshire Terriers) the nose is often dry
- *Acquired* causes include immune-mediated disease, the commonest cause, especially in the West Highland White Terrier (Figure 3.19(a)); systemic diseases (e.g. canine distemper); direct insult (injuries to the head, chemical injury, irradiation); neurogenic; drug-induced (e.g. sulphonamides, topical atropine); metabolic (e.g. hypothyroidism); unknown.

(a) 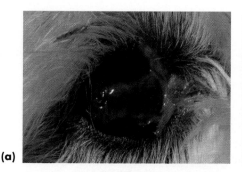 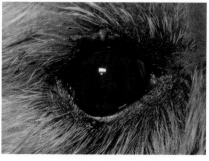 (b)

Figure 3.19 **(a)** Keratoconjunctivitis sicca (dry eye) in a two-year-old West Highland White Terrier, the breed most commonly affected by the immune-mediated type of dry eye in the UK. Both eyes were affected. A profuse and tacky mucoid discharge is adherent to the cornea of the right eye. The Schirmer tear test reading in this eye was 0 mm/minute and 5 mm/minute in the left eye. **(b)** The left eye responded to topical cyclosporin and this treatment was maintained, whereas it was discontinued in the right eye after two months' of treatment brought about no improvement and a parotid-duct transposition was performed. The right eye is illustrated some two years after parotid duct transposition.

Clinical signs
- The eye is usually uncomfortable, rather than frankly painful, although frank pain and corneal ulceration may accompany acute onset KCS
- Disruption of the corneal reflex and lacklustre appearance of the cornea
- Superficial keratitis with neovascularisation, oedema and, eventually, secondary pigmentation; in chronic KCS corneal desiccation (*xerosis*) also occurs
- Diffuse conjunctivitis
- Mucopurulent ocular discharge (yellow or green in colour and of tenacious consistency)
- Secondary bacterial infection
- In neurogenic dry eye the nostril on the affected side, or both nostrils in bilateral cases, are dry and crusty. Acquired KCS of neurogenic origin is sometimes associated with chronic middle ear disease

Diagnosis
- Breed, age and sex; systemic and ophthalmic history including any previous treatment
- Clinical signs
- A Schirmer I Tear Test should *always* form part of the work-up for animals with an ocular discharge, or any indications of ocular surface disease – it is important to test *both* eyes

Medical treatment
- The KCS can be managed medically by careful *cleaning* of the eyes to remove the tenacious discharge, followed by frequent application of a *proprietary ocular lubricant* such as carbomer 980 (polyacrylic acid)
- Preparations containing *mucolytics*, such as acetylcysteine, can be of value initially if excessive amounts of mucin are present

- Topical antibiotic treatment may be necessary in the early stages, as secondary bacterial infection is common
- Drugs that have *immunosuppressive activity* and *stimulate tear production* (e.g. topical cyclosporin) are the most useful, especially for possible *immune-mediated* KCS. A commercial preparation of cyclosporin ointment is available for clinical use and this is now the treatment of choice for most cases of KCS. The drug has a beneficial effect on mucin secretion as well as stimulating aqueous production. Cyclosporin should be applied twice daily for at least six weeks to assess the adequacy of response and the Schirmer tear test repeated during this time. Responsive cases require twice daily treatment for life
- The *parasympathomimetic agent* pilocarpine may be beneficial, by the oral or topical route, in KCS of *neurogenic origin*, but is of no value for immune-mediated types
- *Topical corticosteroids* may be helpful in initial management, provided that no corneal ulceration is present. Some of the proprietary preparations contain ocular lubricants as well as corticosteroids (see Appendix 2)

Surgical treatment – parotid duct transposition

- If the loss of tear production is absolute and permanent, or the owners cannot manage medical therapy, or the clinical signs are not kept under control with medical treatment, then parotid duct transposition should be considered. If the surgeon is not thoroughly familiar with the technique, it is sensible to practise it first or refer the patient.
- Case selection is important, for example an excessively wet eye may result when parotid duct transposition is carried out in greedy animals and, in all cases, it is usual to divide the feeds up over a 24-hour period to provide optimal lubrication.
- Parotid duct transposition is carried out under general anaesthesia and should only be performed after checking that the parotid salivary gland actually produces saliva, that the pH of the saliva is not too alkaline (ideally less than 8.4, from clinical experience) and after discussing the possible postoperative management at some length with the owners.
- Possible immediate complications of parotid duct transposition include those associated with poor case selection and surgical mistakes.
- Chronic postoperative problems include excessively wet eyes and face, periorbital hair loss, skin excoriation and corneal deposition (usually calcium salts). Very rarely, if the results are not satisfactory, the parotid duct can be ligated either to reduce the flow of saliva or stop it altogether.
- If patients are chosen carefully the results of parotid duct transposition are very rewarding (Figure 3.19(b)).

CANINE LACRIMAL SYSTEM PROBLEMS – THE WET EYE

Epiphora is tear overflow resulting from poor drainage, the aetiology is outlined below and epiphora should be distinguished from the excessive lacrimation that is associated with ocular pain (Figure 3.20).

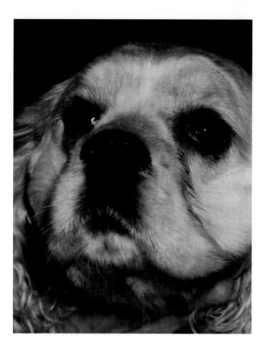

Figure 3.20 Epiphora (tear overflow) in an American Cocker Spaniel. This eight-year-old dog had only recently developed epiphora, so congenital causes can be discounted despite the dog's somewhat imperfect eyelid anatomy. In this case dacryocystitis had developed after conjunctivitis. *Staphylococcus* spp were cultured from material irrigated from the nasolacrimal duct and the condition resolved soon after a course of topical antibiotic drops was instituted.

Aetiology of developmental abnormalities of the nasolacrimal drainage system

Poor or imperfect anatomy

- Long-nosed dogs ('pocket' effect at medial canthus), especially when the dog has both a long nose and small eyes
- Tight apposition between the cornea and eyelid margin, especially if combined with a prominent eye
- Medial canthal entropion
- Hairs on the caruncle
- Distichiasis and trichiasis
- Abnormal location of lacrimal puncta

Imperforate puncta and micropuncta

Imperforate puncta and micropuncta are common, and it is usually the lower punctum that is affected. There is a breed predisposition in the English Cocker Spaniel and Golden Retriever and epiphora is first noticed at an early age. The diagnosis is usually straightforward in that the punctum is either absent or very small, the dog is young and the owners have noted persistent tear staining (unilateral or bilateral) from an early age.

Treatment of imperforate puncta and micropuncta

- Treatment is not always required in mildly-affected cases
- Surgery is used to enlarge existing puncta or to create puncta when they are absent

- With the patient anaesthetised, the correct site is identified by careful inspection or by cannulating the upper punctum and injecting saline or viscoelastic material to raise a bleb in the region of the occluding conjunctiva
- Any occluding conjunctiva is removed with scissors, usually as a single piece
- Topical antibiotic-corticosteroid eye drops are given for three days postoperatively

Aetiology of acquired nasolacrimal problems
- *Internal* blockage may affect nasolacrimal drainage (e.g. foreign bodies and inflammation)
- *External* influences such as nasal and tooth-root problems, space-occupying lesions, surgery and trauma may also produce nasolacrimal obstruction

Treatment of acquired nasolacrimal problems
- Depends on the site of blockage and the cause, so careful investigation is necessary
- Some aspects of investigation and treatment require general anaesthesia
- Foreign bodies such as barley awns can be difficult to remove because of their shape and their tendency to disintegrate. It is important to avoid flushing the foreign body into the narrow intraosseous portion of the nasolacrimal duct and to ensure that all the material has been removed
- Complex cases should be referred

CONJUNCTIVA

The conjunctiva is a thin, variably-pigmented, mucous membrane. It has a rich vascular supply and bright-red, freely-branching blood vessels are visible in the non-pigmented areas. The blood flow is from fornix to limbus. Vessels move with the mobile bulbar conjunctiva and the blood flow is from fornix to limbus. In disease, conjunctival vessels may invade the superficial cornea. Sensory nerve supply is from the ophthalmic division of the fifth cranial nerve and pain fibres are somewhat sparse.

The conjunctiva is freely mobile except for areas of closer attachment at fornix, limbus and eyelid margins. Because of the loose arrangement, *conjunctival oedema (chemosis)* and *subconjunctival haemorrhage* form readily after insult.

Conjunctival epithelium contains goblet cells that contribute mucin to the preocular tear film. There is also a contribution (transmembrane mucin) from surface epithelial cells. The conjunctival stroma is divided into a superficial (*adenoid*) layer and a deep (*fibrous*) layer. Lymphoid tissue is rich in the superficial layer of adults, but may be sparse, or absent, in neonates. Conjunctival-associated lymphoid tissue (CALT) is associated with immune-mediated conjunctival responses.

Palpebral conjunctiva covers the inner surface of the upper and lower eyelids, terminating in the mucocutaneous junction at the eyelid margin and reflecting at the fornices as *bulbar conjunctiva*, which covers the anterior portions of the globe, except for the cornea. *Nictitating conjunctiva* covers both surfaces of the third eyelid.

DISEASES OF THE CANINE CONJUNCTIVA

Epibulbar dermoid (see Cornea, this section pp 109–123)
Conjunctivitis
Conjunctivitis is one of the commonest problems encountered in most species (Figure
3.21), but is unsatisfactorily classified unless the aetiology can be determined. It is
important to remember that conjunctivitis is often a self-limiting disease, that not all
cases require treatment and that, in the dog, it is frequently secondary to some other
problem. In many types of conjunctivitis it is common for the ocular discharge to
persist for several weeks after the acute signs have subsided, a situation that is sometimes exacerbated when ointments are used for treatment because of 'mucus trapping'.
If the eye is comfortable and no longer inflamed the treatment should not be prolonged
solely because of an ocular discharge.

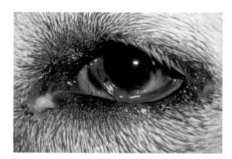

Figure 3.21 Acute conjunctivitis in a dog
(Left eye). There is an ocular discharge and the
eye is uncomfortable and red because of conjunctival hyperaemia. Conjunctival oedema,
most obviously involving the third eyelid, is also
a feature. Despite a comprehensive work-up, the
cause was not established and the acute signs
resolved within seven days without any treatment, although a mild ocular discharge persisted
for some three weeks afterwards.

Aetiology of canine conjunctivitis
- Viral – e.g. distemper virus
- Bacterial – usually Gram +ve cocci
- Parasitic – *Thelazia* spp common in parts of Europe (Italy), Russia, Asia and western
  America
- Mycotic – e.g. blastomycosis (non-temperate climates)
- Immune-mediated and allergic (e.g. atopy is common)
- Physical (common) and chemical (uncommon)
- Preocular tear film abnormalities (common – see earlier)
- Iatrogenic (home remedies, inappropriate therapy); quite common
- Unknown; common

Clinical signs of acute conjunctivitis
- Conjunctival discomfort (probably itchy rather than frankly painful)
- Active hyperaemia (dilatation) of conjunctival vessels (diffuse redness of conjunc-
  tiva) – usually all the conjunctival surfaces are involved (palpebral, nictitating and
  bulbar)
- Chemosis (conjunctival oedema)
- Ocular discharge (serous, mucoid, purulent, haemorrhagic or combinations of these)

Clinical signs of chronic conjunctivitis
- Follicle formation (lymphoid hyperplasia); occasionally the follicles can be localised to specific areas of conjunctiva, such as beneath the third eyelid
- Conjunctival thickening and conjunctival vascular injection
- A persistent discharge; the nature of the discharge can vary

Differential diagnosis
Conjunctivitis is the commonest reason for a red eye in dogs (Figure 3.21). There are, however, a number of other conditions that can present with an acute red eye and they must be distinguished from conjunctivitis. It is helpful to remember that simple conjunctivitis is *not* associated with corneal or intraocular involvement. The brief list below highlights the key ocular features that aid differentiation of *non-traumatic causes of acute red eye* in the dog.
- Keratoconjunctivitis sicca
- Keratitis – corneal involvement, extent and depth of which varies
- Episcleritis and episclerokeratitis – nodular or diffuse, perilimbal oedema ± superficial corneal lipid infiltration
- Scleritis – nodular or, less commonly, diffuse, perilimbal oedema ± deep corneal lipid infiltration ± uveitis
- Anterior uveitis – aqueous flare, iris is oedematous and inflamed, pupil may be constricted
- Glaucoma – non-responsive, dilated pupil, corneal oedema may be present if the intraocular pressure is sufficiently high (>40–50 mmHg)

Protocol for investigation and diagnosis
- History (e.g. unilateral or bilateral, duration, lifestyle, management, treatment, seasonal variation, vaccination status, others at risk or affected)
- Clinical appearance
- Schirmer I Tear Test to check tear production
- Conjunctival scrapes, swabs or cytobrush samples
- Biopsy on occasions
- If ophthalmic stains are to be used to aid diagnosis, they should be applied *after* the samples have been taken

Conjunctival scrapes may be taken for cytology, and swabs or cytobrush samples for culture and sensitivity. In first opinion practice, scrapes and swabs are usually taken only from those cases that do not respond to treatment. Topical anaesthesia is not normally required for sampling. Swabs and cytobrush samples are usually taken from the ventral fornix and palpebral conjunctival region by firm application of a moist sterile swab. Bacteria can often be recovered from the conjunctival sac of normal dogs, so the results should always be interpreted with caution.

In complex or chronic cases, conjunctival biopsy may be performed following topical local anaesthesia. Several drops of proxymetacaine hydrochloride 0.5% should be applied first, then a cotton wool bud soaked in amethocaine hydrochloride 1% is held, for several minutes, against the area to be biopsied. A piece of affected conjunctiva is tented up with small tissue forceps and removed with tenotomy scissors (crushing or distorting the sample should be avoided). The sample is placed flat on very thin card for routine histological fixation so as to avoid distortion.

Canine infectious conjunctivitis
Viral
- Canine distemper virus is the most important cause

- Ocular signs may include bilateral conjunctivitis, ocular discharge, KCS, corneal ulceration, multifocal choriotretinitis, optic neuritis and acute loss of vision
- There is no specific therapy, but the animal should be isolated and nursing care should include adequate cleansing of the eyes and tear replacement therapy

Bacterial
Aetiology and diagnosis
- Although there is a range of possible pathogens, they are most commonly *secondary* to an underlying predisposing problem such as KCS, eyelid abnormalities and contaminated traumatic injuries
- The diagnosis is made on the basis of the history, clinical signs, conjunctival scrapings and swabs
- The most common bacterial pathogens are Gram +ve cocci (*Staphylococcus* and, less commonly, *Streptococcus*). Neonatal conjunctivitis (*ophthalmia neonatorum*) has been described under Eyelids

Treatment
- Successful treatment depends upon establishing and removing the underlying cause
- For Gram +ve organisms, the commonest situation, topical fusidic acid gel is the first choice and topical chloramphenicol (as drops or ointment) is a useful second choice. If Gram −ve bacteria are involved, then gentamicin solution is the agent of choice. For mixed infections, fucidic acid and gentamicin can be used together
- For *confirmed* staphylococcal infection, topical corticosteroids are also appropriate, to lessen the hypersensitivity reaction to staphylococcal toxins

Allergic conjunctivitis
Aetiology and diagnosis
- Variety of causes (e.g. atopy, drug sensitivity, food sensitivity, following insect and arachnid bites, insect stings, hypersensitivity to bacterial toxins and unknown)
- The history can be diagnostic when hypersensitivity reactions are immediate
- Intradermal skin testing will be required for diagnosis of possible atopy

Treatment
- Depends upon identifying and removing the allergen(s). Hyposensitisation is effective in some cases, but the range of possible allergens complicates the situation
- Acute allergic conjunctivitis requires early treatment with corticosteroids
- If allergen(s) cannot be identified, then palliative treatment with topical anti-inflammatories (e.g. sodium cromoglycate or corticosteroids) is indicated
- Note that with the exceptions already stated (atopy and staphylococcal toxins), the routine use of corticosteroids to treat conjunctivitis may obscure the cause, make correct diagnosis difficult, lengthen the time course of the disease and can prevent resolution of the inflammation

Physical causes of conjunctivitis
Aetiology and diagnosis
- Usually a consequence of consistent trauma from dust, cilia or masses which irritate or abrade the conjunctiva
- History and lifestyle may be helpful – an acute unilateral problem might suggest a

conjunctival foreign body, a more chronic problem may relate to the dog's environment, including bedding materials like sawdust
- Chronic conjunctival exposure and irritation can also result from poor eyelid anatomy (e.g. ectropion) and other abnormalities, for example, anatomical entropion can also cause conjunctivitis because of chronic irritation

Treatment
Identify and remove the primary cause

Chemical causes of conjunctivitis
Aetiology and diagnosis
- Various causes (e.g. shampoo, insecticidal sprays, antiseptic skin preparation, acid or alkali burns)
- Identify the cause, check the pH of both the conjunctival sac and the offending chemical

Treatment
- When shampoos and weak acids are involved, use bland ophthalmic ointment after first flushing the conjunctival sac with water
- For any alkalis and strong acids, continue to flush the conjunctival sac with water while seeking urgent specialist help and possible referral. Ask the owner to bring the offending chemical with them whenever possible

'Iatrogenic' and idiopathic causes of conjunctivitis
Aetiology and diagnosis
- It is always worth enquiring if the owner has used home remedies
- It is important to avoid creating iatrogenic problems by inappropriate medication
- Check tear-film distribution and production if there is any suggestion of ocular surface disease
- Take swabs and scrapes if there are any signs of infection (e.g. mucopurulent discharge)

Treatment
- Stop inappropriate treatment
- Check all the conjunctival surfaces carefully. If follicular conjunctivitis is present, then a dry swab can be used to rub the follicles firmly under topical local anaesthesia – an empirical approach that often leads to their resolution

LIMBUS, EPISCLERA AND SCLERA

THE LIMBUS

The limbus is the transition zone between the orderly arrangement of the cornea and the less ordered tissues of the conjunctiva and underlying episclera and sclera (Figure 3.22(a,b)). It may be a site of chronic proliferative disease and neoplasia. The limbus can also be used as a site for surgical entry into the eye as well as being a common site for accidental intraocular penetration.

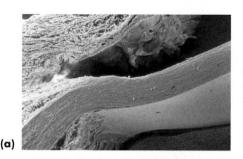 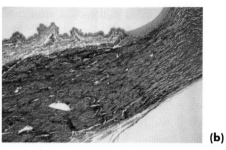

(a)   **(b)**

Figure 3.22(a,b) Scanning electron micrograph (a) and histological section (b) of the normal canine conjunctiva, episclera, sclera limbus and cornea.

   Limbal-based changes are invariably the result of inflammation or neoplasia and should be distinguished from pathology of similar appearance involving the cornea and anterior chamber. For example, multicentric lymphoma may be associated with peripheral corneal and iris infiltration and anterior-chamber involvement. Physical examination of the whole animal may help to differentiate local ocular disease such as episclerokeratitis from generalised disease such as multicentric lymphoma.

Inflammatory problems
Benign proliferation of connective tissue is reasonably common at the limbus. It should be differentiated from cysts and neoplasia.

Treatment
Treatment consists of surface-active topical corticosteroids (e.g. dexamethasone, prednisolone, fluorometholone) combined with complete excision or excisional biopsy. Most limbal inflammations are, strictly speaking, forms of episcleritis and/or episclerokeratitis (see this section, pp 107–108).

Neoplasia
Aetiology and diagnosis
- Pigmented limbal (epibulbar) tumours are usually benign, and the majority can be classified as melanocytomas (Figure 3.23), rather than melanomas, based on their behaviour and histological appearance
- In old dogs the growth rate is invariably slow, whereas in younger dogs it may be rapid
- The German Shepherd Dog is the most commonly affected breed
- Gonioscopy is a useful adjunct to routine ophthalmic examination in these cases

Differential diagnosis
- Limbal pigmented neoplasia should be distinguished from scleral defects (e.g. staphyloma and *scleromalacia perforans*) and post-traumatic uveal prolapse
- Non-pigmented limbal neoplasia should be classified as primary (focal or invasive) or secondary (metastatic) neoplasia and differentiated from inflammatory disease

GENERAL AND CANINE OPHTHALMOLOGY

Treatment

Tumours at this site can be kept under observation if they are static or of slow growth. Those of rapid growth are probably best removed under general anaesthesia by excision. If necessary, a graft (e.g. scleral homograft) can be used to make good the defect and support healing, although a number of different approaches (e.g. cryotherapy, laser photocoagulation, corneoscleral transposition) have also been described. It is unusual to have to sacrifice the eye. If in doubt seek specialist opinion and consider referral.

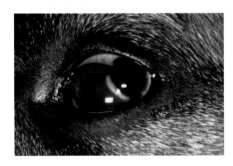

Figure 3.23 Limbal melanocytoma in a German Shepherd Dog. Note the lipid infiltration of the cornea (*arcus*) which is a common feature of most limbal, episcleral and scleral pathology, whether it is neoplastic or inflammatory in origin. The serum lipid and lipoprotein profile was normal.

THE CANINE EPISCLERA

The episclera consists of collagen, blood vessels, some elastic fibres, fibroblasts, melanocytes, phagocytic cells and nerves (both myelinated and unmyelinated). The episclera is most developed between the limbus and the extraocular muscle insertions where it blends superficially with the overlying Tenon's capsule.

Episcleritis

This condition is seen occasionally in dogs and may be diffuse (simple) or nodular and either unilateral or bilateral (Figure 3.24).

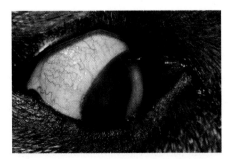

Figure 3.24 Diffuse (simple) episcleritis in a dog. Note the radial configuration of the episcleral vessels. There is faint dorsolateral anterior stromal corneal lipid deposition and more marked paraxial medial lipid deposition. In the latter region lipid deposition has been exacerbated by the presence of a small sebaceous adenoma of the lower eyelid, just visible overlying the corneal lipid. The serum lipid and lipoprotein profile was mildly abnormal, mainly because of an increase in high-density lipoprotein. The eyelid tumour was surgically excised and the episcleritis treated with topical surface-active corticosteroid (fluorometholone).

Clinical signs
- The diffuse form involves the visible 'white' of the eye, the nodular form is most commonly found in the region of the limbus in the palpebral aperture
- Accompanying hyperaemia, both episcleral and conjunctival, is often striking, but the eye is not painful
- The conjunctiva moves freely over the inflamed episclera and this is an easy way of distinguishing the two layers
- Hyperaemia of the episcleral vessels is usually obvious, although there will also be some hyperaemia of the overlying conjunctival vessels
- Corneal oedema and lipid deposition are ubiquitous accompaniments and the depth of corneal involvement is the easiest way of determining the level of inflammation
- If lipid deposition is extensive, particularly in cases of diffuse episcleritis, analysis of the lipid and lipoprotein profile is desirable, as recurrent hyperaemia may simply reflect intermittent raised levels of circulating lipid

Nodular episclerokeratitis
This is a bilateral condition and, in the USA, is most commonly found in Rough Collies and Shetland Sheepdogs. It differs from episcleritis in the more extensive corneal involvement and the fact that similar granulomatous masses are sometimes found at other sites (e.g. eyelids and lip commisures). It resembles nodular episcleritis in consisting histologically of plasma cells, lymphocytes and histiocytes and so treatment regimes for both conditions are similar.

Treatment of episcleritis and episclerokeratitis
- Some forms of diffuse episcleritis are probably ocular manifestations of hyperlipoproteinaemia, so that the clinical signs will resolve if the lipid and lipoprotein profile is restored to normal. Topical corticosteroids will also speed resolution
- For nodular episcleritis and episclerokeratitis, an extended course of topical corticosteroids may be effective, although other regimes including oral corticosteroids ± oral azathioprine, or niacinamide and tetracycline can be used
- Surgical excision, local radiotherapy (e.g. beta-irradiation) and cryotherapy are other possible approaches for the nodular types
- Specialist advice should be sought for more complex cases

THE CANINE SCLERA

The sclera is relatively avascular and has a more compact arrangement of collagen than the overlying episclera. The cell types are similar but sparser. Most of the blood vessels found in the sclera can be regarded as in transit, so that the sclera can be regarded as a relatively avascular tissue.

Scleritis
Scleritis is very rare and is not as obvious as conjunctivitis or episcleritis because the inflamed tissue is located at greater depth.

Clinical signs

- The affected sclera is of darker colour, usually salmon pink, or even purple, rather than bright red
- Rather confusingly, inflammatory changes are also usually present in the overlying conjunctiva and episclera. Phenylephrine 10% will blanch the more superficial vessels and allow the inflamed sclera to be visualised (Figure 3.25(a))
- The anterior, posterior or whole sclera may be involved. Whilst it is most likely to present as a granulomatous inflammation, necrosis may be an additional, if rare, complicating factor (*necrotising granulomatous scleritis*)
- Scleral thickening can be detected on slit-lamp biomicroscopy and/or ophthalmoscopic examination depending on its location. Diagnostic imaging can also be used to demonstrate the scleral thickening
- Uveitis may also be present, typically granulomatous in type and with keratic precipitates as the most obvious feature (Figure 3.25(b))
- Scleritis in the dog is not as intensely painful as it is in human patients; furthermore, it is not associated with generalised immune-mediated collagen disease, but is apparently a local ocular phenomenon

Treatment

Scleritis cases are probably best referred.

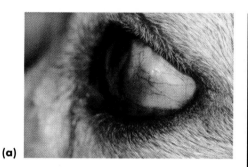

(a)

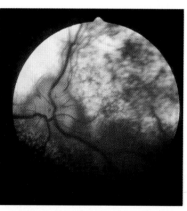

(b)

Figure 3.25 (**a**) Nodular scleritis in a Labrador Retriever. The location of the inflammation was much more clearly defined following the use of topical phenylephrine 10% to blanch the more superficial conjunctival vessels and most of the episcleral vessels. (**b**) Fundus examination of the eye in (a) revealed that posterior nodules were also present as well as some pigmentary disturbance. One of the nodules is apparent to the right of the optic disc beneath an arteriovenous crossing.

CORNEA

ANATOMY AND PHYSIOLOGY

The cornea contains both ectodermal and mesenchymal elements. It consists of an anterior epithelium, basement membrane, *substantia propria*, Descemet's membrane and endothelium and it is normally less than 0.7 mm in thickness. The preocular tear film is inextricably linked with corneal health and any investigations of corneal disease should include assessment of the production, distribution and drainage of the tear film.

The *corneal epithelium* consists of an outer layer of squamous cells, a middle layer of polyhedral, or wing, cells and a single layer of columnar cells, which produce the *basement membrane*. The epithelium is attached to the underlying stroma by hemidesmosomes and anchoring fibrils link the basal epithelium, basement membrane and subepithelial stroma.

The *substantia propria* comprises the bulk of the cornea. It contains some unmyelinated nerves (particularly anteriorly), fibroblasts (keratocytes), regularly-arranged collagen fibrils and ground substance. The fibrils are of uniform size and extend across the entire length of the cornea, from limbus to limbus, as bundles (lamellae) which cross at approximate right angles to each other. The ground substance, a hydrated matrix of proteoglycans, occupies the space between lamellae. The corneal fibroblasts have a slow turnover rate in normal adult cornea and are located in and between the collagen lamellae; they produce both collagen and ground substance. Other cells are less common, but all the cells found in the stroma, including the fibroblasts, are able to move through the tissues in response to stimuli.

Blood vessels and lymphatic vessels are conspicuously absent from the cornea, but they are present in the perilimbal tissues and the limbal vessels contribute to the gaseous and metabolic requirements of the peripheral cornea. The epithelium and endothelium are the most metabolically active parts of the cornea.

Descemet's membrane is the basement membrane of the endothelium. The *corneal endothelium* produces it throughout life, but its own powers of replication are limited in all but young puppies. When endothelial cells die, they are replaced by neighbouring cells spreading to fill the gap. Hence the endothelium thins and Descemet's membrane thickens as the animal ages. The endothelium is a single layer of cells of high metabolic activity and is of critical importance in maintaining corneal deturgescence and corneal clarity by an active pumping mechanism.

CORNEAL WOUND HEALING

Epithelium
Epithelial damage is repaired by corneal epithelial slide (early response – within one hour) and epithelial mitosis (later response – within 24 hours). Limbal stem cells also contribute to the repair process. Phagocytic cells, notably polymorphonuclear leucocytes, gain access to the injured cornea through the tear film. The entire epithelium turns over in seven days, so uncomplicated epithelial healing should not exceed seven days.

Stroma
Stromal damage is repaired with help from the overlying epithelial cells which fill the defect, migration of cells from the limbus and by generation from the stromal elements – fibroblasts derived from resting keratocytes produce collagen and ground substance. The type of collagen that is laid down in damaged stroma is different from the

original collagen in type and orientation, so the transparency of the damaged region is compromised. Neovascularisation is usual when the stroma is damaged by, for example, infection, trauma or chemicals. Clean wounds of the cornea heal by avascular scarring. When neovascularisation accompanies wound healing more fibrous tissue is laid down.

Descemet's membrane

Descemet's membrane rupture is followed by recoil, as Descemet's membrane is elastic. Reduplication of Descemet's membrane can occur from production by the endothelial cells, which slide in over the injured area.

Endothelium

Endothelial damage repairs poorly in most adult species and because of poor, or absent, regenerative abilities it can only respond to insult by spreading more thinly.

CORNEAL OPACIFICATION

Oedema

- Corneal oedema is indicative of corneal damage, and stromal oedema can result after insult to the anterior epithelium or posterior endothelium as well as to the stroma itself. When stromal oedema develops the cornea swells and becomes thicker and its optical properties are compromised.
- Discrete damage to the epithelium will result in a focal area of corneal oedema (e.g. following superficial ulceration), but more widespread injury (e.g. chemical or thermal burns) may result in more diffuse involvement. When diffuse oedema accompanies corneal ulceration it is likely that infection is present.
- Damage to the corneal endothelium will affect the corneal pump mechanism and stromal oedema results. The oedema may be localised (e.g. at the site of contact of an anteriorly luxated lens) or diffuse (e.g. associated with widespread endothelial loss in endothelial dystrophy or with immune-mediated endothelial damage in canine viral hepatitis).
- Other causes of corneal oedema include blunt and penetrating injury and iatrogenic damage caused during intraocular surgery. Severe inflammation (e.g. endophthalmitis) and intraocular neoplasia are often associated with corneal oedema. Glaucoma is an important cause of corneal oedema as the increased intraocular pressure adversely affects the endothelial pump mechanism, and the degree of endothelial damage is directly related to the level of pressure elevation and its duration.

Vascularisation

- The normal canine cornea is devoid of blood vessels, but corneal neovascularisation is a common response to corneal insult.
- Superficial vessels arise from the conjunctival vessels and are readily observed as they cross the limbus, the vessels branch dichotomously and are bright red in colour. Superficial keratitis often accompanies conjunctivitis.
- Deep vessels arise from the ciliary plexus and cannot be observed until they enter

the cornea. These vessels are usually short, dark and straight, occasionally they are so extensive that they form a complete circle (ciliary flush). Deep vascularisation may be associated with a variety of ocular conditions, including keratitis, uveitis, glaucoma, endophthalmitis and intraocular neoplasia.

- Persistence of the pupillary membrane may be associated with intracorneal haemorrhage if vessels connecting the iris and posterior cornea remain patent. Leakage of blood from extensive corneal neovascularisation can also result in intracorneal haemorrhage, as new blood vessels are inherently leaky.
- Vascularisation can enhance corneal healing. Once healing has taken place the vessels narrow and become faint, but permanent, 'ghost' vessels.

Pigmentation

- Posterior pigment deposition may be a feature of congenital abnormalities such as persistent pupillary membrane (PPM) remnants or other types of anterior-segment dysgenesis.
- Acquired corneal pigmentation is commoner, often as a non-specific response to corneal insult. It is associated with pigment proliferation and migration of melanocytes and neovascularisation. The location, extent and depth of pigment deposition often depend on the initiating insult (e.g. medial canthus hairs in brachycephalic dogs).
- Endothelial pigment deposition, encroaching onto the posterior cornea from the limbus, appears to be a feature of ageing in some dogs, it may also be seen when uveal cysts have ruptured and adhered to the cornea and in association with anterior synechiae.
- Pigment deposits on the posterior cornea should be distinguished from keratic precipitates. The latter darken with age and can resemble pigment, but they are usually deposited on the posterior ventromedial cornea and this 'regionalisation' is helpful, as are any accompanying indications of active uveitis or legacies of previous uveitis.

Other causes of corneal opacification

- Foreign bodies
- Xerosis (drying and desiccation)
- Cellular infiltration
- Lipid deposition
- Calcium deposition
- Neoplastic infiltration (e.g. peripheral infiltration by lymphoma)
- Degenerative changes and scarring

CONDITIONS OF THE CANINE CORNEA

A considerable number of corneal conditions have been identified in the dog and only the more important are described here. Congenital conditions include corneal dermoid, which is reasonably common, various types of anterior-segment dysgenesis and rare imperfections of development such as absence, microcornea and megalocornea that are usually associated with globe abnormalities. Acquired problems that are *not* discussed include a presumed epithelial dystrophy identified most commonly in the

Shetland Sheepdog, lysosomal storage disease, calcium keratopathy, immune-mediated disease other than pannus, Florida keratopathy, epithelial inclusion cysts and neoplasia.

Epibulbar dermoid

Dermoids are superficial masses, present from birth, which contain many of the elements of normal hairy skin. They usually involve the cornea and conjunctiva and, less commonly, the eyelids. Dermoids are reasonably common in the dog and are usually unilateral (Figure 3.26(a)).

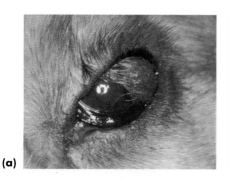 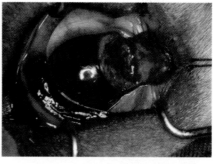

(a) **(b)**

Figure 3.26 **(a)** Epibulbar dermoid in a Cocker Spaniel puppy. The position at the lateral limbus is typical. **(b)** A superficial keratectomy was performed to remove the dermoid and a lateral canthotomy has been used to improve access. A bridle suture allowed the dermoid to be manipulated more easily during removal.

Treatment
- These cases are often referred for corneal surgery (lamellar keratectomy).
- Surgical excision should be performed when the puppy is old enough for routine general anaesthesia. Lateral canthotomy may be required to allow adequate exposure, and good fixation of the dermoid (e.g. a bridle suture) makes surgery simpler. The dermoid is excised from the corneal side at the correct plane of cleavage (i.e. beneath the dermoid, some ¼ of corneal thickness) ensuring that the affected conjunctiva is included in the excision (Figure 3.26(b)).
- Postoperative topical non-steroidal anti-inflammatories (e.g. ketorolac trometamol 0.5%) or corticosteroids (e.g. fluoromethalone 0.1%) can be given, to minimise corneal scarring, once epithelialisation is complete.

Corneal dystrophies

The description corneal *dystrophy* is appropriate for functional and morphological changes occurring bilaterally, but not necessarily symmetrically, in a previously-normal cornea, not caused by disease elsewhere in the eye or elsewhere in the body. To justify the use of the term dystrophy the condition should ideally be of proven inheritance. Although a number of familial canine corneal dystrophies are suspected, their mode of inheritance is poorly understood.

Epithelial basement membrane dystrophy

This form of superficial ulceration (synonyms: recurrent epithelial erosion, indolent ulceration) is not uncommon and is associated with abnormal adherence of the corneal epithelium to the underlying stroma. Certain breeds are over-represented, although other factors, such as age and previous ocular insult, may also be of relevance. Whilst it most frequently presents as a unilateral condition, both eyes are potentially at risk in the course of an animal's life. The predisposing factors are poorly understood and any possible mode of inheritance is unknown.

Clinical findings

- Commonest in older dogs (6–7 years), particularly in the Boxer (should also check for distichiasis in this breed) and Pembroke Corgi
- The ulcer produces moderate pain accompanied by blepharospasm and lacrimation
- The appearance of the ulcer is quite characteristic in that it is always superficial, does not incite inflammation, shows little if any tendency to resolve, and is surrounded by a rim of non-adherent corneal epithelium (Figure 3.27(a))
- The ulcer is fluorescein positive

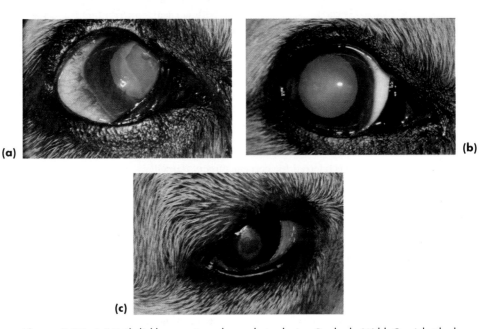

(a) (b)

(c)

Figure 3.27 **(a)** Epithelial basement membrane dystrophy in a Pembroke Welsh Corgi that had received a variety of topical treatments over a period of months to no effect. Retroillumination is a useful ancillary technique to demonstrate the apparent edge of the ulcer and the extensive abnormal surrounding area. Note the complete lack of any vascularisation or other inflammatory response. **(b)** Within a week of chemical cautery with liquefied phenol the eye in (a) was free of pain and the cornea had re-epithelialised. **(c)** The cautery must extend beyond the areas of abnormal epithelial adhesion as illustrated here in another Pembroke Welsh Corgi.

Differential diagnosis

- Superficial corneal ulcers have a variety of causes (see Ulcerative Keratitis, this section, pp 117–120) and the aetiology should be investigated in all cases that present with epithelial loss in order to differentiate them from epithelial basement membrane dystrophy.
- Qualitative and quantitative tear-film deficiencies must always be considered in the presence of corneal disease, especially so when the superficial cornea is involved.
- Tear-film distribution and corneal sensitivity should be assessed if the underlying cause of superficial corneal disease is not apparent.
- Other dystrophic conditions of the canine cornea may occur. For example, in the Shetland Sheepdog, multiple grey-and-white, ring-shaped opacities primarily involving the epithelium may constitute a form of epithelial dystrophy, or may simply be a manifestation of tear-film dysfunction. Affected dogs usually respond to topical cyclosporin, suggesting that the latter hypothesis is more likely.

Treatment of epithelial basement membrane dystrophy

A number of different types of treatment have been reported, including chemical cautery, punctate and grid keratotomy and superficial keratectomy. Of these techniques, chemical cautery is the safest in inexperienced hands as both keratotomy and keratectomy can result in complications, such as corneal scarring and even corneal perforation, when performed by those unfamiliar with corneal surgery. A major advantage of chemical cauterants is that they can be applied under topical local anaesthesia and there is no need for a general anaesthetic (Figure 3.27(c)).

Chemical cautery

Possible chemical cauterants include liquefied phenol (80% w/w of phenol:20% w/w water), pure trichloracetic acid and 6% aqueous iodine solution. Phenol is a most effective agent in the treatment of primary persistent corneal erosions. Unfortunately, in common with other benzene derivatives, there is some concern about its potential carcinogenic effects.

- Chemical cautery is performed in the conscious, non-sedated dog following topical anaesthesia (e.g. proxymetacaine hydrochloride 0.5%)
- No more than 2 ml of the selected cauterant should be poured carefully into a small container. A tiny pledget of cotton wool is grasped using Halstead's mosquito forceps, wound tightly around the closed jaws of the forceps and moistened by dipping the tip of the forceps into the cauterant
- The cauterising agent is applied with precision, starting at the rim of loosened epithelium and working outwards to the true edge of the erosion (the region where the epithelium is properly attached to underlying stroma) and just beyond. The cauterised areas will become greyish because phenol precipitates protein (Figure 3.27(c))
- After cautery the eye is flushed with sterile water or saline, although such is the precision of application that this is not really necessary
- In addition to its cauterising action phenol also has local anaesthetic, antiseptic and bactericidal properties, so there is no need to provide any further treatment after cautery
- Phenol cautery is simple, cheap and effective, although a mild inflammatory response may be associated with healing

If the problem does not resolve within a few days of initial treatment it is usually because of inadequate cautery or misdiagnosis. For example, the cautery may not have extended to the region of normal epithelial adhesion, or the dog may have some other primary problem, or an additional problem, such as distichiasis or ectopic cilia.

Grid keratotomy

Grid keratotomy is best performed under general anaesthesia, although the adjunctive application of topical anaesthetic will allow a lighter plane of anaesthesia.
- The loose corneal epithelium is removed as described for chemical cautery using a sterile dry cotton swab
- A 25-gauge hypodermic needle is used to create a grid pattern of microsurgical incisions, some 1–2 mm apart, at a depth not exceeding 0.3 mm
- The grid pattern should extend some 2–3 mm beyond the area of abnormal epithelial adhesion

Crystalline stromal dystrophy (see under Lipid Deposition, this section, pp 121–122)
Corneal endothelial dystrophy
Clinical findings
- This is a rare condition, associated with degeneration of the corneal endothelial cells. The breeds most commonly affected in the UK are the English Springer Spaniel (early onset) and the Boxer (later onset). In the USA the condition is most frequently reported in the Boston Terrier, Chihuahua and Dachshund.
- Bilateral stromal oedema is the most constant feature. The two eyes are often dissimilar in the early stages and at this stage the condition is not painful. Many cases progress to *bullous keratopathy* and loss of the normal corneal profile (*keratoglobus*) (Figure 3.28). Discomfort, or frank pain, is likely at this stage.

Treatment

Specialist advice should be sought, as referral for penetrating keratoplasty may be an option in early cases and thermokeratoplasty a means of achieving pain relief in later cases.

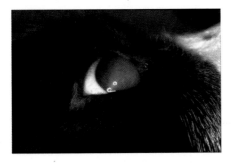

Figure 3.28 Endothelial dystrophy in a young English Springer Spaniel. The right eye is illustrated, and both eyes were affected. In addition to stromal oedema there is *bullous keratopathy* and the corneal profile is abnormal (*keratoglobus*). There was also a single distichium on the upper eyelid.

Keratitis

Inflammation of the cornea (keratitis) is a common condition with a multiplicity of causes in dogs. Keratitis is best classified according to aetiology and is broadly classified into ulcerative and non-ulcerative types. Direct mechanical trauma (see below) is the commonest cause of canine ulcerative keratitis.

Ulcerative keratitis
Aetiology
Preocular tear-film defects
Keratoconjunctivitis sicca (see earlier)

Direct mechanical trauma
- Claws and teeth
- Foreign bodies
- Eyelid tumours
- Eyelid abnormalities (e.g. entropion, absence or partial absence of eyelid)
- Ectopic cilia and, less commonly, distichiasis and trichiasis
- Aberrant hairs (e.g. nasal folds)

Irritants
- Thermal injuries
- Ultraviolet light
- Alkalis and acids

Immune-mediated disease
Both local and systemic causes (rare as a cause of ulcerative keratitis)

Neurogenic
Nerve damage (e.g. neuroparalytic – VIIth cranial nerve; neurotrophic – Vth cranial nerve)

Dystrophic
See under Corneal Dystrophies, this section, p. 113

Other
Note that bacteria (e.g. *Pseudomonas aeruginosa*) can only become established if there is pre-existing epithelial damage, so that bacterial keratitis is a *secondary*, rather than a primary, problem.

Clinical signs of ulcerative keratitis
- Pain, blepharospasm and excessive lacrimation
- Corneal oedema (implies infection if diffuse, as does stromal loss)
- Vascularisation is usually associated with chronicity
- Ocular discharge may replace initial excessive lacrimation
- The ulcer can be delineated by careful examination and following the application of fluorescein (Figure 3.29(a,b)). It is the exposed corneal stroma that takes up the stain, intact anterior epithelium and Descemet's membrane do not

Diagnosis of ulcerative keratitis
- Accurate history, including duration of the clinical signs and any previous treatment

- Meticulous examination of both eyes and their adnexa with adequate magnification is essential
- Check that tear production of both eyes is normal (likely to be excessive, but occasionally it is reduced in the affected eye if tear production is abnormal). The Schirmer tear test is performed *before* any other preparations are applied to the eye
- Corneal scrapings and swabs for culture should be taken early in the course of disease and before treatment has altered the initial presentation. Topical local anaesthesia is necessary. Sample from the edge of the ulcer, as this is where organisms will be replicating if infection is present
- The results of Gram staining may enable appropriate antibiotic therapy to be selected, but note that Gram +ve organisms are often easily found and may not always be of great significance. Gram −ve organisms are likely to be of significance if any can be found
- It is essential to use ophthalmic stains such as fluorescein to aid diagnosis, but *after* swabs and scrapes have been taken. Excess stain should be rinsed away with sterile saline and the eye examined as soon as possible after fluorescein application so as to avoid false positives

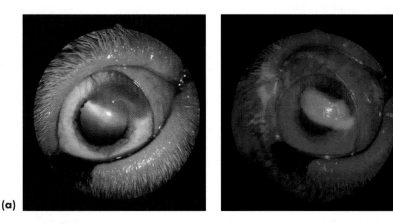

(a)   **(b)**

Figure 3.29(a,b) Ulcerative keratitis in a Boxer. Delineation of the ulcer (a) is obvious after staining with fluorescein (b) and the ulcer is clearly superficial. A single short extra lash on the upper eyelid was the cause. The lash, like most of the coat hair, was white and this made it difficult to see against the white background of the conjunctiva without good magnification.

Basic management of ulcerative keratitis
- Identify and eliminate the primary problem (e.g. ectopic cilium)
- Address any secondary complications (e.g. infection)
- Assist healing (e.g. appropriate selection of topical drugs, pedicle graft)
- Monitor the situation carefully to ensure that the ulcer is healing, rather than progressing

Superficial corneal ulceration (loss of epithelium ± anterior stroma only)
- Uncomplicated ulcers heal quickly and without scarring if epithelium only is

involved. A faint scar will remain if there has been stromal involvement. Topical antibiotic is not always required, particularly if the cause has been established and eliminated (e.g. ectopic cilium).

- Protection during healing is not usually required, however, a therapeutic soft contact (bandage) lens (TSCL) or third eyelid flap can be used for those cases in which pain relief and protection are needed. A bandage lens can be put in after applying topical local anaesthetic and the edge of the lens should reach some 2 mm beyond the limbus. The lens may be left *in situ* for up to six weeks. A general anaesthetic is needed for the placement of third eyelid flaps, and the ulcerative lesion is less-easily monitored as it is hidden from sight. TSCLs provide a useful and preferable alternative to third eyelid flaps, but should be avoided when there is keratoconjunctivitis sicca, active ocular surface infection, serious eyelid dysfunction, hypoaesthesia (an anaesthetic cornea) or uveitis.

Deep corneal ulceration (loss of approximately half or more of the corneal thickness)

- Deep ulceration may be an immediate result of the initial injury or a later complication. If there is any likelihood of corneal perforation then healing must be aided by support from a graft (e.g. free conjunctival graft, conjunctival pedicle graft, porcine submucosal graft). A rotation conjunctival pedicle graft is the most commonly used means of support (Figure 2.14(a–g), p. 45), as it brings a blood supply direct to the damaged region. It is probably the treatment of choice. The graft is placed with the patient under general anaesthesia and it is usually left *in situ* for at least four weeks before it is sectioned, following the application of topical local anaesthetic. It is important to warn owners that the graft will become white and necrotic once it has been sectioned and it is axiomatic that sectioning does not take place until healing is complete.
- Full-thickness complications will need primary repair and may also require keratoplasty techniques. Such cases should be referred if microsurgical facilities and expertise are not available.
- Intensive treatment with topical antibiotic solution (proprietary preparation or specially made up fortified solution) will be required for the management of deep corneal ulcers.
- Deep corneal injuries are invariably accompanied by uveitis, and symptomatic treatment of the uveitis with topical atropine sulphate 1% must accompany treatment.
- Anticollagenases, such as acetylcysteine or EDTA, are of largely unproven benefit in the treatment of complicated ulcerative keratitis, and careful removal of necrotic tissue is a more rational approach. Ascorbic acid (vitamin C) has proved useful in human patients for treating the stromal lysis that follows alkali burns and may be given orally. Whole fresh serum is easy to obtain from the patient and is an empirical and readily available topical therapy for any situation where collagenases and proteases complicate the situation. Acetylcysteine (5–10%) may be used in conjunction with fresh serum to prevent collagenolysis.
- If the ulcer progresses despite treatment, the patient is best referred before perforation occurs.

Antibiotic selection

- If bacterial infection is proved or suspected then an appropriate topical antibiotic should be selected. For most Gram +ve infections, topical chloramphenicol can be used; for most Gram −ve infections gentamicin is effective. For mixed infections, a triple preparation containing, for example, polymixin B, neomycin and gramicidin, is useful. For confirmed *Pseudomonas aeruginosa* infection gentamicin is the drug of choice. On the rare occasions when gentamicin-resistant *Pseudomonas aeruginosa* infection is encountered, ciprofloxacin can be used

- Topical rather than systemic therapy is always the route of choice for corneal infections
- Ointments and suspensions can be used to treat ulcers with epithelial loss only; they should not be used in situations where they can become incorporated in the healing tissues, or when there is full-thickness perforation
- Proprietary solutions are the treatment of choice for uncomplicated ulcers up to mid-stromal depth
- Fortified liquid preparations should be reserved for complicated ulcers and for when corneal penetration has occurred (see Appendix 2, pp 333–344)

Points to note in the treatment of ulcerative keratitis
- *Local anaesthetics* should *never* be used as part of treatment regimes, as their action is of short duration only and they are epitheliotoxic. If pain is marked then systemic analgesics should be given.
- Topical *corticosteroids* should *not* be used to treat ulcerative keratitis as they can adversely affect the reparative functions of epithelial cells and fibroblasts and also enhance stromal collagenolysis. The only exception to this rule is the carefully-monitored treatment of certain rare immune-mediated corneal problems.
- Topical *non-steroidal inflammatory agents* (e.g. ketorolac trometamol 0.5%) may be used with caution when significant uveitis accompanies ulcerative keratitis. They appear not to cause collagenolysis, but may delay epithelialisation.

Chronic superficial keratoconjunctivitis (pannus)
Aetiology
- An immune-mediated problem
- Certain breeds are susceptible, most commonly the German Shepherd Dog, but also Belgian Shepherd Dog, Border Collie, Dachshund and gaze hounds such as the Greyhound and Lurcher
- Predisposing factors include ultraviolet light, altitude and smoke

Clinical findings
- In the UK, dogs first present with pannus at approximately 3–5 years of age
- The condition usually produces mild ocular discomfort
- Some or all of the conjunctival limbus (follicular hyperplasia), cornea (initially infer-otemporal/ventrolateral pink-grey fibrovascular infiltration, but will extend across the whole cornea if untreated) and third eyelid (follicular hyperplasia with depigmentation) may be involved (Figure 3.30)
- Involvement of the third eyelid alone is sometimes separately classified as *plasmacytic conjunctivitis*, a *plasma cell infiltrate*, or *plasmoma*, but it is treated in the same way as pannus. The condition is usually bilateral
- Corneal pigmentation and lipid deposition may complicate the presentation, but corneal ulceration is not usually present

- Note that the roughened nature of the infiltrate can lead to false positives after fluorescein application unless excess stain is rinsed away gently with saline or water
- Pannus is essentially a superficial, subepithelial, fibrovascular infiltration in which lymphocytes and plasma cells predominate

Treatment
- The clinical appearance can be largely reversed by topical application of cyclosporin. Topical cyclosporin ointment 0.2% applied once or twice daily is the treatment of choice, especially as it appears to reduce the degree of corneal pigmentation. A side effect of no clinical relevance is that it will also increase tear production.
- A surface-active preparation such as fluorometholone, or other topical corticosteroid such as prednisolone, betamethasone, or dexamethasone, can also be used in the early stages of treatment to achieve a quick resolution of clinical signs. For example, the corticosteroid preparation should be applied at least five times daily for five days, then four times daily for four days, then three times daily for three days, then two times daily for two days, then once daily for one day. Long-term topical corticosteroids are not usually indicated and cyclosporin can be introduced as the dose of corticosteroid is tapered off.
- Note that recurrence is likely when either of the above treatment regimes is stopped, almost universally so in the commonly-affected susceptible breeds. In most cases, therefore, treatment should be maintained for life once the diagnosis has been made. The treatment regime is varied to take into account known predisposing factors such as ultraviolet light.
- Surgery (superficial keratectomy) is required only in the very rare instances of those dogs that remain blind despite medical therapy, usually because of extensive pigment deposition. Topical treatment should be started as soon as possible after surgery to prevent rapid reversion to the preoperative state.

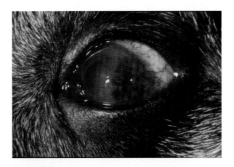

Figure 3.30 Chronic superficial keratoconjunctivitis (pannus) in a German Shepherd Dog. There was fibrovascular infiltration of the lateral quadrant of the cornea and also some third eyelid involvement in the form of follicular hyperplasia and pigment loss.

Lipid deposition in the cornea
Crystalline stromal dystrophy
Crystalline stromal dystrophy (Figure 3.31) is a relatively common condition in some breeds (e.g. Cavalier King Charles Spaniel) in which lipid is deposited in a central or paracentral position in the corneal stroma of both eyes, without any sign of inflammatory response. In a proportion of cases the lipid and lipoprotein profile is abnormal, in others, temporary variations occur during oestrus, pregnancy or lactation and,

in the remainder, there are no discernible abnormalities. Additional factors, such as distichiasis, may modify the local appearance.

In some breeds the condition is likely to be inherited, and in others a familial tendency is demonstrable. Crystalline stromal dystrophy may be a consequence of an inherent metabolic defect in the corneal fibroblasts, possibly a temperature-dependent enzyme defect, and slit-lamp examination with maximum magnification often indicates panstromal accumulation of lipid material in the fibroblasts. The grossly apparent axial and paraxial crystalline appearance is associated with fibroblast death and liberation of the accumulated lipid material.

It should be noted that the central cornea is more than 3°C cooler than the peripheral cornea, so the central cornea would be preferentially affected by a temperature-dependent enzyme defect.

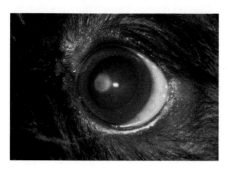

Figure 3.31 Crystalline stromal dystrophy in a Cavalier King Charles Spaniel. Both eyes were affected. Note the typical crystalline appearance and axial position of the gross lesion. The dog was normolipoproteinaemic.

Lipid keratopathy
Lipid keratopathy (Figure 3.32) is the deposition of lipid within the cornea of one or both eyes. The appearance is very variable. Vascularisation is a constant feature of lipid keratopathy and it may precede or follow the predominantly-stromal lipid deposition. Lipid keratopathy may be a complication of ocular inflammation, and some affected animals, but by no means all, have plasma hyperlipoproteinaemia (usually raised high density lipoprotein cholesterol).

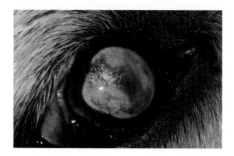

Figure 3.32 Lipid keratopathy in a Golden Retriever that had been scratched by a cat when he was a puppy. The eye had subsequently become phthitic. Low intraocular pressure is one of many factors that can enhance lipid deposition, and phthitic eyes have very low intraocular pressure. The dog also had mild hyperlipoproteinaemia (mainly affecting cholesterol).

Arcus lipoides corneae (corneal arcus)
Arcus lipoides corneae or corneal arcus (Figure 3.33(a,b)) is bilateral peripheral corneal lipid deposition. The condition in dogs is always associated with plasma hyper-

lipoproteinaemia, most commonly secondary to a problem such as primary acquired hypothyroidism.

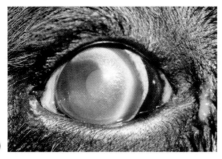 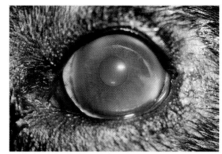

(a) **(b)**

Figure 3.33(a,b) *Arcus lipoides corneae* (corneal arcus) in a Rottweiler. The dog had primary acquired hypothyroidism and was hyperlipoproteinaemic (both cholesterol and triacylglycerides were raised). Peripheral lipid deposition was present in both eyes, but the right eye (a) was first to become involved, and the lipid has a more crystalline appearance than that of the left eye (b).

Management of corneal lipid deposition

- As local and systemic factors can be involved, both must be considered in assessing the management options. In general, progressive corneal opacification, any indications of active ocular inflammation, any ocular manifestations of hyperlipoproteinaemia (e.g. lipaemic aqueous, *lipaemia retinalis*), or any signs of systemic disease, are indications for detailed investigation
- The total serum or plasma cholesterol and triacylglyceride levels and lipoprotein profile should be analysed. Total cholesterol and triacylglyceride values alone provide insufficient information
- Systemic disease should be diagnosed and treated
- Dietary manipulation (e.g. low fat, high fibre) may be used to modify the evolution of the corneal opacity if no other abnormalities are established. Most of the lipid-lowering drugs currently used in human medicine are not applicable to management of dyslipoproteinaemia in the dog
- Any ocular inflammation must also be investigated and treated, as should any potential exacerbating factors such as distichia
- Other factors that may affect the potential for lipid deposition, but are not amenable to treatment, such as ocular hypotension (reduced intraocular pressure) must be taken into account

UVEAL TRACT (IRIS, CILIARY BODY AND CHOROID)

ANATOMY AND PHYSIOLOGY OF THE IRIS

The *iris* is the most anterior part of the uveal tract, and functions as a movable diaphragm in front of the lens. It consists of a cellular anterior border layer, which is a modification of the loosely-arranged stroma that lies beneath it. The iris sphincter muscle is located in the pupillary portion of the stroma. Two layers of epithelial cells form the posterior part of the iris. The anterior epithelium consists of an epithelial apical portion and a muscular basal portion, the iris dilator muscle, which projects into the iris stroma. The posterior surface of the iris consists of very heavily pigmented epithelial cells. Iris musculature and the epithelial layers are of neuroectodermal origin, and the stroma is of mesenchymal origin.

Iris colour depends on the number of melanocytes in the stroma and the thickness of the anterior border layer. The anterior surface is grossly divisible into a central (pupillary) zone and a peripheral (ciliary) zone, separated by the collarette. The pupillary zone of the iris is usually darker and thinner than the ciliary zone and the differences are obvious in most dogs.

Control of pupil size
The main function of the sphincter and dilator muscles is to control pupil size under different lighting conditions. The *sphincter muscle* encircles the iris at the pupillary zone and pupil constriction is mediated by the parasympathetic branches of the oculomotor nerve. Pupillary constriction regulates the amount of light that enters the eye, increases the depth of focus for near vision and reduces optical aberrations.

The *dilator muscle* controls pupillary dilation and consists of radially orientated fibres that pass from close to the pupil towards the root of the iris. Dilation is mediated by postganglionic sympathetic nerves.

ANATOMY AND PHYSIOLOGY OF THE CILIARY BODY

The *ciliary body* is located posterior to the iris and anterior to the choroid and is roughly triangular in cross section, its base facing the anterior chamber and its apex merging with the choroid. The ciliary body can be divided into the *pars plicata* and *pars plana*, the latter extending to the edge of the retina, a zone known as the *ora ciliaris retinae*. The stroma, ciliary muscles and blood vessels are of mesenchymal origin, the epithelium originates from neuroectoderm. The ciliary body serves to anchor the zonular fibres of the lens. Ciliary muscles are poorly developed in domestic animals and there is little dynamic accommodation of the lens in consequence.

Aqueous production
Aqueous is produced from the non-pigmented epithelium of the *pars plicata* of the ciliary body. The rate of aqueous production equals that of outflow, thus maintaining a relatively constant intraocular pressure.

ANATOMY AND PHYSIOLOGY OF THE CHOROID

The *choroid*, a highly-vascularised structure, is situated between the retina and the sclera. The energy requirements of the outer retina are served by diffusion of glucose and oxygen from the *choriocapillaris* vessels. The outer retina is exposed to near arterial levels of oxygen because of the high rate of blood flow through the choroid.

The choroid consists of:

1 A poorly-developed basal complex known as Bruch's membrane, adjacent to the retinal pigment epithelium

2 The *choriocapillaris*, a network of highly fenestrated capillaries, linked to the large vessels of the stroma

3 A cellular tapetum located in the dorsal choroids, which increases visual sensitivity by reflecting light back through the photoreceptors. The fine vessels (choroidal arterioles) that traverse the tapetum to link the blood vessels of the stroma and the *choriocapillaris* are such an obvious feature of fundus examination that they are referred to as the 'stars of Winslow'

4 The stroma (fibrocytes, melanocytes, elastic fibres and collagen fibres) and blood vessels

5 The *suprachoroidea* (heavily-pigmented connective tissue) adjoins the *lamina fusca* of the inner sclera

CONGENITAL AND DEVELOPMENTAL ABNORMALITIES OF THE IRIS

Colour variations

Normal variations in the colour of the iris are common in dogs of different breeds and coat colour. Some of these variations are illustrated later together with photographs of the normal fundus. The two eyes of the same animal may differ and there may also be variations of colour in the same eye. Colour differences are termed heterochromia. Ocular heterochromia may be the only manifestation of colour dilution, or may be part of more widespread colour dilution, especially in *merle animals*. Sub-albinism refers to a lack of normal pigmentation and manifests as a blue iris. It is reasonably common in dogs.

Congenital colour variations should be distinguished from acquired ones – in patients with chronic or previous uveitis it is common for the iris to become darker and lose fine structural detail.

Merle animals

A range of ocular abnormalities may be encountered in merle animals of any species. Mildly-affected animals have heterochromia and iris hypoplasia (incomplete iris development) often with abnormal pupil position (*correctopia*) and shape (*dyscoria*). Persistent remnants of the pupillary membrane and iris colobomas are also common. Severe ocular defects, often multiple in nature, are more likely to be encountered in animals which are homozygous for the merle trait; they include microphthalmos, retinal dysplasia, optic nerve hypoplasia and cataracts. Affected animals are also likely to be congenitally deaf. The combination of a white coat, blue eyes and deafness in animals is analogous to Waardenburg's syndrome in humans.

Persistent pupillary membrane

Persistent pupillary membrane (PPM) is the most obvious and common example of faulty differentiation of the anterior segment, and is a result of failure of the normal process of atrophy of the vascular arcades (*tunica vasculosa lentis anterioris*) and associated mesenchymal tissue (Figure 3.34). Remnants of the pupillary membrane may be

GENERAL AND CANINE OPHTHALMOLOGY

found as an isolated defect or in conjunction with other abnormalities (anterior segment dysgenesis and multiple ocular defects). Persistent pupillary membrane may be inherited in the Basenji and possibly in other breeds.

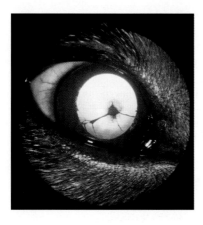

Figure 3.34 Persistent pupillary membrane in a cross-bred puppy. Note that the remnants arise, predominantly, from the iris collarette.

Clinical features
Persistent pupillary membrane remnants often arise from the collarette region of the iris. They may run across the face of the iris ± span the pupil ± attach to the anterior lens capsule ± attach to the posterior cornea. They should be distinguished from acquired adhesions (synechiae).

Incomplete iris development
There is a range of appearances, from apparent absence of the whole iris (*aniridia*) which is very rare, to incomplete iris development (*hypoplasia*) or absence of a portion of the full thickness of the iris (*coloboma*) which are uncommon (Figure 3.35). Iris hypoplasia and colobomatous defects should be differentiated from acquired iris atrophy.

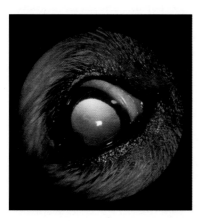

Figure 3.35 Atypical colobomatous defect of the iris (2 o'clock) in a Shetland Sheepdog. This was an incidental finding as the dog had actually been referred because of an epitheliopathy. Note the disruption of the camera flash on the ocular surface.

ACQUIRED ABNORMALITIES OF THE UVEAL TRACT

Iris pigmentation

Discrete hyperpigmentation and pigment proliferation on the iris surface can occur as a phenomenon of ageing and is usually of no clinical significance in such cases (Figure 3.36). However, all unexplained changes of pigmentation should be observed carefully over time, as it is not usually possible to differentiate focal pigmented lesions on the basis of a single clinical examination alone. Malignancy may be associated with proliferation, elevation and iris infiltration. *Iris freckles* are of no clinical significance and consist of focal accumulations of normal, but hyperplastic, melanocytes. *Iris nevi* represent proliferations of abnormal melanocytes and are of significance as they can undergo malignant transformation. *Iris neoplasia*, most commonly melanoma, should always be considered in the differential diagnosis; malignancy is associated with rapid enlargement.

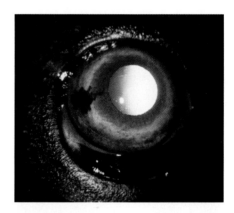

Figure 3.36 Benign melanosis in a Labrador Retriever. Note the superficial nature of the pigment.

In breeds such as the Cairn Terrier *diffuse ocular melanosis*, associated with proliferation of melanocytes, is recognised as a breed-related problem in middle-aged and older dogs. The large numbers of pigment-laden cells that accumulate can cause an insidious secondary glaucoma and the prognosis for retention of long term vision is poor (Figure 3.37).

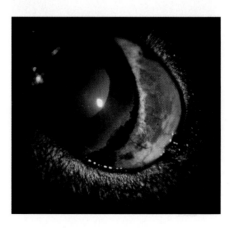

Figure 3.37 Diffuse ocular melanosis and secondary glaucoma in a Cairn Terrier.

GENERAL AND CANINE OPHTHALMOLOGY

Eversion of the heavily-pigmented posterior pigment epithelium of the iris, visible at the pupillary border, is termed *ectropion uveae* and is most commonly seen following previous iris inflammation. Note that poorly-pigmented eyes may have a pigmented ruff at the pupil margin as a normal feature of colour dilution.

Pre-iridal fibrovascular membranes (PIFMs)

Neovascularisation of the iris surface occurs when angiogenic factors, released as a feature of, for example, chronic uveitis and intraocular neoplasia, stimulate production of blood vessels by the iris stroma. The abnormal blood vessels can be a source of haemorrhage into the anterior chamber, resulting in the formation of peripheral anterior synechiae and subsequent secondary glaucoma. Neovascularisation is most readily observed in a lightly-pigmented iris and may not be obvious in the dark iris found in most breeds of dog.

Iris atrophy

Senile iris atrophy is observed most commonly in breeds such as the Miniature and Toy Poodle (Figure 3.38), but it can also follow trauma, chronic uveitis and glaucoma. The atrophy can result in full-thickness defects, including loss of the iris sphincter muscle, and is associated with poor pupil constriction in such cases. In some instances the atrophy is restricted to certain sectors of the iris, for example the pupillary margin (Figure 3.39).

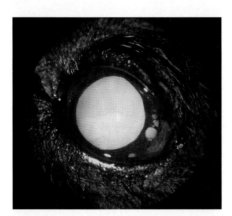

Figure 3.38 Senile iris atrophy in an aged Miniature Poodle. There are a number of full-thickness iris defects in the pupillary zone of the iris, and it is possible to see the lens equator through the defects. The ciliary zone does not appear to be affected on gross inspection. The dog also had generalised progressive retinal atrophy with secondary total cortical cataract.

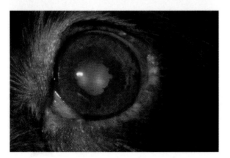

Figure 3.39 Senile iris atrophy in an old English Springer Spaniel. The pupillary margin is affected and there is also a cortical cataract and a benign cystic lesion on the upper eyelid.

Iridociliary cysts

Although iridociliary cysts can be of developmental origin, they are most commonly observed as an acquired phenomenon. They may be a feature of ageing or follow uveitis or appear for reasons unknown. The cysts are of variable size and intact cysts are usually free-floating and can be transilluminated with a bright light even when they are heavily pigmented (Figure 3.40). Sometimes the cysts rupture, leaving remnants on the anterior face of the lens or the posterior surface of the cornea. They should be differentiated from primary tumours of the iris and ciliary body and from metastatic tumours.

In some breeds, notably the Great Dane and Golden Retriever, there is an association between iridociliary cysts, uveitis and secondary glaucoma and suspected cases should be referred early.

Treatment

- Any underlying abnormalities such as uveitis should be addressed
- No treatment is usually required for iris cysts, although multiple cysts that obstruct the visual axis can be treated by needle puncture and extraction, or using non-invasive laser therapy
- In those breeds in which iridociliary cysts are associated with uveitis it is sensible to seek early specialist advice.

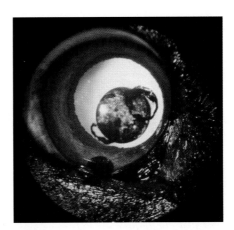

Figure 3.40 Iridociliary cysts in a Labrador Retriever. These cysts usually arise from the posterior face of the iris and are often found in ageing Labrador Retrievers; they are invariably of no clinical significance.

Synechiae

These are adhesions that form as a result of iris inflammation and they should be differentiated from persistent pupillary membrane (PPM) remnants. The formation of *anterior* synechiae, adherence of the iris to the cornea, is a common complication of corneal penetrating injury (Figure 3.41). The formation of *posterior* synechiae, adherence of the iris to the anterior lens capsule, is a likely sequel to anterior uveitis. Peripheral anterior synechiae involve the iridocorneal angle and are usually associated with iris inflammation especially that associated with the formation of pre-iridal fibrovascular membranes.

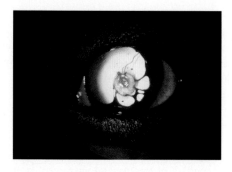

Figure 3.41 Anterior synechiae in a Border Collie that had been scratched by a cat when he was a puppy. No treatment had been given and the dog has been left with a large and deep corneal facet, anterior synechiae, an irregular pupil and a darkened iris. Note that the adhesions arise from the pupillary border and attach on the posterior cornea.

Canine uveal neoplasia
Primary neoplasia

The majority of primary tumours of the uveal tract arise from the iris and ciliary body rather than the choroid and are usually benign with little tendency to metastasise. The commonest primary intraocular neoplasm is the *melanoma* (Figure 3.42) and most anterior uveal melanomas are unilateral, circumscribed and benign. Choroidal melanomas, the commonest site in human eyes, are very rare. Primary iris melanoma is over represented in the Labrador Retriever in the UK. Melanomas can cause secondary intraocular disease such as uveitis and glaucoma and, rarely, they metastasise to distant sites.

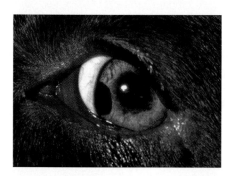

Figure 3.42 Iris melanoma in a Labrador Retriever. The melanoma is most obvious medially and extends from about 7 o'clock to 9 o'clock, but note that there are also pigmentary changes in the dorsomedial quadrant of the iris.

Ciliary body tumours (*adenoma* and *adenocarcinoma*) (Figure 3.43) are the most frequently reported primary ciliary body tumours and are usually unilateral. Other primary anterior uveal tumours are rare: they include fibrosarcoma, medulloepithelioma, haemangioma, haemangiosarcoma and leiomyosarcoma.

Diagnosis
- History and clinical appearance. The owner should be questioned about changes of appearance and growth pattern
- The iris should be examined carefully under magnification
- Transillumination of the eye, scleral depression techniques, gonioscopy and ultrasonography
- Thoracic and abdominal imaging

- Samples such as aspirates may yield diagnostic cytology, but interpretation may be difficult. Needle biopsy and histology of the tumour are appropriate diagnostic aids. Lymph node biopsy should be undertaken if lymphadenopathy is a feature

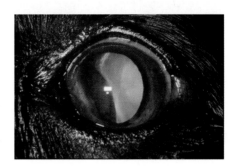

Figure 3.43 Ciliary body adenoma in an old Labrador Retriever. The tumour is quite discrete and has interposed itself between the lens and the iris. Note also the tumour extension into the anterior chamber ventrally. There is secondary cataract formation as well as senile nuclear sclerosis of the lens.

Differential diagnosis of iris melanoma
- Acquired hyperpigmentation – benign localised changes, diffuse changes associated with chronic uveitis, breed-related hyperpigmentation (e.g. diffuse ocular melanosis in the Cairn Terrier)
- Uveal cysts – smooth and usually free-floating spheres that can be transilluminated with a bright light even when they are heavily pigmented. Ultrasonography will differentiate a fluid-filled cyst from a solid mass

Management of iris melanoma
- The abnormal region of the iris should be kept under careful observation and left alone if there is no indication of growth
- For those masses that demonstrate a temporal increase in size, laser ablation, or local excision is effective and such cases may require referral
- For those melanomas that produce secondary complications, most commonly glaucoma, the whole eye should be removed and this decision is made easier if the eye is blind or intractably painful
- If local excision or globe removal is undertaken, the tissues or globe should be submitted for histopathology

Secondary neoplasia
- Secondary neoplasia may involve the uveal tract, and *lymphoma* (Figure 3.44) is the most common secondary tumour to affect the eye and orbit. Ocular involvement follows lymphadenopathy as the most frequently diagnosed clinical sign
- Haemangiosarcoma is probably the next most common secondary tumour after lymphoma, and may present with hyphaema as the most obvious ocular feature
- Other metastatic tumours include adenocarcinoma, fibrosarcoma, rhabdomyosarcoma, osteosarcoma, phaeochromocytoma, seminoma, transmissible venereal tumour and malignant melanoma

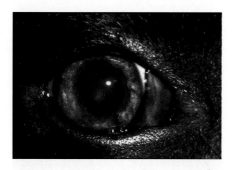

Figure 3.44 Multicentric lymphoma in a German Shepherd Dog. Early invasion of the iris usually involves the ciliary zone, rather than the pupillary zone and in this dog the medial iris shows signs of tumour infiltration. The infiltration is much more obvious in such cases if the anterior chamber is viewed from the side. There was also some ill-defined haemorrhage from the iris.

Diagnosis
- History, ocular signs and clinical signs
- The ocular manifestations are variable; there is not only infiltration of the uveal tract by the tumour, but there may be associated generalised abnormalities such as anaemia, thrombocytopaenia and disseminated intravascular coagulation, all of which can present with ocular manifestations
- Haematology and biochemistry profiles, together with appropriate tests (e.g. lymph node and bone marrow biopsy) where indicated

Management
- Treatment depends upon the type of tumour and the stage of development. Malignant lymphoma is the commonest type of disseminated neoplasia that is treated routinely and responds well to chemotherapy; the earlier the diagnosis and treatment the better the success
- Chemotherapy is also the commonest approach adopted for other disseminated tumours judged to be treatable
- Referral should be considered for the management of all types of complex tumour

Miscellaneous conditions
Histiocytosis
Histiocytosis is an example of immunoproliferative disease that is remarkably similar to malignant lymphoma; the same chemotherapy protocol is used for management.

Granulomatous meningoencephalitis
Granulomatous meningoencephalitis (GME) is an inflammatory disease in which there is proliferation of reticuloendothelial cells and involvement of the central nervous system, optic nerves and globes. The ocular manifestations usually involve the posterior segment and anterior uveitis is unusual.

Canine uveitis
It is inevitable that the inflammatory boundaries in uveitis are not as distinct as the terminology would suggest. In addition, ocular changes in bilateral cases are rarely symmetrical, as they may reflect different time courses in the pathogenesis (Figure 3.45(a,b)). Anterior uveitis may involve the iris (*iritis*) or both the iris and the anterior part of the ciliary body (*iridocyclitis*). Intermediate uveitis mainly involves the posterior part of the ciliary body and the region of the *ora ciliaris retinae* (*pars planitis*). Posterior uveitis involves the choroid (*choroiditis*), but close association of the retina

means that inflammation of both choroid and retina (*chorioretinitis*) is the usual situation. *Panuveitis* is inflammation of the entire uveal tract – iris, ciliary body and choroid (Figure 3.45(c)). In addition to what is described below, some aspects of uveitis are reviewed with diseases of the fundus.

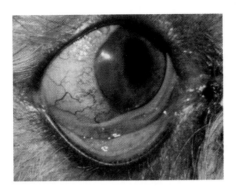

Figure 3.45(a) Acute/subacute uveitis in a dog. Both eyes of this Bearded Collie were involved and the uveitis was probably a sequel to immune-mediated inflammatory bowel disease. The dog was antinuclear antibody positive. Pain, blepharospasm, lacrimation and photophobia were prominent. In the right eye there is a more acute presentation, with perilimbal hyperaemia, subtle pancorneal opacification, aqueous flare and sparse keratic precipitates, reduced anterior chamber depth, loss of iris detail and pupil constriction. The intraocular pressure measured with an applanation tonometer (Mackay Marg) was 7 mm of mercury.

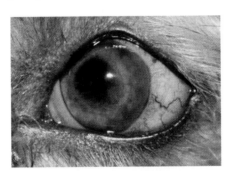

Figure 3.45(b) Uveitis has been present for longer in the left eye and the uveitis is less acute. Hyperaemia is more diffuse and corneal oedema is more obvious, otherwise the changes are similar. It was possible to examine the posterior segment of both eyes after intensive topical treatment for 60 minutes with a mydriatic cycloplegic (atropine) and corticosteroids (prednisolone acetate). Examination of the posterior segment revealed vitiritis, chorioretinitis and optic neuritis, confirming panuveitis. On the basis of the history and ocular findings medical treatment was adjusted to include systemic immunosuppressive agents (corticosteroids and azathioprine).

Clinical signs of acute uveitis (Figures 2.21(a,b), p. 55)
- Unilateral/bilateral involvement
- Pain, photophobia, blepharospasm and increased lacrimation*
- Variable effects on vision, from no effect to blind

* Readily identifiable key features

- Inflammation hyperaemia, as perilimbal hyperaemia or more diffuse redness*
- Hypotony, sometimes so obvious that digital tonometry can be used to confirm the low intraocular pressure*
- Corneal oedema (usually subtle, occurs because of endothelial dysfunction)
- Aqueous flare (protein-rich aqueous produces a Tyndall light-scattering effect, which can most easily be detected with a slit beam of light)
- Hyphaema, or hypopyon in some cases, although hypopyon is more a feature of chronicity
- Iris swelling and loss of iris detail*
- Anterior chamber may be shallower than normal (related to the inflammatory changes in the iris)
- Synechiae (adhesions) may form rapidly
- Miosis, the pupil is constricted because of ciliary spasm, there may be a sluggish or incomplete response to bright light*
- Inflammatory debris on the anterior lens capsule
- Vitritis
- Active chorioretinitis ± vascular changes
- Choroidal effusion
- Choroidal haemorrhage
- Optic neuritis

Clinical signs of chronic uveitis (Figures 3.46(a,b))
- Mild ocular discharge may be present
- Keratic precipitates/mutton-fat precipitates on posterior surface of the cornea*
- Hyphaema or hypopyon
- Corneal oedema and corneal neovascularisation may be present in some cases
- Gross iris changes, such as alteration in colour (usually darker), iris bombé, post-inflammatory iris cysts*
- Pupil changes because of synechiae formation – the pupil is irregular in shape and may be partially reactive or immobile*
- Neovascularisation of the iris
- Pigment deposition on the lens (iris rests), inflammatory debris on the lens, cataract or lens luxation*
- Cobblestone effects in the fundus, pigment proliferation, focal and/or diffuse hyperreflectivity*
- Retinal detachment
- Optic atrophy
- Glaucoma (a complication of posterior synechiae or peripheral anterior synechiae)

Diagnosis
- Patient details, ocular and systemic history (including vaccination), plus details of any previous treatment
- Complete physical examination should always be performed, neurological examination may also be required
- Ophthalmic examination of both eyes and their adnexa. Bilateral uveitis can indicate systemic involvement, but one eye may be affected before the other

* Readily identifiable key features

- Diagnostic imaging techniques can be useful, and thoracic radiography may be needed if neoplasia suspected
- If the cause is not obvious, routine haematology, blood biochemistry, serodiagnosis and, if possible, specific diagnostic tests should be performed whenever practicable
- Other samples are sometimes required (e.g. for culture, cytology, histopathology) by paracentesis, aspiration or biopsy

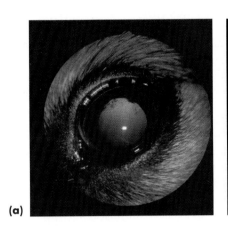 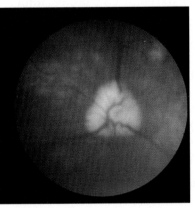

(a)   **(b)**

Figure 3.46 **(a)** Chronic uveitis. The pupil is slightly irregular and the iris darkened. Iris rests (pigment deposition on the lens) are present on the anterior lens capsule. **(b)** The fundus displays the typical 'cobblestone' appearance of chronic uveitis. Chronic vitritis is also present, so that the vitreous is hazy.

GENERAL PRINCIPLES OF TREATMENT FOR CANINE UVEITIS

Corticosteroids
Topical corticosteroids
Prednisolone acetate 1% is currently the preparation of choice for anterior uveitis, and topical application is the route of choice. Initially one drop is applied to the eye up to five times daily, and treatment should be tapered off over a period of some 5–10 days, when the uveitis has resolved.

Subconjunctival corticosteroids
Subconjunctival injections delivered beneath the dorsal bulbar conjunctiva are painful, so this route is used less commonly than others in the conscious patient. Its advantage is that one injection lasts for 2–3 weeks. The disadvantages, aside from the pain of injection, include the risk of accidental ocular penetration, continuing absorption in the face of complications, variable intraocular concentrations (accurate deposition is difficult and absorption of the drug can be variable) and occasional granuloma formation at the site of injection. Dexamethasone and betamethasone are both suitable preparations. Dose rate is 0.75–2.0 mg per eye according to the dog's size.

Systemic corticosteroids
Oral prednisolone is indicated for the treatment of intermediate and posterior uveitis.

Both topical and oral corticosteroids will be required for the treatment of panuveitis and for immune-mediated types of uveitis. Higher dose rates are selected when immunosuppression is the prime purpose of treatment (2 mg/kg prednisolone every 12 hours) and lower dose rates may be used when anti-inflammatory effects are primarily required (1 mg/kg of prednisolone every 12 hours). Treatment should be tapered off when the condition has resolved and not stopped abruptly.

Non-steroidal anti-inflammatory drugs (NSAIDs)
Topical NSAIDs
NSAIDs available as topical preparations include diclofenac sodium 0.1%, flurbiprofen sodium 0.03% and ketorolac trometamol 0.5%. Although these drugs are mainly used in cataract surgery, they also have an important anti-inflammatory role in situations where corticosteroids would be contraindicated, and ketorolac trometamol is commonly selected for this purpose.

Systemic NSAIDs
Carprofen (4 mg/kg i/v or s/c initially, followed by oral treatment at a dose rate of 2 mg/kg) is usually selected to control mild to moderate pain and inflammation. It is most effective when given prior to inflammation and pain (e.g. preoperatively), so its indications are more limited in the treatment of unanticipated inflammations.

NSAIDs and corticosteroids should not be used concurrently because of their potential adverse effect on the gastrointestinal tract.

Cytotoxic drugs
These systemic preparations (e.g. azathioprine) are occasionally used in cases of presumed immune-mediated uveitis, often in conjunction with immunosuppressive doses of systemic corticosteroids.

Mydriatic cycloplegics
Usually atropine 1% alone is sufficient, but phenylephrine 10% can also be used initially when pupillary dilation is difficult to achieve. The patient's progress should be monitored closely and the aim is to eliminate pain (by relaxing ciliary spasm) and to reduce the risk of synechiae formation. Once the pupil has dilated, mydriatic cycloplegics can be applied only as often as is necessary to maintain this state. The patient should be monitored carefully for potential complications, particularly glaucoma.

NON-INFECTIONS CAUSES OF CANINE UVEITIS

Reflex
This is the transient and mild uveitis that can follow an ocular surface or corneal insult. It is mediated by an axon reflex within the trigeminal nerve and is usually self-limiting.

Associated with keratitis (see also Section 2, p. 57)
Ulcerative keratitis and corneal insult (e.g. chemical injury) can both be associated with uveitis, which may be transient or sustained.

Trauma (see also Section 2, pp 35–49)

Transient reflex uveitis associated with minor corneal insult is common, but sustained uveitis will accompany deep keratitis and more serious corneal injury. Hypopyon is often present as a feature of deep keratitis.

The uveitis that follows penetrating or blunt traumatic injury may become complicated by secondary problems such as glaucoma, cataract and *phthisis bulbi*. Endophthalmitis is also possible following traumatic injury, because of the high risk of infection being introduced into the eye by direct inoculation.

Uveitis associated with lens damage (see also Section 2, p. 48)

Lens-induced uveitis occurs when there is a breakdown of the normal T-cell tolerance to lens proteins. It is usually a consequence of traumatic rupture of the lens capsule, for example from a penetrating claw injury or a gunshot wound. The release of antigenic lens protein initiates a *phacoclastic uveitis*. Phacoclastic uveitis tends to be very intense in dogs, and short-term complications include the development of persistent uveitis, glaucoma or fulminating endophthalmitis.

Small puncture wounds in the lens capsule may seal, and such cases can be managed medically, but, when there is likely to be extensive or sustained release of lens contents, surgery to remove the antigenic lens protein, usually by phacoemulsification, should be undertaken without delay. Because the examination, assessment and management of lens damage can be difficult, early referral is advised.

Slow leakage of soluble lens protein though an intact lens capsule, as, for example, leakage associated with hypermature cataracts, produces a low-grade *phacolytic uveitis* that may be treated symptomatically (Figure 3.47).

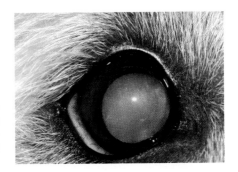

Figure 3.47 Uveitis associated with hypermature cataract in a dog. The iris of this eye was slightly darker than that of the fellow unaffected eye. The total cataract is not of uniform appearance.

Immune-mediated uveitis

The *uveodermatological syndrome* in dogs has been compared with the Vogt-Koyanagi-Harada syndrome in humans, and in both species the disease is a possible example of an autoimmune reaction against melanocytes. Breeds at risk include the Japanese Akita, Chow Chow and Samoyed.

Clinical signs

- Depigmentation of the lids, muzzle, rhinarium, skin and whitening of the hair
- Acute, usually bilateral, panuveitis that may precede or follow mucocutaneous

involvement and skin and hair changes. The ocular inflammation is often intense, painful and sustained
- Complications include degenerative changes in the retina and optic nerve and secondary glaucoma

Diagnosis

Diagnosis is based on the characteristic clinical signs and supplementary tests such as skin biopsy, because the primary disease process is associated with destruction of dermal, as well as uveal, melanocytes.

Treatment

- Should be started as early as possible and maintained long term, as the management can be difficult and the prognosis guarded. Many of these cases are best referred for initial assessment
- Combination of immunosuppressive doses of systemic corticosteroids (oral prednisolone 1–2 mg/kg/day initially, with gradual reduction to the lowest dose which prevents recurrence) and immunosuppressive drugs such as azathioprine (oral dose of 2 mg/kg/day, reducing after 3–5 days)
- The uveitis must also be treated locally with topical applications of corticosteroid (prednisolone acetate 1% some five times daily for the first 5–10 days) and atropine 1% (as frequently as is necessary to achieve and maintain pupil dilation)
- If there is any suspicion of secondary glaucoma, the animal should be hospitalised and the intraocular pressure monitored
- Even with early and aggressive treatment the prognosis is guarded, so management requires specialist help

CANINE UVEITIS ASSOCIATED WITH INFECTION

Systemic viral disease

Infectious canine hepatitis

Infectious canine hepatitis (canine adenovirus type I) is the most important viral cause of canine uveitis. The initial clinical signs consist of a mild, usually unilateral, uveitis, with photophobia, that occurs during the acute phase of clinical illness, followed by a much more severe keratouveitis 1–3 weeks after infection, in a proportion of cases.

Ocular signs
- In addition to the usual clinical features of iritis, the most striking ocular sign is corneal oedema ('blue eye'), as a result of a delayed hypersensitivity response that damages the corneal endothelium. The corneal oedema is usually unilateral. If the corneal damage is severe enough, bullous keratopathy and keratoglobus can develop. In some animals there is slow resolution of the corneal oedema, which clears from the limbus towards the centre over a period of weeks. In other animals, however, the corneal opacity persists.
- The intraocular pressure is lower than normal in most cases, but rises if secondary glaucoma supervenes. A substantial rise in intraocular pressure may produce permanent globe enlargement (hydrophthalmos), especially in young dogs.

Treatment
The treatment of infectious canine hepatitis is symptomatic (as outlined earlier under general principles) and supportive.

Canine herpes virus
Canine herpes virus is an occasional cause of neonatal death in litters of puppies. Ocular signs include severe panuveitis, keratouveitis and chorioretinitis and survivors may be severely visually impaired or blind.

Canine distemper virus
Canine distemper virus infection is frequently associated with chorioretinitis and optic neuritis, especially in dogs with neurological signs (see under Fundus, this section, pp 138–142).

Rickettsial diseases
The tick-borne diseases, *monocytic ehrlichiosis* or tropical canine pancytopaenia (*Ehrlichia canis*), *Rocky Mountain spotted fever (Rickettsia rickettsii)* and *infectious cyclic thrombocytopaenia (Ehrlichia platys)* have all been reported as causes of uveitis in tropical and sub-tropical zones.

Monocytic ehrlichiosis is the most important disease in this group. After the acute phase of infection, some dogs eliminate the organism, while others become subclinically infected so that chronic disease can develop years later. Although not endemic in the UK, subclinically infected dogs imported into the country pose a risk.

Clinical signs
- All these tick-borne rickettsial diseases are associated with vasculitis and thrombocytopaenia. Serious bleeding problems, especially epistaxis and ocular haemorrhage, are most likely to be associated with monocytic ehrlichiosis and this infection should be considered in the differential diagnosis of intraocular haemorrhage.
- Uveitis, vasculitis and intraocular haemorrhage are common ocular findings in tick-borne disease. Severe ocular haemorrhage, retinal detachment and secondary glaucoma are common complications.

Treatment
- Doxycycline is usually the drug selected for treating acute rickettsial infections (5 mg/kg twice daily for 14 days). Sub-clinical infections are less-successfully treated and imidocarb dipropionate (5 mg/kg intramuscularly once, repeated at 14–21 days) is probably the treatment of choice.
- The uveitis is treated symptomatically.

Bacterial infections
Leptospirosis
Leptospirosis is caused by a number of potential serovars, and the kidney is usually the main target organ in dogs. The zoonotic implications of infection should be explained to the owner.

Clinical signs and diagnosis
- Vasculitis, endotheliitis and renal failure, disseminated intravascular coagulation

- Uveitis seems most likely to occur after a latent period following previous acute infection
- The diagnosis is usually confirmed from the clinical signs, urinalysis and serology

Treatment
- Acute leptospiral infection can be treated with penicillin and its derivatives and tetracyclines can be used for follow-up therapy to eliminate the carrier state
- Doxycycline is an alternative drug for treatment of the acute infection and as follow-up therapy
- Supportive care is required for those cases with renal disease
- The uveitis is treated symptomatically

Systemic bacterial infections
Systemic bacterial infection may also be associated with uveitis, and it is the posterior uvea that is most likely to be involved in blood-borne infection; examples include salmonellosis and tuberculosis. Uveitis can be initiated by circulating toxins and is thus associated with a variety of conditions that result in toxaemia or sepsis. The commonest associations are with endocarditis, dental disease and pyometritis.

Local bacterial infections
Direct introduction of pathogens such as *Pasteurella multocida* following a penetrating injury may be a cause of exogenous uveitis with complications such as abscessation or endophthalmitis.

Fungal and algal infections
These disseminated infections are only likely to be seen in dogs that have been imported into the UK from non-temperate climates, or in severely immunocompromised animals. Ocular involvement, notably posterior uveitis and panuveitis, is often an obvious feature of infection and lesions are typically granulomatous or pyogranulomatous in type. Examples of systemic mycoses include *blastomycosis, cryptococcosis, coccidioidomycosis, geotrichosis, aspergillosis* and *histoplasmosis. Prototothecosis* is a rare disease caused by colourless algae.

Specialist advice should be obtained with regard to the specific diagnosis and management of these conditions, relapse is common and most cases are best referred.

Parasitic infection
Leishmaniasis
Leishmaniasis is caused by a diphasic protozoan parasite. Old World leishmaniasis is caused by *Leishmania donovani infantum* and New World leishmaniasis by *Leishmania donovani chagasi*. Clinical disease develops in a high proportion of infected dogs after an incubation period of several months to several years. Leishmaniasis is an endemic problem in many parts of the world, but may also occur in dogs that have been imported to the UK. It is a difficult condition to treat effectively as the relapse rate is high. The zoonotic implications should be discussed before considering treatment, and it is sensible to seek specialist advice from a referral centre when treatment is contemplated.

Clinical signs
- Chronic emaciation and non-pruritic skin disease
- Periocular lesions, including blepharitis
- Ocular lesions include conjunctivitis, keratitis, scleritis, keratouveitis and uveitis

Diagnosis
- History of visiting an endemic area
- Clinical signs
- Serology
- Identification of causative organism from lymph node or bone marrow aspirates, or biopsy specimens

Toxoplasmosis
Toxoplasmosis, caused by the protozoan parasite *Toxoplasma gondii*, is unusual in dogs, and most of the ocular lesions encountered in clinical practice are associated with chronic and sub-clinical infection. Concurrent disease may well be present on the rare occasions when generalised toxoplasmosis develops.

Clinical signs
Anterior and posterior uveitis, scleritis and optic neuritis, less commonly, extraocular myositis

Diagnosis
- Serological testing may be indicative of active infection if a fourfold increase in antibody levels can be demonstrated in paired serum samples
- Histopathological identification of the organism

Treatment
- Oral clindamycin, 12.5 mg/kg twice daily for 3–4 weeks
- Symptomatic treatment of the uveitis
- Relapse is possible, so regular follow up is necessary

Neosporosis
Neosporosis caused by *Neospora caninum* shares similarities with toxoplasmosis, but can be differentiated, as the two *protozoan* organisms do not crossreact serologically. Most cases occur in very young dogs and ascending paralysis is the classical clinical presentation. Any accompanying uveitis is generally mild. Treatment is as for toxoplasmosis.

Parasitic larvae
Migrating metazoan parasitic larvae may provoke uveitis of differing intensities. For example, canine *toxocariasis*, *angiostrongylosis* and *filariasis* have all been reported as causes of uveitis. Working Border Collies demonstrate a high incidence of chorioretinopathy lesions that have been ascribed to previous infestation with *Toxocara canis*.

Aberrant *Angiostrongylus vasorum* larvae may provoke a range of responses, from minimal to severe granulomatous uveitis, if they reach the eye. The most spectacular ocular manifestation is undoubtedly the free nematode or nematodes within the eye. Because of the uveitis they elicit it is usual to remove aberrant larvae from the anterior chamber surgically, and such cases are usually referred.

Dirofilaria immitis is not endemic in the UK, but may be encountered in animals imported from the Americas and parts of Europe. Ocular signs include anterior uveitis with varying degrees of corneal oedema. It is also possible to detect aberrant dirofilaria in the anterior chamber of some cases.

Intraocular diptera larvae *(ophthalmomyiasis interna)* that are thought to penetrate the eye through the conjunctiva are also a potential cause of uveitis. *Ophthalmomyiasis interna* may present as anterior uveitis in the acute phase of invasion by the dipteran larva, but is more likely to be an incidental finding in the chronic stage of infection when fundus examination reveals typical curvilinear criss-crossing tracts.

ANTERIOR CHAMBER AND AQUEOUS HUMOUR

The anterior chamber is the space delineated by the posterior surface of the cornea, the anterior surface of the iris and the anterior surface of the lens in the pupillary aperture. It is normally filled with clear aqueous humour.

Production and drainage of aqueous humour

The intraocular pressure is a consequence of the balance between aqueous production and drainage, but may be affected by other factors, such as ocular rigidity.

Aqueous resembles an ultrafiltrate of plasma and is produced by the processes of the *ciliary body*. Aqueous traverses the posterior chamber (the space between the anterior surface of the lens and the posterior surface of the iris), passes through the pupil and enters the anterior chamber. The majority of aqueous outflow in the dog occurs through the iridocorneal angle, the so-called conventional route. The iridocorneal angle consists of the pectinate ligament and the sponge-like tissue of the trabecular meshwork. Aqueous drains across these structures to the avascular aqueous plexus and thence to the scleral venous circulation.

Blood–aqueous barrier

The blood–aqueous barrier consists of the endothelium of the iris and ciliary vessels and the non-pigmented ciliary epithelium. Breakdown of the blood–aqueous barrier results in modification of the aqueous humour composition, primarily by increased quantities of protein.

EXAMINATION

- Examination of the anterior chamber and aqueous humour requires good lighting, preferably with a focussed light beam and magnification. Most information is obtained when the examination is performed in a darkened room and when the light source is shone from as many different angles as possible. A slit beam is particularly useful in the assessment of aqueous transparency and anterior chamber depth.
- It is important to note the transparency of the aqueous humour as well as the details of posterior cornea, iris and anterior lens. The depth of the anterior chamber

should also be assessed with a narrow beam of light shone across the anterior chamber.

- Gonioscopy (examination of the iridocorneal angle) may also be required, but because there is bewildering normal variation, it is a technique best performed in referral centres.
- In a very small number of cases, anterior chamber paracentesis is useful for differentiation of anterior chamber infiltrates, but interpretation of aspirates can be difficult, so requirements should be discussed with a pathologist before taking samples.

ABNORMALITIES OF THE CANINE ANTERIOR CHAMBER AND AQUEOUS HUMOUR

Anterior chamber and aqueous involvement are secondary to disease elsewhere, and the appropriate parts of the notes should be consulted for further details.

Inflammation
Aqueous flare
Protein-rich aqueous scatters light (Tyndall effect), and aqueous flare is best appreciated in the dark utilising a narrow slit beam and magnification.

Cellular infiltrates
Most common are keratic precipitates (KPs). If large enough they are called mutton fat precipitates. Because of the thermal currents within the anterior chamber that influence aqueous circulation, they usually end up adhering to the ventral (inferior) corneal endothelium, particularly ventromedially.

Hypopyon
White cell infiltrates, commonly sterile, are most commonly associated with deep corneal ulceration and uveitis. Hypopyon is usually whitish in colour and located in the ventral aspect of the anterior chamber. Hypopyon should be distinguished from chylomicrons (*lipaemic aqueous*) and anterior chamber infiltration by neoplastic cells.

Lipaemic Aqueous
Triacylglyceride-rich lipid in the aqueous humour is a possible ocular manifestation of systemic hyperlipoproteinaemia. A pre-existing uveitis will increase the likelihood of lipid leakage because of the breakdown of the blood–aqueous barrier. The lipid is only visible if triacylglyceride levels are abnormally high (>2.5 mmol/l); raised cholesterol levels do *not* alter aqueous appearance. If there is hypertriglyceridaemia alone, the aqueous appears turbid, but if chylomicrons are also raised the aqueous may appear milky white. In both primary chylomicronaemia (e.g. Miniature Schnauzer) and secondary hypertriglyceridaemia or chylomicronaemia (e.g. animals with diabetes mellitus) triacylglyceride-rich or chylomicron-rich aqueous is a possible ocular manifestation (Figure 3.48). The whole of the anterior chamber is turbid or opaque. Fundus examination can also be useful, in both fasting and non-fasting animals, as lipaemia retinalis is commoner than lipaemic aqueous in animals with raised serum triacylglycerides.

Normolipoproteinaemia (especially normal levels of triacylglycerides) and effective control of uveitis can be critical to the success of elective procedures such as cataract surgery in susceptible breeds, and preoperative preparation is key to the management of such cases. Routine preoperative screening should include measurement of serum or plasma triacylglycerides, as well as cholesterol, and investigation of any underlying causes of hyperlipoproteinaemia. If no underlying treatable causes can be found, then a low-fat–high-fibre diet, with fish oil supplementation, for life, should be instituted. A low-fat diet and good control of diabetes mellitus, together with careful perioperative and postoperative management of intraocular inflammation, will reduce the postoperative complications in animals at risk.

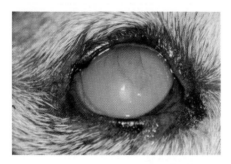

Figure 3.48 Lipaemic aqueous in a Miniature Pinscher with chylomicronaemia secondary to diabetes mellitus. Only the right eye was affected, and this eye had mild kerato-uveitis and a healing ulcer.

Haemorrhage (hyphaema)

Hyphaema, haemorrhage in the anterior chamber, is not uncommon. It is important to establish the cause of any intraocular haemorrhage (Figure 3.49).

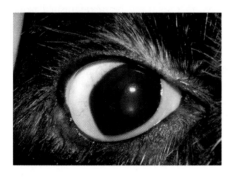

Figure 3.49 Hyphaema associated with immune-mediated thrombocytopaenia in a Cocker Spaniel. Compare this photograph with Figure 2.23 and note that there are no signs of uveitis and the visible mucous membranes are very pale. The dog also had petechiation of the oral mucous membranes.

Differential diagnosis of intraocular haemorrhage
Congenital and developmental conditions
- Collie eye anomaly
- Persistence of the primary vitreous and persistent hyperplastic primary vitreous

Acquired conditions
- Trauma
- Severe inflammation
- Chronic glaucoma
- Neoplasia
- Systemic hypertensive disease
- Immune-mediated disease (e.g. thrombocytopaenia, auto-immune haemolytic anaemia)
- Clotting defects – genetic and acquired (e.g. warfarin [coumarin] poisoning)
- Sepsis
- Disseminated intravascular coagulation (DIC)

Neoplasia

On the basis of ophthalmic examination alone it may be impossible to distinguish inflammatory exudates from neoplastic infiltrates within the anterior chamber. Both inflammation and neoplasia may be unilateral or bilateral (Figure 3.50(a,b)). The patient's history and the results of physical examination may help in differentiation, as may paracentesis.

(a) 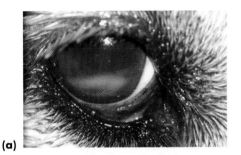 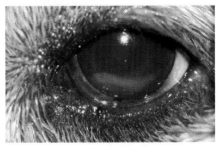 **(b)**

Figure 3.50(a,b) Blood-tinged neoplastic cells in the anterior chamber of a Golden Retriever with multicentric lymphoma, both eyes were involved.

Clinical approach to anterior-chamber opacities
- Careful examination of the whole animal, as well as both eyes. The changes that are observed in the anterior chamber reflect pathology elsewhere (e.g. breakdown of the blood–aqueous barrier, metastatic neoplasia)
- Ultrasound examination ± other imaging techniques, particularly if the anterior chamber is opaque
- Laboratory examination may be useful (e.g. plasma lipid and lipoprotein profile)
- Direct sampling can be helpful, but the techniques of obtaining the material and interpretation of the samples require skill

Differential diagnosis of a 'white' anterior chamber
- Hypopyon
- Neoplastic cells
- Chylomicronaemia

GLAUCOMAS

Glaucoma is a consequence of an abnormally high and usually sustained increase of intraocular pressure (IOP). The increase is sufficient to damage the eye and vision and the underlying abnormality is invariably defective aqueous drainage. It is increasingly recognised that many of the damaging effects are a consequence of ischaemia and subsequent necrosis. Glaucoma is a challenging condition that may result in acute vision loss and severe pain and the prognosis, even in specialist hands, is usually guarded.

There are a number of causes and it is better to consider the glaucomas as a group, rather than a specific condition. These cases often constitute complex ocular emergencies, so it is crucial to be able to recognise the acute clinical signs. Unless there are facilities for accurate monitoring of intraocular pressure and assessment of the iridocorneal angle, all acute glaucoma cases should be referred as a matter of urgency.

CANINE GLAUCOMA

Clinical features of acute glaucoma (Figure 2.24, p. 58)
- Pain (usually very head shy), blepharospasm and increased lacrimation*
- Globe is of normal size but feels very tense*
- Episcleral congestion (vessels run at right angles to the limbus)*
- Redness may not be confined to episcleral vessels alone, may also have distended conjunctival vessels. A 'brush border' of corneal vessels may also be apparent at a relatively early stage
- Corneal oedema (steamy, bluish cornea) especially if the IOP is greater than 45–50 mm Hg*
- Unresponsive, mid-dilated to dilated pupil (because of oculomotor nerve neuropraxia)*
- Vision loss in affected eye (inability to negotiate a maze, absence of tracking response, loss of consensual pupillary light reflex, loss of dazzle reflex, loss of menace response)
- Lens luxation may also be present

Confirmation of glaucoma
- The breed of dog is often highly relevant (see below)
- Tonometry – the intraocular pressure of both eyes should be measured. Normal IOP in the dog is 10–25 mm Hg. IOP, in canine cases with acute angle closure glaucoma, regularly exceeds 50 mm Hg
- Gonioscopy – examination of the drainage angle of both eyes with a goniolens to assess the state of the iridocorneal angle

Clinical features of chronic glaucoma (Figure 3.51(a–c))
- Blindness and persistent pain
- Globe usually permanently enlarged because of stretching of the ocular coats – this happens more readily in young animals than adults*

* Readily identifiable key features

- Corneal vascularisation (deep brush border peripheral vessels advance axially with chronicity)*
- Thinning of Descemet's membrane (Haab's striae or Descemet's streaks) – grey lines, rather like a snail track crossing the cornea
- Corneal ulceration because of exposure keratopathy and inadequate blink
- Equatorial staphyloma – scleral thinning, of dark blue colour, posterior to the limbus
- Iris atrophy – iris can be readily transilluminated
- Cataract
- Lens subluxation or luxation (but note that this may also be a primary event – see below)
- Increased tapetal reflectivity, attenuation of retinal blood vessels, retinal and optic atrophy, loss of vision
- Cupping of the optic disc, the *lamina cribrosa* is a weak region of the sclera
- Intraocular haemorrhage, which may be recurrent
- *Phthisis bulbi* is much less common than globe enlargement, but may supervene in some chronic cases

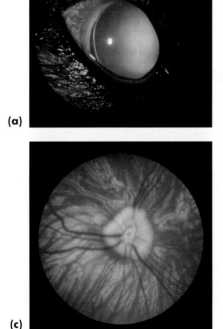

(a)

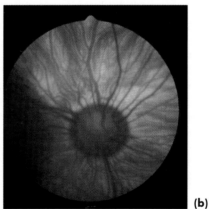

(b)

(c)

Figure 3.51(a–c) Chronic glaucoma. The eye is painful and red, the pupil widely dilated and the globe slightly enlarged. Characteristic Haab's striae (thinning of Descemet's membrane) are present and the lens has become subluxated (a). Fundus examination indicates cupping of the optic nerve head (b) and the change of optic nerve head shape is very obvious when this eye is compared with the fellow, unaffected eye (c).

* Readily identifiable key features

GENERAL AND CANINE
OPHTHALMOLOGY

PRIMARY GLAUCOMA

In this type of glaucoma there is no other recognised antecedent ocular disease process, and primary glaucoma is thought to be hereditary. It is invariably a bilateral condition, although the two eyes are not usually affected simultaneously. There are two forms: that associated with goniodysgenesis (abnormal drainage angle development) and open angle. For an up-to-date list of affected breeds see *In Practice Supplement on Hereditary Eye Disease*.

Goniodysgenesis

This is the commonest cause of primary glaucoma in dogs in the UK. It most commonly involves the drainage angle only, but more complex presentations are infrequently encountered in some types of anterior-segment dysgenesis. Affected breeds include the Basset Hound, Bouvier des Flandres, Great Dane, Samoyed, Siberian Husky, spaniels (English and American Cocker, English and Welsh Springer) retrievers (Flatcoated, Golden and Labrador) and terriers (Dandie Dinmont and Welsh).

'Open-angle' glaucoma

This is the type seen in the Norwegian Elkhound and possibly other breeds, including the Miniature and Toy Poodle in the UK. In the USA it has also been well documented in a laboratory strain of Beagle. It is rare, but may be under-diagnosed.

Management of primary glaucoma

- Seek immediate referral to a specialist centre
- Both surgical and medical treatment may be needed (see Management of Glaucoma, this section, pp 150–151).
- Long term management may include prophylactic treatment of the second eye before any clinical signs of raised IOP are present

SECONDARY GLAUCOMA

Abnormal elevation of IOP associated with recognisable antecedent, or concurrent, eye disease. May be unilateral. Some types, notably primary lens luxation, are breed-associated, others are not.

Lens-associated

Lens-induced uveitis

Lens-induced uveitis with secondary glaucoma usually occurs because of a penetrating injury to the lens and consequent release of lens protein (phacoclastic uveitis).

Primary lens luxation (PLL)

Primary lens luxation is the commonest cause of secondary glaucoma in the dog. The lens may also luxate as a complication of other types of glaucoma, so advice should be sought if unsure.

- Terrier breeds are susceptible to primary lens luxation (Jack Russell Terrier, Wire and Smooth Fox Terrier, Sealyham Terrier, Tibetan Terrier, Miniature Bull Terrier

for example). PLL has also been recorded in the Border Collie, in which it is uncommon. The Shar Pei is rarely affected
- The condition has been shown to be an autosomal recessive in the Tibetan Terrier and is due to an inherent weakness of the lens zonules (*suspensory ligament*). It is probably inherited in similar fashion in other susceptible breeds and should *always* be considered as a possible diagnosis in young adult terriers (usually 3–6 years) with ocular redness or pain
- The condition is essentially bilateral, although only one eye may be affected at initial presentation
- When the lens has moved anteriorly, or is causing pupil block, secondary glaucoma results and the lens should be removed as a matter of urgency (i.e. as an emergency referral)
- Posterior lens luxations do not necessarily produce glaucoma and surgery in such cases can be delayed, because lens removal in this position is technically difficult and may not be necessary unless the lens moves
- The majority of luxated lenses move anteriorly with time

Clinical signs of lens luxation (Figure 2.25, p. 59)
- Glaucoma in most cases, therefore usual clinical signs with pain, photophobia, blepharospasm, lacrimation, redness and dilated unresponsive pupil*
- Greyish strands of prolapsed vitreous may be apparent in pupillary aperture
- The lens is not in its normal position. Look for signs such as instability of the lens (*phacodenesis*), abnormal location of the lens, aphakic crescent, refractile ring at lens equator*
- Localised corneal oedema if the lens is contacting the cornea, more extensive corneal oedema if the intraocular pressure exceeds 40–50 mm Hg*
- Trembling of the iris (*iridodenesis*) is pathognomonic; it occurs because the iris has lost the support of the lens*
- May appear to be a unilateral problem, but early signs (e.g. vitreous prolapse or lens subluxation) or actual lens luxation may be present in the other eye, so always look carefully at *both* eyes

Inflammatory
- Following uveitis (a result of, for example, pre-iridal fibrovascular membrane formation; inflammatory debris, fibrin or haemorrhage in the filtration angle or trabecular meshwork; iris swelling)
- Adhesions may be in the form of posterior synechiae (iris to lens), if they ring the entire circumference iris bombé is present
- Adhesions may be peripheral anterior synechiae (iris base to corneoscleral tissue), usually because of pre-iridal fibrovascular membranes
- Anterior synechiae (iris to cornea) are not usually extensive enough to produce secondary glaucoma
- Secondary glaucoma associated with uveitis and multiple iridociliary cysts is an unusual problem in the Golden Retriever and Great Dane

* Readily identifiable key features;

Neoplastic
- Variety of primary intraocular tumours (most commonly melanoma). Metastases from primary tumour elsewhere (most commonly mammary adenocarcinoma)
- Glaucoma is a consequence of fibrovascular membrane formation, blood–aqueous barrier breakdown, inflammatory material and solid tumour or tumour cells obstructing the drainage angle

Traumatic
- Blunt, non-penetrating trauma may result in extensive hyphaema, complicated by glaucoma
- Penetrating trauma may result in glaucoma as a complication of inflammation associated with the injury and the disruption of the normal intraocular relationships

Haemorrhagic
Extensive haemorrhage may compromise the drainage angle with subsequent glaucoma. Note, however, that recurrent haemorrhage may itself be a feature of chronic glaucoma.

Pigment-associated
The Cairn Terrier and occasionally other breeds of dog (e.g. Labrador Retriever, Boxer) are subject to a form of abnormal pigment deposition, termed *diffuse ocular melanosis*, in middle-aged and older dogs. Glaucoma may develop when accumulated pigment-filled epithelioid cells, presumed to be melanocytes, block the drainage angle.

Diagnosis of secondary glaucoma
Breed, history, aetiology and clinical signs

Management of secondary glaucoma
- Seek early expert advice as to initial treatment and subsequent management. All cases will require referral for initial assessment if the practice lacks facilities for accurate measurement of intraocular pressure. The majority of cases will require early referral if there is a possibility of restoring and retaining vision
- The underlying cause must be identified and, whenever possible, treated
- Surgical and medical options are available, often a combination of both is needed

MANAGEMENT OF GLAUCOMA

Summary of surgical techniques available for glaucoma management
- Aqueous outflow can be increased by means of bypass procedures that provide an alternative aqueous outflow pathway. Bypass can be achieved with or without the aid of drainage implants; medium to long-term results are better if implants are used.
- Patients with primary lens luxation invariably require surgery to remove the luxated lens by intracapsular extraction. When the lens is subluxated, phacoemulsification may be the treatment selected for removal of the lens contents
- Patients with lens luxation secondary to primary glaucoma rarely benefit from lens

removal, as the eye is often blind and enlarged by the time the lens luxates. Enucleation is the preferred option for permanently blind and painful eyes with this pathogenesis
- Aqueous production can be reduced using laser cyclophotocoagulation or cyclocryotherapy. The former technique tends to be used in sighted eyes and the latter in blind eyes as an alternative to enucleation
- For end-stage glaucoma where eyes are painful and permanently blind, irrespective of whether they are enlarged or not, enucleation is the most simple and effective choice

Medical management of acute glaucoma
Osmotic agents
- Mannitol 20% is usually used as an emergency therapy to reduce IOP rapidly in acute glaucoma and also during surgical intraocular procedures
- Mannitol is administered intravenously at a dose rate of 1–2 g/kg over 20–30 minutes, and will produce ocular hypotension within minutes
- When used prior to intraocular surgery, mannitol should be used some 30–60 minutes prior to surgery for maximum effect. Repeat in six hours if necessary
- State of hydration should be monitored, particularly in small dogs, and considerable caution should be exercised if there is pre-existing renal disease

Carbonic anhydrase inhibitors
- Usually used as part of long-term management
- Topical carbonic anhydrase inhibitors (dorzolamide and brinzolamide) work well for moderate increases of IOP
- There appear to be no systemic side effects, which represents a considerable advance on previous treatments
- For dorzolamide, one drop three to four times daily is required for 24-hour control and, for brinzolamide, one drop two to four times daily in the same time period

Prostaglandin analogues
- These drugs increase uveoscleral outflow, but should be used with caution when there is a possibility of uveitis
- The best known is latanoprost, which is expensive, but it is used only once or twice daily. Travaprost is an alternative choice used at the same application rate
- They may be used in conjunction with topical carbonic anhydrase inhibitors and are usually reserved for the more severe cases of glaucoma
- Both agents are very effective at lowering the IOP, albeit with intense pupil constriction as a side effect of treatment in dogs

LENS

EMBRYOLOGY

The lens develops from surface ectoderm, and four distinct stages are apparent:
1 Formation of the lens placode
2 Formation of the lens vesicle

3 Formation of the primary lens fibres
4 Formation of the secondary lens fibres

Primitive vascular supply

- The hyaloid system (HA) extends from the developing retina to the posterior aspect of the lens where it divides into a capillary network that invests the lens, known as the *tunica vasculosa lentis* (TVL)
- The posterior part of the vascular system disappears some 2–3 weeks after birth, whereas the anterior part of the system has degenerated by 3–4 weeks after birth. For most of the animal's life, therefore, the lens is avascular
- Any parts of the primitive vascular system remaining *in situ* eight weeks after birth will persist for life

FEATURES OF THE LENS

- Biconvex structure made up of lens fibres, contained within an elastic capsule. In the adult lens there is a single layer of epithelial cells beneath the anterior lens capsule
- The lens grows throughout life by the production of lens fibres from epithelial cells in the equatorial region. The epithelial cells turn inward and elongate to become secondary lens fibres. Old fibres are compressed centrally into a solid nucleus while younger ones form a softer cortex
- Avascular, but metabolically active
- Naturally-occurring lens tumours are unrecognised in the dog
- Consists of approximately 65% water and 35% protein. Soluble proteins (*crystallins*) predominate with lesser quantities of insoluble *albuminoids*. The insoluble proteins increase as the lens ages, with concomitant decrease in the soluble proteins

EXAMINATION

- In the normal animal, pen light and slit lamp examination of the lens following topical application of one drop of mydriatic (tropicamide) will reveal details of the anterior and posterior lens sutures, the corticonuclear junction and Mittendorf's dot. Mittendorf's dot is located the posterior lens capsule, beneath and between the ventral suture lines, which marks the original attachment of the hyaloid artery.
- In older animals, *nuclear sclerosis*, a normal feature of ageing that affects the lens nucleus, is apparent (Figures 3.52(a,b) and 3.53). The lens appears grey on naked eye examination and with distant direct ophthalmoscopy refractive rings at the nuclearcortical interface can be delineated clearly. Senile nuclear sclerosis should be differentiated from the true opacities of *cataract* in which lens opacities appear as black silhouettes with distant direct ophthalmoscopy.

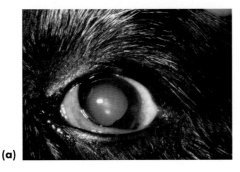
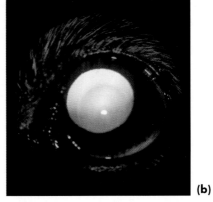

(a)

(b)

Figure 3.52(a,b) Senile nuclear sclerosis in an aged Collie Cross. Gross appearance (a) and appearance with distant direct ophthalmoscopy (b). The distinction of the nuclearcortical interface and the lack of any true opacity are particularly clear with the latter technique. Note that benign melanosis of the iris is also present.

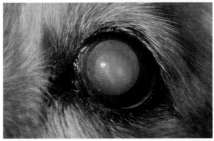

Figure 3.53 Senile nuclear sclerosis of the lens and equatorial cataract (peripheral vacuoles) in an old Miniature Long-Haired Dachshund.

CATARACT

Cataract is defined as any opacity of the lens and/or the lens capsule and is a common problem in the dog.

Classification (applies to all species)
- Time of onset (e.g. congenital, juvenile, senile)
- Location (e.g. capsular, subcapsular, equatorial, cortical, nuclear, axial, polar)
- Degree of maturation (e.g. incipient, immature, mature, hypermature, Morgagnian)
- Aetiology (e.g. primary and secondary inherited, traumatic, metabolic, nutritional, toxic, radiation-induced, electrocution, complicated). Complicated cataracts accompany or follow other ocular disease, such as neoplasia, or inflammations, such as uveitis

Developmental canine cataract
Developmental cataracts are almost certainly congenital (i.e. present from birth) but they will only be apparent when the eyelids open after birth. They may be inherited,

or more commonly, non-inherited (as a reaction to intrauterine influences, e.g. teratogens).

Clinical findings
Can occur at any stage of lens formation, be unilateral or bilateral and may or may not be associated with other ocular anomalies (e.g. microphthalmos, nystagmus, persistent pupillary membrane, iris abnormalities, persistent hyperplastic primary vitreous, retinal dysplasia).

Inherited canine cataract
Primary
Primary inherited cataract is associated with no other ocular abnormality and is a relatively common cause of canine cataract; both congenital and acquired types are recognised (Figure 3.54). For an up-to-date list of affected breeds see *In Practice Supplement on Hereditary Eye Disease.*

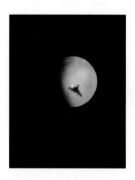

Figure 3.54 Primary inherited cataract in a Golden Retriever. Posterior polar subcapsular cataract is a common type of inherited cataract in a number of breeds. The photograph approximates to the view obtained with distant direct ophthalmoscopy and the cataract appears as a black silhouette (compare this appearance with that in Figure 3.52(b)).

Secondary
Secondary inherited cataract is associated with other ocular abnormality, for example, generalised progressive retinal atrophy, retinal dysplasia, persistent pupillary membrane, persistent hyperplastic primary vitreous and multiple ocular defects. The luxated lens of animals with primary lens luxation can also become secondarily cataractous.

Acquired cataract
- *Traumatic:* blunt and penetrating injuries
- *Metabolic:* e.g. diabetes mellitus is a common cause of rapid-onset total bilateral cataract
- *Nutritional:* e.g. hand rearing on milk substitutes
- *Toxic:* e.g. drug-induced and teratogenic
- *Radiation and electrocution*
- *Complicated:* e.g. following severe ocular inflammation

Management of cataracts
Potential cataract patients should be referred as early as possible in order to allow accurate assessment and simplify the surgery.

- Cataract surgery is the *only* means of treatment at present and is a specialist procedure
- It is wise to refer cataract cases early for specialist assessment (e.g. fundus examination, diagnostic imaging, electroretinography). Hypermature cataracts, for example, are not ideal for surgery as the leakage of lens protein produces low-grade uveitis (Figure 3.47, p. 137)
- Diabetic cataracts can rapidly become hypermature, therefore affected patients should be referred as early as possible, provided their diabetes is under effective control
- Certain types of cataract are likely to be unsuitable for surgery. For example, cataracts secondary to other inherited eye diseases such as generalised progressive retinal atrophy (GPRA), post-traumatic cataracts and some types of cataract secondary to, or associated with, uveitis
- Prior to referral, the patient should be examined carefully, especially for other adnexal and ocular abnormalities (e.g. eyelid infections, eyelid tumours, distichiasis, KCS, uveitis, GPRA) and for systemic disease (e.g. diabetes mellitus)
- Cataract surgery is an elective procedure, so the patient can be prepared thoroughly
- The patient should be of good temperament and easily handled
- The age of the patient is not a contraindication

VITREOUS

Embryologically, development of the vitreous occurs in three stages:
1 The *primary vitreous* forms initially, mainly as a primitive mesodermal vascular hyaloid system, which gradually disappears as the eye matures
2 The *secondary vitreous* forms the definitive adult vitreous
3 The *tertiary vitreous* forms the lens zonule
In the normal adult eye, Cloquet's canal is all that remains of the primary vitreous.

The vitreous fills the posterior cavity of the eye; it is a transparent, semi-fluid hydrogel which is almost 99% water. Collagen fibrils make up the framework of the vitreous and the collagen content varies between species. Hyaluronic acid interacts with the collagen network, both to stabilise the system and to produce a type of molecular sieve. This means that the normal vitreous excludes large molecules and impedes others.

CONGENITAL ANOMALIES OF THE CANINE VITREOUS

Persistent primary vitreous
Anterior remnants
- Persistent hyaloid remnants, sometimes with a network of branching ghost vessels, are normal findings in puppies of a few weeks of age. Hyaloid remnants may not be obvious without a slit lamp.
- A small spiral tag, or a focal lens opacity (Mittendorf's dot), inferonasal to the confluence of the posterior suture lines, is usually all that is apparent in adults. These remnants may not be apparent without a slit lamp.

- Persistence of an extensive hyaloid system in the adult is abnormal and may be associated with congenital posterior capsular cataracts.

Posterior remnants

The posterior part of the hyaloid artery may persist, usually extending from the central optic disc into the posterior vitreous within Cloquet's canal. It may or may not contain blood.

Persistent hyperplastic primary vitreous (PHPV)

- In this condition there is failure of regression of the foetal vasculature and fibroblastic hyperplasia of mesodermal tissue within the posterior vascular tunic of the lens. The result is a plaque of fibrovascular tissue on the posterior surface of the lens, with an attached hyaloid stalk, presenting as *leukocoria* (a white pupil) and interfering with vision (Figure 3.55(a,b)).
- Hereditary PHPV has been described in the Dobermann and Staffordshire Bull Terrier. It is pleomorphic in both breeds and usually bilateral. For an up-to-date list of affected breeds see *In Practice Supplement on Hereditary Eye Disease*.

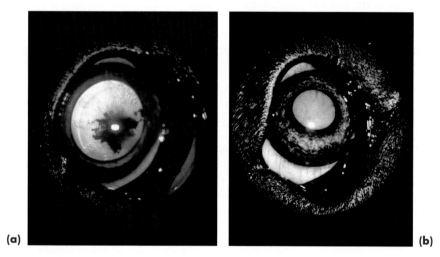

(a)   **(b)**

Figure 3.55 **(a)** Unilateral persistent hyperplastic primary vitreous with intralenticular haemorrhage in an English Mastiff puppy. **(b)** Total cataract developed in the same eye some months later.

Differential diagnosis of leukocoria

Congenital and developmental

- Congenital and early-onset cataract
- Congenital non-attachment and early detachment of the retina
- Persistent hyperplastic primary vitreous and other vitreous abnormalities
- Endophthalmitis

Acquired

- Cataract

- Retinal detachment
- Severe vitritis (active inflammation)
- Endophthalmitis
- Chronic degenerative changes of the vitreous (e.g. asteroid hyalosis – see below)
- Neoplasia

ACQUIRED CONDITIONS OF THE CANINE VITREOUS

Syneresis
Vitreal liquefaction is known as *syneresis*. It is a degenerative process associated with ageing and disease.

Asteroid hyalosis
- Asteroid hyalosis is an occasional finding in dogs with no previous history of ocular or generalised disease. The condition usually affects only one eye, but can affect both, and is more frequently encountered in older animals
- The asteroid bodies are calcium soaps (calcium-lipid) attached to the vitreous fibrillar framework, so that they move with eye movement but return to their original position when the eyes are still
- The opacities usually have little or no effect on vision, and the majority are of no clinical significance

Synchysis scintillans (Figure 3.56)
- This condition is also known as *cholesterolosis bulbi*. The numerous scintillating crystals that are present in the vitreous are indeed cholesterol, but the condition is not associated with systemic dyslipoproteinaemia
- The vitreous is liquefied and the crystals swirl around the vitreous cavity when the eyes move and settle ventrally (inferiorly) when movement stops
- The condition is not uncommon and is seen in association with a variety of ocular insults and diseases (e.g. after intraocular haemorrhage and other inflammatory and degenerative eye conditions)
- There is no obvious effect on vision, the condition is non-progressive and treatment is not required

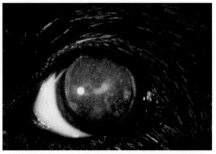

Figure 3.56 Unilateral *synchysis scintillans* in an old Border Collie. This eye had suffered an intraocular haemorrhage some years previously when the dog was kicked by a cow.

Vitreous inflammation

• The vitreous can become secondarily involved in the inflammations of neighbouring tissues, especially as there is no defined barrier between the aqueous humour and vitreous or the vitreous and retina
• Vitreous inflammation (*vitritis*) encompasses a wide range of clinical appearances, from a few scattered inflammatory cells to vitreal abscessation (*endophthalmitis*)

Vitreous haemorrhage

• The clinical appearance varies according to the location and amount. At worst, the whole eye appears red as the haemorrhage also fills the anterior chamber
• Fresh blood is readily identified. In time (over months or years), and providing that no fresh haemorrhage occurs, there is some clearing of the optical pathway and the resorbing blood becomes darker

Summary of the causes of intraocular haemorrhage

• Blunt and penetrating ocular injury
• Congenital intraocular anomalies (e.g. Collie eye anomaly, retinal dysplasia, persistent hyperplastic primary vitreous)
• Neoplasia (e.g. primary tumours such as adenocarcinoma and secondary tumours such as haemangiosarcoma and lymphoma)
• Systemic hypertension
• Clotting disorders and vasculopathies
• Inflammatory eye disease (e.g. uveitis, chorioretinitis)
• Chronic glaucoma
• Toxins and generalised diseases (e.g. sepsis)
• Iatrogenic – as a result of surgery, inappropriate or prolonged drug use (e.g. drugs affecting platelets)

OCULAR FUNDUS

A number of diseases affecting the ocular fundus are inherited or of suspected inheritance. For an up-to-date list of affected breeds see *In Practice Supplement on Hereditary Eye Disease*.

NORMAL GROSS APPEARANCE OF THE FUNDUS (Figures 3.57–3.60)

Tapetum

The ocular fundus is that part of the posterior segment of the eye viewed with an ophthalmoscope, and the normal canine fundus shows many variations in appearance. In most dogs, the fundus is divided into tapetal and non-tapetal areas with the optic nerve head (ONH) or optic disc usually located at the junction between the two. Fundus variations relate to age, breed and size of dog as well as to eye colour and coat colour – the colour variants are related to the amount of pigmentation.

In merle dogs and animals with sub-albinotic eyes, the tapetum is usually absent (*atapetal*) and the lack of pigment in these colour-dilute animals allows details of both retinal and choroidal vessels to be viewed against the creamy white background of the sclera. A number of other breeds are atapetal and the entire fundus has a non-tapetal appearance being dark and non-reflective, although sometimes islets of tapetal tissue are apparent dorsal to the ONH.

When a tapetum is present, it is located in the dorsal half of the fundus and is of almost triangular shape, with the base located ventrally. Tapetal colour can be shades of yellow, orange, green or blue.

In puppies there is no tapetum, but differentiation of the future tapetal and non-tapetal regions is apparent from about four weeks of age onwards, and the fundus is of adult appearance by about four months of age.

The highest cone density is found in the *area centralis*, which is a region devoid of large blood vessels situated lateral and slightly dorsal to the ONH. Rods are the predominant photoreceptors in the canine retina.

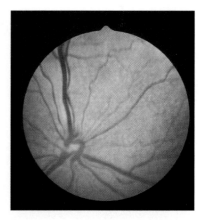

Figure 3.57 Normal Border Collie puppy, six weeks of age (left eye). The eye is still immature and the developing tapetum is of blue-grey colouration; the adult tapetal colour was yellow in this dog. Note that the optic nerve head is round as it is unmyelinated at this stage.

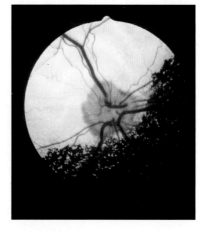

Figure 3.58 Normally pigmented eye of an adult Border Collie ocular fundus. The optic nerve head is located in the tapetal fundus close to the border of the tapetal and non-tapetal fundus. The retinal vasculature is clearly distinguished and there is an incomplete venous circle on the optic nerve head. The optic nerve head is myelinated and the physiological pit can be seen as an obvious dark spot at almost the centre of the optic nerve head.

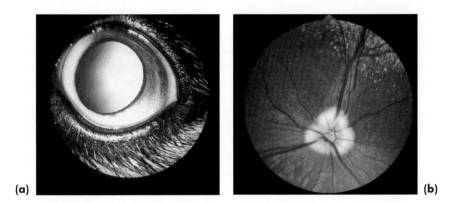

Figure 3.59(a,b)   Partially-pigmented eye in a crossbred dog. The variation of pigmentation of the iris (a) is reflected in the fundus (b).

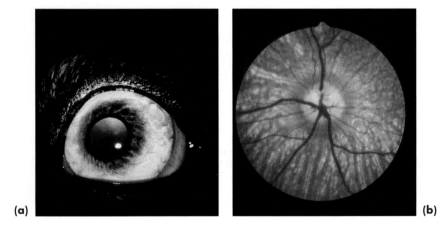

Figure 3.60(a,b)   Subalbinotic eye of a Border Collie. Iris (a) and ocular fundus (b). There is no tapetum and, in addition to the superficial retinal vessels, the underlying choroidal vessels are clearly visible.

Optic nerve head (ONH)

The ONH is approximately circular in puppies, but postnatal myelination produces a change of shape, so that most of the variations seen in adult dogs are related to the degree of postnatal myelination. Excessive myelination is referred to as *pseudopapilloedema* and is most likely to be observed in the Golden Retriever and German Shepherd Dog. A small round depression, the physiological pit, is usually apparent in the centre of the ONH and represents the origin of the hyaloid vasculature. A rim of pigment may surround the ONH in some animals and in those dogs with a small ONH a distinct reflective surround, known as *conus*, is a normal variant.

Blood vasculature

The dog has a holangiotic retinal blood supply. There are usually some 3–4 primary retinal veins and satellite arterioles located on the retinal surface. It is possible to distinguish these vessels as the arterioles are of smaller diameter and lighter colour than the veins. Smaller vessels cannot be so readily distinguished.

The arterioles, some 15–20 in number, radiate peripherally from their peripapillary origin, whereas veins and venules can be traced to a complete, or incomplete, venous circle on the surface of the ONH. Choroidal vessels (predominantly choroidal arterioles), perforating the tapetum to supply the retina, may be viewed against the tapetal background as fine dots ('stars of Winslow'). In colour-dilute dogs in which the fundus lacks pigment and there is no tapetum, the choroidal vessels can be seen radiating from the ONH in an organised spoke-like fashion.

NORMAL HISTOLOGY OF THE RETINA

The *retina* has ten layers: the outermost layer, the retinal pigment epithelium, which lies next to the choroid, is derived from the outer layer of the optic cup (ectoderm) whereas the remaining nine layers, the neurosensory retina, develop from the inner layer of the optic cup (also ectoderm). The pigment epithelium is pigmented except over the tapetum, as is the case in all animals with a tapetal fundus.

Retinal layers

1 Retinal pigment epithelium (RPE)
2 Photoreceptors (rods and cones)
3 External limiting layer
4 Outer nuclear layer
5 Outer plexiform layer
6 Inner nuclear layer
7 Inner plexiform layer
8 Ganglion cell layer
9 Optic nerve fibre layer
10 Internal limiting layer

1 = retinal pigment epithelium
2–10 = neurosensory retina

DEVELOPMENTAL CONDITIONS OF THE CANINE RETINA AND CHOROID

Collie eye anomaly (CEA) (Figs. 3.60 and 3.61)

- Inherited congenital condition.
- The key feature of choroidal hypoplasia is inherited as a single autosomal recessive trait
- Affects the Rough Collie, Smooth Collie, Shetland Sheepdog, Border Collie and Lancashire Heeler. The incidence in the first three breeds is very high (Figures 3.61 and 3.62(a,b))

GENERAL AND CANINE
OPHTHALMOLOGY

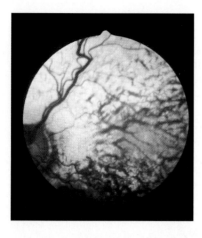

Figure 3.61 Collie eye anomaly in a six-week-old Border Collie puppy (left eye). The choroidal hypoplasia forms a very obvious 'pale patch' lateral to the optic nerve head.

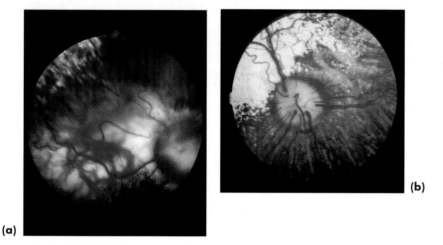

(a)

(b)

Figure 3.62 **(a)** Collie eye anomaly in a Rough Collie. In the right eye there is a large papillary colobomatous defect and an extensive area of choroidal hypoplasia ('pale patch') adjoining it. **(b)** In the left eye there is also choroidal hypoplasia lateral to the optic nerve head and a small peripapillary coloboma ventrally.

Clinical signs

- The condition is almost always bilateral and the two eyes are usually dissimilar.
- Easiest to diagnose in 5–6 week-old puppies; the tapetum has not developed in puppies of this age and so choroidal hypoplasia is more obvious. It is important to stress the value of examination of 5–6 week-old puppies, for later development of the fundus may obscure the mild lesion and lead to the erroneous supposition that the animal is genotypically and phenotypically normal, whereas it is, in fact, only phenotypically normal. The inappropriate designation of 'go normal' has been applied to dogs of this type.
- Most dogs show no obvious visual disability, but some animals (<10%) are

obviously visually impaired or blind, usually because of intraocular haemorrhage or retinal detachment.

- The classical feature of CEA is a 'pale patch' of choroidal hypoplasia ± retinal and scleral involvement. The extent of the hypoplasia is variable, but, irrespective of size, always involves an area lateral to the optic disc. The retinal vessels may be of bizarre appearance (excessive tortuosity, preretinal vessels) and any visible choroidal vessels in the affected areas are abnormal.
- Colobomas, if present, are located in or near the optic nerve head. They may be the only observable abnormality when postnatal development has obscured minor areas of choroidal hypoplasia.
- Intraocular haemorrhage and retinal detachment are the major reasons for visual impairment and blindness. Fortunately, they are an uncommon complication.

Treatment
There is no treatment for CEA, so advice to breeders is crucial.

Retinal dysplasia (RD)
- Retinal dysplasia may be inherited and there are two types: total and multifocal (focal and geographic lesions)
- Breeds affected by *total retinal dysplasia* (TRD) in the UK include the English Springer Spaniel, Labrador Retriever, Bedlington and Sealyham Terrier (Figure 3.63(a,b))
- *Multifocal retinal dysplasia* (MRD) in the UK is most commonly seen in Spaniel breeds (American Cocker, Cavalier King Charles and English Springer), Hungarian Puli, Golden and Labrador Retrievers and is inherited as an autosomal recessive trait in the breeds that have been studied (Figure 3.64)
- *Geographic retinal dysplasia* in the UK is most likely to be encountered in the Cavalier King Charles Spaniel, Golden Retriever and Labrador Retriever (Figure 3.65)
- Retinal dysplasia can also be non-inherited, and is either present from birth or induced in early perinatal life by, for example, infection, irradiation, intrauterine trauma, drugs and toxins

Clinical signs
- The clinical signs of retinal dysplasia (RD) are variable and may alter (remodelling)
- Total retinal dyplasia (TRD) is associated with congenital non-attachment and infundibular detachment of the retina, and affected animals are blind at an early age
- In animals with multifocal retinal dysplasia (MRD), both focal and geographic, vision is not usually affected, but haemorrhage is occasionally observed from abnormal retinal vessels in dogs with the geographic type. Multifocal lesions should be differentiated from inactive post-inflammatory chorioretinopathy lesions

Treatment
There is no treatment for RD, but advice to breeders and litter screening is important for the inherited types.

GENERAL AND CANINE OPHTHALMOLOGY

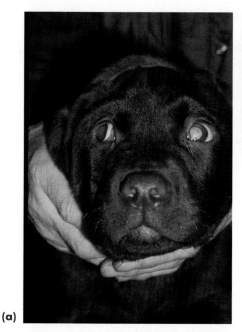

(a)

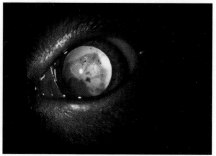

(b)

Figure 3.63(a,b) Total retinal dysplasia in a Labrador Retriever puppy. The non-attached retina is obvious behind the lens. Both eyes were involved and the puppy was blind.

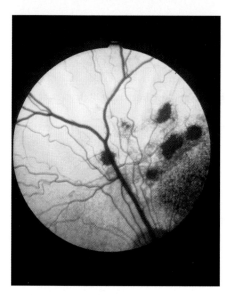

Figure 3.64 Multifocal retinal dysplasia in an English Springer Spaniel with the multifocal type of retinal dysplasia. If it were not for the presence of vermiform lesions, the focal dysplastic areas could easily be confused with inactive chorioretinopathy lesions.

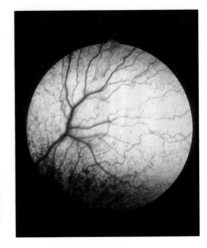

Figure 3.65 Geographic type of multifocal retinal dysplasia. A Cavalier King Charles Spaniel with the geographic type in the typical location some distance dorsal to the optic nerve head and involving the dorsal primary blood vessels.

ACQUIRED CONDITIONS OF THE CANINE RETINA AND CHOROID

Generalised progressive retinal atrophy (GPRA)
- Many different types in this group, e.g. photoreceptor dysplasia (early onset) and photoreceptor degeneration (later onset)
- The breeds most commonly affected in the UK are the English Cocker Spaniel, Miniature Long-haired Dachshund, Miniature and Toy Poodle and Labrador Retriever
- GPRA is inherited as an autosomal recessive trait
- Electroretinography (ERG) is a sensitive method for early diagnosis

Clinical signs and ophthalmoscopic appearance (Figure 3.66)
- The clinical features include progression from night blindness (*nyctalopia*) to day blindness (*hemeralopia*) and eventual total blindness
- Bilateral and symmetrical retinal changes
- Tapetal hyperreflectivity and attenuation of the retinal blood vessels
- Patchy depigmentation of the non-tapetal fundus (NTF)
- The pupillary light response is gradually lost as the condition advances. Also note that it may still be present when no functional vision remains
- Secondary cataracts are common in advanced cases
- Secondary atrophy of the optic nerve can be observed in advanced cases

Treatment
There is no treatment, but prevention by selective breeding is a realistic aim.

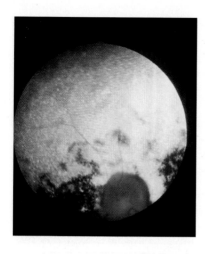

Figure 3.66 Generalised progressive retinal atrophy (progressive rod–cone degeneration) in a Toy Poodle. The fundus changes were bilateral and symmetrical, with attenuation of the retinal vessels, retinal hyperreflectivity and pallor of the optic nerve head.

Retinal pigment epithelial dystrophy (RPED)

- Retinal pigment epithelial dystrophy, originally known as central progressive retinal atrophy (CPRA), is a condition in which the primary defect lies with the retinal pigment epithelium (RPE). Autofluorescent lipopigment (*lipofuscin*) accumulates within the amelanotic RPE of the tapetal fundus.
- This condition has been described in the Briard, collie breeds (Border, Smooth and Rough), Cocker Spaniel, Golden and Labrador Retrievers and Polish Lowland Sheepdog.
- ERG is not helpful as an early diagnostic tool.
- In some of the breeds studied in detail the condition appears to be an example of the inherited lysosomal storage disease ceroid lipofuscinosis.

Clinical signs and ophthalmoscopic appearance (Figure 3.67(a,b))

- Poor vision in bright light or daylight and affected dogs often collide with stationary objects. There is usually a slow and progressive loss of central vision and the changes are bilateral, but not usually symmetrical
- Retinal changes occur from about 14 months of age onwards, but the age at which clinical signs are apparent is quite variable, ranging from 2–6 years of age
- The early ophthalmoscopic features consist of small light-brown spots within the tapetal fundus. Later in the evolution of the condition, the spots increase in number and coalesce (cobweb-like)
- Tapetal hyperreflectivity and attenuation of the retinal vessels are obvious later features
- The pupillary light response may remain normal and is not always lost
- Some dogs retain partial vision, whereas others become blind

Treatment

- Vitamin E deficient diets have produced lesions of similar appearance in experimental animals, and there may be an association between low plasma vitamin E levels and the development of RPED

- Vitamin E has anti-oxidant properties that help to prevent damage from free radicals and may also have a primary role in the maintenance of normal retinal function
- It is possible that vitamin therapy may be of value in the early stages of disease
- There is no treatment for dogs with established fundus changes

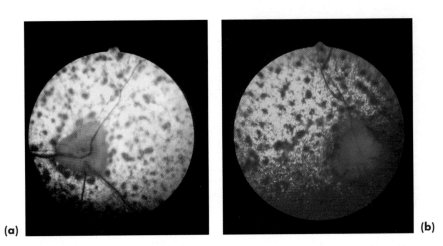

(a)   **(b)**

Figure 3.67(a,b) Retinal pigment epithelial dystrophy in a Cocker Spaniel. The changes were bilateral, but not symmetrical. The right eye has been photographed in white light. The fellow (left) eye has been photographed in blue light to reduce the flashback from the hyperreflective retina.

Sudden acquired retinal degeneration (SARD)

- Sudden onset of blindness with bilateral, dilated, fixed pupils and, initially, no detectable ophthalmoscopic abnormality. Ophthalmoscopically visible retinal degeneration occurs within weeks or months
- Total extinction of the ERG at the outset of blindness is pathognomonic and distinguishes SARD from optic and retrobulbar neuritis and most types of CNS neoplasia
- Essentially an uncommon disease of rather overweight adult dogs, especially female (6–14 years)
- There may be sub-clinical hepatopathy and hyperadrenocorticism
- Affected animals should be subjected to laboratory screen and their blood pressure should be checked – any systemic disease detected can be treated

Management of SARD

No treatment is available at present to restore vision or prevent the retinal changes, but it is important to differentiate SARD from other potential causes of sudden blindness, some of which may be amenable to treatment.

Inflammatory conditions of the fundus

Active

Active fundus inflammation (Figure 3.68) is associated with some or all of vasculitis, perivascular cuffing and poorly defined opacities near blood vessels, pre-retinal exudates, vitritis and optic neuritis. Animals with bilateral optic neuritis are blind. Active inflammation is usually less obvious than inactive and is not observed with anything like the same frequency.

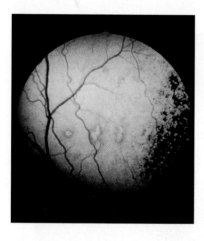

Figure 3.68 Active inflammation of the ocular fundus in a Labrador Retriever with distemper. Multiple focal lesions were present in the tapetal fundus of both eyes and the dog also had neurological signs.

Inactive

Inactive post-inflammatory lesions (Figures 3.69 and 3.70) consist of either focal or diffuse changes in the tapetal and non-tapetal fundus. In the tapetal fundus, there may be sharply-demarcated hyperreflective foci of variable size. Pigment-cell proliferation results in pigment placed centrally in such foci. Disseminated inflammation can produce changes in the whole of the tapetal fundus.

In the non-tapetal fundus, focal and, less commonly, diffuse depigmentation is apparent. The blood vessels crossing affected areas are sometimes tortuous and constricted and perivascular pigment may be present.

Other possible findings include retinal detachment, vitreal changes and optic atrophy. Inactive chorioretinopathies are a common finding in many breeds of dog, especially working Border Collies.

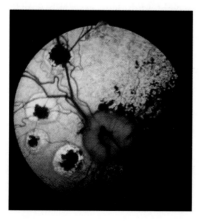

Figure 3.69 Inactive inflammation (focal chorioretinopathy) of the ocular fundus in a Border Collie. There was a history of heavy roundworm infestation (*Toxocara canis*) as a puppy. Only one eye was affected.

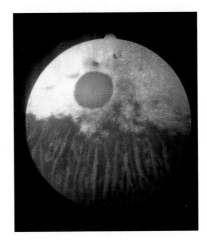

Figure 3.70 Inactive inflammation (diffuse chorioretinopathy) of the ocular fundus in a Border Collie. This is the end stage of severe retinal degeneration, irrespective of the cause. In addition to the panretinal degeneration there is gross vascular attenuation and optic nerve atrophy and the eye is blind.

Aetiology and diagnosis

- Establishing the cause of active fundus inflammation is not always easy
- The causes of fundus inflammation have been summarised under Uveitis (this section, pp 132–135)
- Complete physical examination, blood samples (routine haematology, serum proteins, biochemistry and serology) and specific tests, if available, are best undertaken when the inflammation is active
- Imaging techniques are sometimes helpful if the ocular media are cloudy and if retinal detachment is suspected

Treatment
Depends on finding the cause

Retinal detachment
The embryological intraretinal space remains throughout life, and the neuroretina is only loosely attached to the retinal pigment epithelium, so that the two may separate to produce a retinal detachment. The retina is firmly attached (or inserted) at the *ora ciliaris retinae* and also around the optic nerve head, and the gel-like consistency of the normal vitreous helps to hold the retina in place.

Causes of retinal detachment
Congenital
For example, associated with CEA, RD, PHPV and multiple ocular defects. There is a range of presentations, from congenital non-attachment to detachment.

Traumatic
For example, blunt trauma. Retinal tears may be produced because of the different rates at which the vitreous and the coats of the eye change shape. Retinal tears and holes usually result in a *rhegmatogenous detachment*.

Intraocular problems

For example, the development of fibrous vitreoretinal adhesions following severe inflammation may produce a *traction detachment*. The retina is also more likely to detach in the presence of severe vitreal degeneration and syneresis.

Intraocular and extraocular space-occupying lesions

For example, choroidal tumours and extraocular tumours can push the retina off, resulting in a *solid detachment*.

Systemic problems

Systemic hypertension (primary and secondary) is associated with the accumulation of subretinal fluid, which lifts the retina off. Initially there are bullous detachments and later, without treatment, there is total detachment. Detachments as a consequence of systemic hypertension are examples of *serous* or *exudative detachment* (Figure 3.71). The subretinal fluid has the composition of a transudate initially, but later may become more exudative in nature.

Systemic hypertension is also associated with changes in choroidal and retinal vasculature and retinal haemorrhage. Causes of secondary systemic hypertension include renal disease, hypothyroidism, hyperadrenocorticism, phaeochromocytoma and diabetes mellitus.

Other causes of serous detachment include the uveodermatological syndrome and severe inflammation (e.g. systemic mycoses and parasitic infections such as toxoplasmosis).

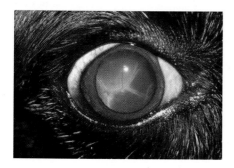

Figure 3.71 Total retinal detachment in a Collie Cross with hyperadrenocorticism and associated systemic hypertensive disease.

Anomalies and abnormalities of retinal vasculature
Developmental

Changes of colour, calibre and tortuosity may be present in the retinal vessels of animals with congenital heart disease and shunts.

Acquired

Anaemia, cyanosis, hyperviscosity, polycythaemia, ocular ischaemia, systemic hypertension, diabetic retinopathy and lipaemia retinalis can *all* be recognised ophthalmoscopically (Figures 3.72(a,b) and 3.73).

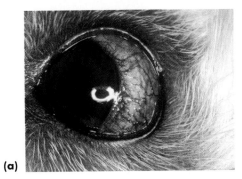

(a)

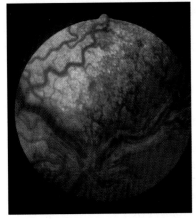

(b)

Figure 3.72(a,b) Hyperviscosity syndrome in a Toy Poodle with the congenital heart disease tetralogy of Fallot. The external eye (a) and fundus (b) are illustrated. The dog was cyanotic and compensatory polycythaemia was the reason for the hyperviscosity.

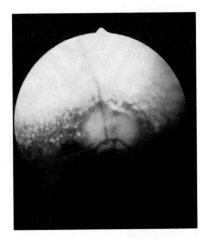

Figure 3.73 Autoimmune haemolytic anaemia in an Old English Sheepdog. Note the extreme pallor of the retinal vessels, giving a spurious impression of attenuation.

Retinal haemorrhage (see vitreous haemorrhage, this section, pp 155–158)

OPTIC NERVE

The shape, size and colour of the canine optic nerve head is variable. The variation can largely be related to the age of the animal and the extent of medullation (i.e. non-myelinated and round in young puppies). The optic nerve head (optic disc, or papilla) is the bulbar portion of the optic nerve. The retrobulbar and cranial portions of the nerve cannot be examined ophthalmoscopically. Congenital anomalies of the optic nerve head are rare and include aplasia, hypoplasia and coloboma.

ACQUIRED ABNORMALITIES OF THE CANINE OPTIC NERVE

Optic neuritis or papillitis (intraocular)

History, ophthalmoscopic signs and diagnosis (Figure 3.74(a,b))

- An uncommon problem which presents as sudden blindness or defective vision. May be unilateral, or bilateral
- Affected eyes are blind during the active inflammation, with an impaired or absent PLR and a fixed dilated pupil
- Optic nerve head appears enlarged and hyperaemic; the normal physiological pit is absent
- Focal haemorrhages may be present within or surrounding the optic nerve head
- Peripapillary retinal oedema or detachment
- May be cellular infiltrates in posterior vitreous
- Normal ERG

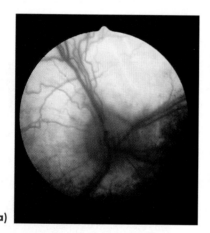 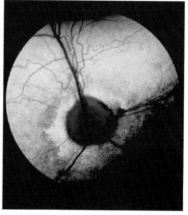

(a)   (b)

Figure 3.74(a,b) Optic neuritis in a Collie Cross with toxoplasmosis. Active stage of inflammation (a) and the same eye after treatment (b). The pathological conus (reflective halo surrounding the optic nerve head) apparent in (b) indicates the extent of the peripapillary oedema during the active phase.

Treatment
See Retrobulbar optic neutritis p. 173.

Aetiology
- Systemic disease, e.g. distemper, toxoplasmosis, leptospirosis
- Local disease, e.g. orbital cellulitis, orbital abscess
- Trauma, e.g. to globe or orbit
- Neoplasia, e.g. retrobulbar neoplasia
- Neurological, e.g. granulomatous meningoencephalitis (GME)
- Toxic and metabolic
- Idiopathic, presumed immune mediated

Retrobulbar optic neuritis (retrobulbar)
Ophthalmoscopic signs
- Uncommon, dilated pupil (unilateral or bilateral) and blindness but the optic nerve head appears normal
- Normal ERG

Differential diagnosis of retrobulbar optic neuritis
- SARD
- Disorders of the central nervous system

Treatment of optic neuritis (both intraocular and extraocular)
- Urgent referral necessary if the diagnosis is in doubt
- Drug treatment for optic neuritis and retrobulbar optic neuritis is the same
- High levels of systemic corticosteroids (usually oral prednisolone at 1–2 mg/kg each 24 hours)
- Rapid response to therapy gives better prognosis than failure to respond, but, for all cases, the prognosis is guarded, as permanent damage occurs rapidly and relapses are common
- Monitor carefully and check for systemic or CNS involvement
- A region of peripapillary hyperreflectivity or even optic atrophy may develop as a sequel to optic neuritis and the animal may recover vision, be partially sighted or blind

Optic nerve neoplasia
- Primary tumours (e.g. glioma, meningioma, astrocytoma) are rare, but an expanding brain tumour may compress the intracranial optic nerve
- Meningioma is the commonest primary tumour and can involve the optic nerve by primary neoplastic transformation of cells within the optic nerve sheath, or secondary extension of intracranial neoplasia
- Infiltration of the optic nerve by tumour cells can also occur, most commonly in animals with lymphoma

Oedema of the optic nerve (papilloedema)
Papilloedema is a *clinical sign*, not a diagnosis, and is usually the result of raised intracranial pressure.

Aetiology
- Congenital or acquired hydrocephalus
- Intracranial and extracranial space-occupying lesions which may be infectious, inflammatory or neoplastic in origin
- Ischaemia (e.g. severe systemic hypertension)

Clinical signs and ophthalmoscopy
- Unusual, affected animals usually have gross neurological signs (e.g. behavioural changes and locomotor problems)
- May be associated with visual disturbance, including vision loss, depending on the aetiology
- Swollen optic nerve head, with an indistinct and elevated margin (Figure 3.75)

- May be venous engorgement and increased tortuosity of the retinal vessels. The retinal vessels may deviate as they cross the margins of the optic nerve head

Differential diagnosis
- Differentiate from optic and retrobulbar neuritis
- Differentiate from pseudopapilloedema, a normal variant as a consequence of marked myelination of the optic nerve head that is common in German Shepherd Dogs and Golden Retrievers
- Vision may be affected and so may the pupillary light response, reflecting the underlying aetiopathology, rather than any specific feature of papilloedema

Treatment
Remove the primary cause, if possible

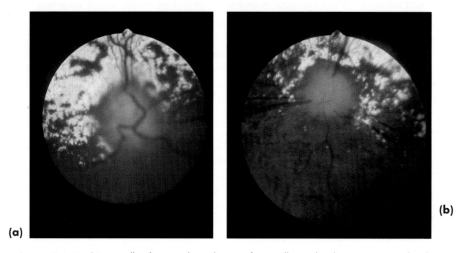

(a)

(b)

Figure 3.75(a,b) Papilloedema in the right eye of a Papillon with a brain tumour in the chiasmal region. Optic atrophy was present in the left eye of the Papillon in Figure 3.75.

Optic nerve atrophy
- The end stage of severe insults such as inflammation, chronic optic nerve oedema and ischaemia (Figures 3.70 and 3.75(b))
- The changes may not develop for some weeks after the initial insult or disease process
- Optic atrophy is quite frequently a complication of eyeball prolapse, so a suitable guarded prognosis should be given in such cases, even when the eye has been replaced rapidly into the orbit

Ophthalmoscopic signs
The optic nerve head usually appears pale and shrunken (loss of myelin results in a round optic nerve head, rather like that of a puppy or cat) and the eye is blind.

Treatment
There is no treatment.

Cranial nerve supply to the eye and adnexa (see Appendix 4)

SECTION 4
FELINE OPHTHALMOLOGY

INTRODUCTION

The cat has a relatively large eye (Figure 4.2(a,b)), which is well adapted to vision in dim light, because of good light-collecting features such as a large cornea and lens, a rod-dominated retina and a *tapetum cellulosum*. The eyes are placed frontally, and about 67% of the optic nerve fibres cross at the optic chiasma, so there is reasonable binocular vision. This compares with a 50% crossover in humans and a 75% crossover in the dog.

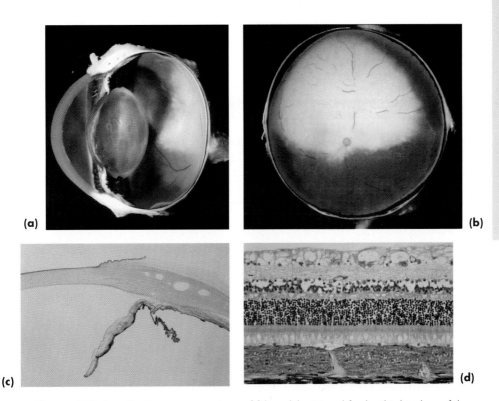

(a)   (b)

(c)   (d)

Figure 4.1(a,b,c,d) Gross cross specimen of feline globe (a) and fundus (b), histology of the cornea, limbus, iris and ciliary body (c), retina and choroid (d) (with acknowledgements to J. R. B. Mould).

FELINE OPHTHALMOLOGY

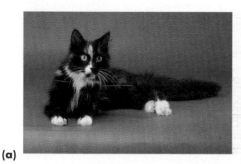

(a)

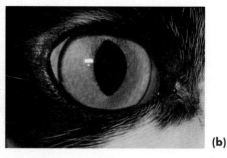

(b)

Figure 4.2(a,b) In the cat illustrated in (a) the eyes were normal and the subtle anisocoria (inequality of pupil size) was of central origin (diffuse inflammation). In (b) a normal external eye is shown.

ANATOMICAL DIFFERENCES FROM THE DOG

- There are no true eyelashes, and modified skin hairs close to the upper eyelid margin serve in this capacity
- The third eyelid has both striated and smooth muscle, so that there is some voluntary control over its movements
- The cornea almost fills the palpebral aperture, the third eyelid is unobtrusive and there is little visible bulbar conjunctiva
- It is possible to view the drainage angle directly without needing to use a goniolens
- The iris is generally less heavily pigmented than that of the dog, and the distinction between the pupillary and ciliary zones is not always clearly defined
- The pupil is round when dilated and a vertical slit when constricted
- The tapetum is larger and more reflective than that of the dog, and the *iridocytes* (tapetal cells) are rich in riboflavin
- The optic nerve head is almost always unmyelinated, so it is round in shape and slightly recessed

The combination of voluntary control over third-eyelid movement, a very effective pupil-constriction mechanism and a reflective tapetum make it essential to examine the cat's eye, and the fundus especially, with as low a light intensity as possible. This is also the case if a mydriatic is used. Subtle fundus lesions will be obscured if the light is too bright because of the mirror-like effect of the tapetum. As emphasised previously, physical and neurological examination may be just as important as ophthalmic examination in determining if the eyes and their adnexa are normal (Figure 4.2a,b).

The common feline ocular and adnexal conditions, and those that are important to recognise because of the serious implications of misdiagnosis, are summarised in Box 4.1.

Box 4.1   Common and important feline ocular and adnexal conditions

- All types of trauma
- Congenital eyelid defects, such as medial lower eyelid entropion (Persian cats) and, less commonly, partial absence in all breeds (*colobomas*)
- Conjunctival problems such as *ophthalmia neonatorum* (including its complications, e.g. *symblepharon*) and conjunctivitis (usually of infectious origin – *Chlamydophila felis* or FHV-1)
- Ulcerative keratitis (including herpetic keratitis), proliferative keratoconjunctivitis and corneal sequestrum
- Uveitis from a variety of causes, especially uveitis of infectious origin – FIP, FeLV, FIV, toxoplasmosis – as well as idiopathic and traumatic
- Neoplasia, notably squamous cell carcinoma (usually eyelids), iris melanoma and the many potential ocular manifestations of lymphoma
- Common generalised problems with ocular manifestations include systemic hypertensive disease and taurine deficiency. Less common, but important to recognise, are dysautonomia, various types of lysosomal storage disease and hyperlipoproteinaemia (hypertriglyceridaemia and chylomicronaemia)

GLOBE AND ORBIT

- As in the dog there is an open orbit, and the supraorbital ligament completes the bony orbital rim laterally
- The globe fits snugly in the orbit, and there is little extraorbital fat

Globe proptosis and prolapse
- Orbital/periorbital trauma may result in orbital haemorrhage, fracture of the bony orbit/zygomatic arch/mandible and *proptosis* (forward displacement of the globe) or *prolapse* (displacement of the globe from the orbit)
- Proptosis may be a complication of orbital haemorrhage, especially when there is damage to the orbital rete
- Globe prolapse is less likely in cats than dogs, as the eye is set quite deeply within the well-defined orbit. Considerable force is required to dislocate the globe from the orbit in most breeds of cat, the Persian cat being an exception
- It is important to check for other injuries, such as facial fractures, particularly involving the lower jaw
- The technique for globe replacement is substantially similar to that in dogs. The prognosis for retention of vision is *very* poor and almost 100% of cats will not retain long-term vision in the affected eye

Enucleation
- The encircling skin incision must be closer to the lids than is necessary in the dog, especially so at the medial canthus, where skin mobility is limited.

- Visualisation of the deep orbit is less easy in cats than dogs, so the optic nerve is clamped blind and it is *most important* to avoid excessive traction on the globe and optic nerve during removal.
- Excessive traction while the optic nerve is intact may cause damage to the other optic nerve via the optic chiasma, so that the fellow eye is blinded at the time of surgery.
- Otherwise the surgery is similar to that in the dog.

Orbital neoplasia
Clinical signs
Some 90% of orbital tumours in cats are *malignant*. Orbital tumours are often of epithelial origin (usually squamous cell carcinoma), or reach the orbit by extension from neighbouring tissues (e.g. from the eye into the orbit, along the optic nerve into the orbit, from the nose into the orbit) (Figure 4.3). Tumours may also reach the orbit as a result of spread (metastasis) from elsewhere (e.g. multicentric lymphoma).

Management
All cases are best referred if there is a prospect of retaining a functional eye, or if the extent (and nature) of the tumour is unclear. Orbital tumours in cats are difficult to manage and the prognosis is usually grave.

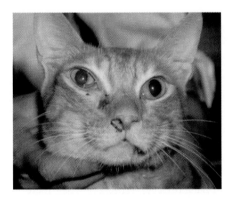

Figure 4.3 Orbital neoplasia in a Domestic Shorthair. There is prominence of the third eyelid and dorsolateral deviation of the right globe. Taken in conjunction with the haemorrhagic discharge from the right nostril, the primary site of the space occupying mass is most likely to be nasal with orbital extension through the medial orbital wall. The tumour was subsequently confirmed as a nasal adenocarcinoma at postmortem examination.

EYELIDS

CONDITIONS OF THE THIRD EYELID (NICTITATING MEMBRANE)

Generalised disease
Dysautonomia
Dysautonomia (an autonomic polygangliopathy) may be associated with unilateral or bilateral third eyelid prominence, although dilated pupils and absence of the pupillary light response are the most constant ocular features.

FELINE OPHTHALMOLOGY

Chronic diarrhoea

Chronic diarrhoea is sometimes associated with a self-limiting, bilateral, third eyelid protrusion. The cause is unknown. Viral disease has been suggested, but never proved. Debility, weight loss and reduction in the amount of retrobulbar fat, do not produce the obvious third eyelid prominence seen in the dog.

Prominence of the third eyelid – summary of causes
- *Anatomical*: e.g. small eye
- *Pain*: produces globe retraction and consequent protrusion of the third eyelid
- *Inflammation and infection*: extensive symblepharon formation may be associated with enophthalmos and third eyelid prominence
- *Systemic and generalised problems*: e.g. tetanus, dysautonomia and chronic diarrhoea
- *Primary and secondary neoplasia*: very rare
- *Retrobulbar space occupying lesions*: e.g. inflammation and orbital neoplasia
- *Horner's syndrome*: third eyelid prominence, together with enophthalmos, narrowing of the palpebral fissure, ptosis and miosis
- *Drug-induced*: e.g. phenothiazine tranquillisers

CONDITIONS OF THE UPPER AND LOWER EYELIDS

Ophthalmia neonatorum
The eyelids of neonatal kittens remain fused for some time after birth (usually 4–12 days). Occasionally, infection behind the closed eyelids results in neonatal conjunctivitis (*ophthalmia neonatorum*), which is invariably caused by feline herpes virus (FHV-1).

Clinical signs and complications
- Swelling behind the closed eyelids often with escape of pus medially (Figure 4.4(a))
- Other signs of FHV-1 infection as, for example, respiratory disease
- The inflammation caused by FHV-1 is severe and may result in symblepharon, occluded lacrimal puncta, keratoconjunctivitis sicca, corneal ulceration, perforation, endophthalmitis and panophthalmitis

Treatment
- The eyelids can be opened with a blunt-tipped probe or blunt-tipped tenotomy scissors as described previously in the dog. The eyelids should be eased open starting in the region of the medial canthus, working from medial to lateral, and carefully cleaning away any purulent material (Figure 4.4(b))
- A short course of topical antibiotic will be required and any ocular discharge should be removed before antibiotic is applied
- Adequate supportive care should be provided
- If the condition is not treated promptly, the severity of the inflammation results in complications (Figure 4.4(c))

FELINE OPHTHALMOLOGY

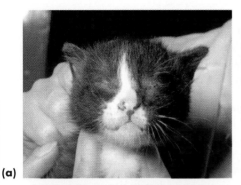 **(a)**

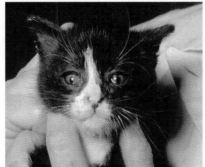 **(b)**

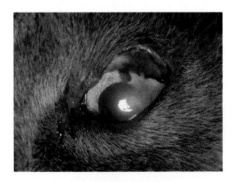 **(c)**

Figure 4.4 (a) *Ophthalmia neonatorum* caused by feline herpesvirus (FHV-1). There was considerable swelling behind the fused eyelids and beads of pus escaped from the medial aspect. This kitten and the others in the litter were systemically ill and had respiratory disease. **(b)** All the kittens received nursing care, their eyelids were opened prematurely and they received topical antibiotic for any secondary bacterial infection. **(c)** Only one kitten had developed complications prior to referral, in the form of globe rupture and secondary endophthalmitis.

Symblepharon (see under Conjunctiva, this section, pp 189–90

Agenesis and coloboma

Complete (*agenesis*) or partial (*coloboma*) absence of the eyelid or eyelids is not uncommon in cats (Figure 4.5).

Figure 4.5 Partial absence of the upper lateral eyelid. This is the usual site of eyelid colobomas in the cat and is sometimes much more subtle, consisting only of a poorly-defined or incomplete eyelid margin. When the defect is large, secondary corneal pathology is inevitable. Corrective blepharoplastic surgery is required.

Management

• Treatment consists of cleaning and ocular lubrication until the animal is old enough for surgery

FELINE OPHTHALMOLOGY

- Repair may be effected by a number of techniques, depending upon the extent of the defect. Cases with large defects that cannot be repaired by primary closure should be referred. In some breeds, such as the Burmese, eyelid defects may be associated with dermoids

Entropion

Entropion is relatively uncommon in cats and is usually a result of chronic inflammation, or of spastic type associated with pain. Persian cats are the exception, as they may have congenital entropion, usually of the lower medial eyelid, which may require corrective surgery (Figure 4.6).

Treatment

- Differentiate spastic entropion from anatomical entropion by applying topical local anaesthetic – spastic entropion disappears, anatomical entropion persists
- Perform surgical correction for anatomical (Hotz-Celsus technique) and cicatricial (Y-to-V technique) types of entropion. Treat the underlying cause for spastic types.

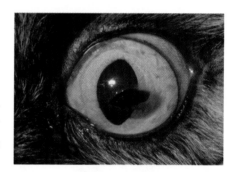

Figure 4.6 Entropion affecting the lower medial eyelid in a Persian Cat. This is the commonest site for anatomical entropion and, in this case, is associated with the formation of a corneal sequestrum.

Meibomianitis

Meibomianitis (Figure 4.7), chronic inflammation of the meibomian glands, can cause inspissation of meibomian lipid and consequent formation of *chalazia* when the glands become overloaded and rupture. The condition is most likely to present as lipogranulomatous conjunctivitis. Cystic glandular changes are also seen occasionally, especially in Persian cats.

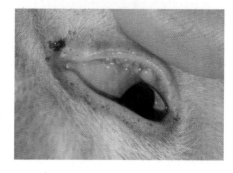

Figure 4.7 Meibomianitis (chronic lipogranulomatous conjunctivitis) in a Domestic Shorthair. Lipid histochemistry of biopsy material indicated large quantities of lipid associated with the meibomian glands.

Treatment
Usually the removal of the inspissated material by curettage after incising the palpebral conjunctiva is curative.

Eyelid neoplasia
Eyelid tumours are uncommon, and histopathology should always be undertaken. *Squamous cell carcinoma* is the most frequently encountered eyelid neoplasm, especially in white cats and those with non-pigmented lids (Figure 4.8). These tumours are often locally invasive, but are also potentially metastatic, so careful examination of the whole animal is mandatory. Animals with extensive eyelid involvement should be referred.

Management
- Squamous cell carcinoma responds to a variety of treatments, including local radiotherapy and surgical excision combined with blepharoplasty. Local radiotherapy on its own can be very effective, as is excision combined with cryosurgery and radiotherapy
- For other eyelid tumours (e.g. *mast cell tumours*) wide-based excision and blepharoplasty is usually the treatment of choice
- All feline eyelid tumours should be submitted for histopathology

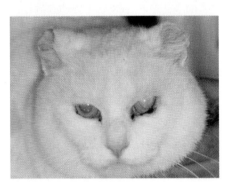

Figure 4.8 Squamous cell carcinoma in a white Domestic Shorthair. Both the lower eyelids are involved and the tips of both ears have already been amputated because of squamous cell carcinoma.

LACRIMAL SYSTEM

- In cats the Schirmer tear test 1 (STT 1) reading is usually lower than in dogs, usually 12 mm ± 5 mm over one minute. In normal cats less than a year of age it may be very low: readings as low as 0 are sometimes obtained.
- Investigative procedures involving nasolacrimal drainage require a general anaesthetic, as the puncta are small and can easily be damaged

THE WET EYE

- The cat is much less frequently affected than the dog
- *Epiphora* (tear overflow) is the commonest presenting sign, and the problems tend

to be resolved into those with increased tear production and those with inadequate tear drainage
- Topically-applied fluorescein 1% does not always appear at the ipsilateral nostril, as the nasolacrimal duct is short and fluorescein may enter the oropharyngeal region and be swallowed
- It may be easier to tilt the head downward and examine the ipsilateral nostril, rather than attempting to identify fluorescein in the oropharyngeal region
- Fluorescein is most readily observed using blue light in the dark

Tear distribution problems
Agenesis and colobomatous eyelid defects are the commonest reason for poor tear film distribution.

Increased tear production
Any painful eye condition may increase tear production. Follicular conjunctivitis may cause sufficient irritation to increase tear production when follicles are prominent on the inner surface of the third eyelid. Very rarely, increased production can be caused by inflammation of the lacrimal or nictitans gland.

Inadequate tear drainage
Congenital problems
- Absence or atresia of the lacrimal puncta; the upper and/or lower punctum is affected and other eyelid anomalies may also be present
- Anatomical imperfection is a possible cause of tear-drainage problems. Flat-faced cats such as the Persian are often severely affected (combination of shallow orbit, prominent globe, shallow lacrimal lake and occlusion of the nasolacrimal duct associated with brachycephalic conformation). Anatomical imperfection may also result from trauma or surgery

Acquired problems
- Loss of punctum ± canaliculus through destruction as a result of inflammation or previous surgery. Punctal occlusion in cats with symblepharon formation is reasonably common, but is not readily amenable to surgery, as adhesions reform
- Blockage of any part of the nasolacrimal system occurs because of problems within the system (e.g. foreign bodies, dacryocystitis), or external influences, such as nasal and tooth-root problems, space occupying lesions and trauma

THE DRY EYE – UNDERPRODUCTION AND ABNORMALITIES OF TEARS

The feline tear film has received little study to date, and it is assumed that, as in the dog, the commonest clinical problem is a lack of aqueous production resulting in keratoconjunctivitis sicca (KCS).

Keratoconjunctivitis sicca
Clinical signs and aetiology
- Disruption of the corneal reflex and lacklustre appearance of cornea, superficial

vascular keratitis, xerosis (corneal desiccation), recurrent ulceration and diffuse conjunctivitis may all be seen (Figure 4.9)
- In most cases there is a tenacious ocular discharge, but this is less conspicuous in cats than dogs, especially in the early stages
- STT 1 values <5 mm/min, but remember that values are generally lower than those of dogs
- Feline herpes virus-1 (FHV-1), symblepharon formation and dysautonomia should be ruled out

Treatment
- Tear replacement therapy in most cases
- Parotid duct transposition is rarely used, but is a useful surgical alternative in selected cases

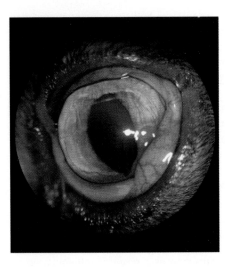

Figure 4.9 Keratoconjunctivitis sicca in a Domestic Shorthair. The cornea is of slightly lacklustre appearance and the camera flash is disrupted. A tacky ocular discharge and chemosis are present. The condition was unilateral and the cause unknown.

CONJUNCTIVA

In the normal cat there is very little exposed conjunctiva. It is usually confined to part of the nictitating conjunctiva and a small area of bulbar conjunctiva visible at the lateral canthus.

DISEASES OF THE CONJUNCTIVA

Epibulbar dermoid
Epibulbar dermoids may be the result of incomplete fusion of the eyelids, with displacement of skin elements into the dermoid. In cats they are usually located on the skin or conjunctiva in the region of the lateral canthus, but they may be found at other sites, and corneal involvement is also encountered. Certain lines of Birman cats show a genetic predisposition, and combined eyelid defects and dermoids in the Burmese cat may also be inherited.

Treatment
Surgical excision, as described previously for the dog (Section 3, pp 101–105).

Symblepharon

Conjunctival adhesion of the palpebral, bulbar or nictitating conjunctiva, to each other or to the cornea, is termed *symblepharon* and, whilst very rare in dogs, it is extremely common in cats (Figure 4.10). Symblepharon is most frequent following neonatal infection, particularly that caused by feline herpes virus. Less commonly, severe conjunctival inflammation, chemical and thermal injuries can cause this problem at any age.

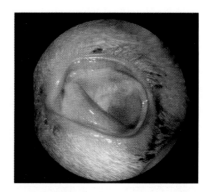

Figure 4.10 Symblepharon formation in a young Siamese cat. The adhesions are extensive and have obliterated the dorsal and ventral fornices as well as occluding the upper and lower puncta. Note the 'conjunctivalisation' of the cornea as a consequence of destruction of the limbal stem cells during the acute phase of inflammation. The cat had suffered from severe conjunctivitis (presumed FHV-1) as a kitten and both eyes were affected.

Clinical features
• The adhesions are usually between the upper and lower eyelids and third eyelid, upper and lower eyelids and bulbar conjunctiva ± cornea (i.e. all the epithelium-covered tissues of the ocular surface)
• The fornix is often obliterated, so the nasolacrimal puncta may also be non-functional and tear production may also be affected because of occlusion of lacrimal gland ductules
• Symblepharon is usually seen as a distinct entity, but may also occur in conjunction with other ocular defects such as microphthalmos

Treatment
• Surgical section of the symblepharon is simple, but the adhesions usually reform rapidly and corneal opacities may be more marked than they were originally. These disappointing results reflect the pathogenesis, notably the destruction of limbal stem cells at the time of acute inflammation. In consequence, corneal epithelium cannot be generated for repair and conjunctival epithelium resurfaces the cornea, causing 'conjunctivalisation' of the cornea
• The clinical picture is of ocular surface failure, characterised by conjunctival overgrowth, corneal epithelial defects, vascularisation and scarring
• Therapeutic soft contact lenses delay the postoperative complications, but do not prevent them. It is therefore sensible to avoid surgery in most cases

FELINE OPHTHALMOLOGY

- Animals with poor or absent vision, impaired eyelid and globe mobility may benefit from complex blepharoplastic procedures and such cases should be referred
- Limbal autograft transplantation offers the most rational future treatment for a variety of ocular surface disorders, including symblepharon

Chemosis
As the cat has a loosely-arranged conjunctiva, conjunctival oedema (chemosis) may be of spectacular appearance and a ubiquitous accompaniment to many types of conjunctival disease. In addition to addressing the underlying problem it is important to prevent conjunctival desiccation.

Subconjunctival haemorrhage
This is commonest in cats after blunt or penetrating trauma (see Section 2, pp 40–41).

Conjunctival neoplasia
Conjunctival neoplasia is rare
The commonest neoplasm to encroach on the conjunctiva is squamous cell carcinoma (Figure 4.8). Primary conjunctival tumours include papilloma, adenoma, adenocarcinoma, basal cell tumour, haemangioma, haemangiosarcoma, lymphoma, neurofibroma, neurofibrosarcoma, fibroma, fibrosarcoma and malignant melanoma. Tumours that can metastasise to the conjunctiva include lymphoma (Figure 4.11) and adenocarcinoma.

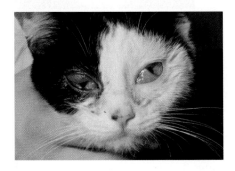

Figure 4.11 Infiltration of the conjunctiva by lymphoma. Bilateral prominence of the third eyelid, more marked on the left than on the right, suggests that there is also orbital infiltration in this cat.

Management
- As many conjunctival tumours in cats are potentially malignant, it is important to assess tumours carefully to make sure that complete excision is a realistic possibility and exfoliative cytology or histopathology should always be performed
- Squamous cell carcinomas may require local radiotherapy, or a combination of surgery, radiotherapy or cryotherapy and reconstructive eyelid surgery for effective cure. Many cases will require referral
- For other types of primary neoplasia the treatment is usually surgical excision, debulking, or biopsy combined with other therapy (e.g. radiotherapy, cryotherapy, laser therapy)
- For secondary neoplasia, treatment other than palliative treatment may not be a realistic option

CONJUNCTIVITIS

The diagnosis of conjunctivitis is not difficult, but effective management depends upon establishing the precise aetiology. It is important to emphasise that respiratory tract viruses are widespread in the cat population, so the isolation of potentially pathogenic viruses should correlate with the clinical presentation and history. The history should include an assessment of the cat's age, vaccination status and lifestyle and whether there are other cats at risk or affected. Clinical appearance may be helpful, but is likely to be remarkably similar with a range of different causes, so laboratory confirmation of infectious causes is of value.

Aetiology
• Infectious agents – *Chlamydophila felis* (formerly known as *Chlamydia psittaci* var. *felis*) is the commonest cause of infectious conjunctivitis in cats in the UK. Respiratory tract viruses such as FHV-1 and, possibly, calicivirus may also be causes of conjunctivitis (Figures 4.12 and 4.13)
• Tear-film abnormalities
• Other causes of conjunctivitis are less common in cats, but note the possibility of allergy (e.g. to topically-applied drugs in particular), trauma and foreign bodies

FELINE OPHTHALMOLOGY

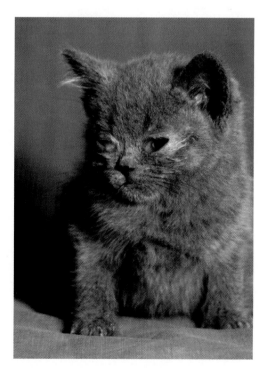

Figure 4.12 Feline herpes virus (FHV-1) in a kitten. Ocular and respiratory signs were present.

FELINE OPHTHALMOLOGY

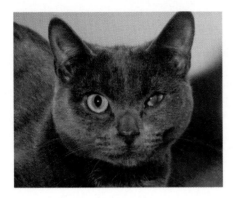

Figure 4.13 Infectious conjunctivitis caused by *Chlamydophila felis* in a young cat. This typically presents as a unilateral problem, and in this cat, at this early stage, is affecting the left eye only.

Clinical signs
- Active hyperaemia of conjunctival vessels and conjunctival inflammation
- Chemosis
- Ocular discharge (serous, mucoid, purulent, haemorrhagic and combinations of these)
- Variable degrees of irritation, blepharospasm, excessive lacrimation and pain
- Chronic changes include follicle formation, conjunctival thickening, ulceration and persistent discharge (Figure 4.14)

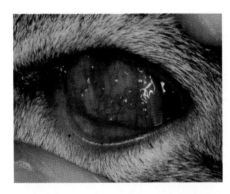

Figure 4.14 Chronic follicular conjunctivitis of unknown cause in a Domestic Shorthair. There were also follicles beneath the eyelids (including the third eyelid) and these can be a source of chronic corneal irritation long after the initiating cause has gone.

Protocol for investigation and diagnosis
- As for the dog, except that *both* conjunctival and oropharyngeal swabs should be taken for virus isolation, preferably using a wire-handled nasal swab for the oropharyngeal sample
- Combined viral and chlamydial transport medium (VCTM) should be used for viral and chlamydial isolation

Differential diagnosis
- Redness of the eye is not synonymous with conjunctivitis and may occur in a number of other situations. For example, as a consequence of haemorrhage after trauma, as

a local manifestation of impeded venous return with an orbital mass, as part of a systemic vascular response or associated with cardiovascular disease
- Conjunctival infiltration by a tumour, most commonly lymphoma, can be confused with conjunctivitis and biopsy may be required for accurate diagnosis

INFECTIOUS CONJUNCTIVITIS

Viral
Feline herpes virus type 1 (FHV-1) (Figure 4.12)
- The most important virus associated with ocular disease in cats
- In neonates (up to four weeks of age) a cause of *ophthalmia neonatorum*
- Usually the whole litter is affected, but the severity may vary between kittens
- Complications of neonatal infection may be severe and include symblepharon formation as a result of conjunctival epithelial necrosis, corneal ulceration, corneal perforation, keratoconjunctivitis sicca, occluded lacrimal puncta and obliteration of the fornices (because of symblepharon), endophthalmitis and panophthalmitis
- In young kittens, infection is usually associated with respiratory signs (rhinitis, tracheitis, bronchopneumonia)
- Acute, usually bilateral, conjunctivitis is the most frequent ocular manifestation in older kittens and cats
- Initially the ocular discharge is serous, but becomes purulent within a week of the onset of the clinical signs
- Most cases also show signs of upper respiratory tract infection
- Uncomplicated infections usually take some two weeks to resolve.
- Some 80% of infected cats become latently infected, and any form of stress in later life may produce a relapse; virus may be shed intermittently and chronic asymptomatic carriers are common
- Recrudescence of infection is likely in chronically infected cats and any form of stress (e.g. re-homing, cat shows, introduction of new cats, lactation, general anaesthesia and surgery), endogenous immunosuppression (e.g. FeLV and FIV) and exogenous immunosuppression (e.g. corticosteroids, cyclosporin and chemotherapy) may produce a relapse
- The clinical signs in chronically affected cats are diverse; they include epiphora, low-grade conjunctivitis and ulcerative and non-ulcerative keratitis

Feline calicivirus (FCV)
- Feline calicivirus is a much less common cause of viral conjunctivitis than FHV-1 and there is some doubt as to whether it is a genuine conjunctival pathogen
- Cats of any age are affected, but FCV infection is commoner and more severe in young kittens
- Ocular signs may be associated with other pathogens
- Clinical signs of infection largely relate to the effects of the virus on the upper respiratory tract, typically producing rhinitis and a serous nasal discharge
- Vesicles that rupture to produce clearly delineated ulcers are commonly found in the mouth (e.g. tongue and oral mucosa)
- Asymptomatic carriers are common, and, since the virus is excreted constantly, it is relatively easy to confirm infection in animals with clinical signs

Diagnosis of viral conjunctivitis
- Clinical signs
- Virus isolation from conjunctival swabs and oropharyngeal swabs
- PCR (polymerase chain reaction) provides the most sensitive and specific test for viral identification and the detection of asymptomatic carriers
- Intermittent excretion of FHV-1 means it is difficult to confirm infection in many cases, whereas calicivirus is excreted constantly
- Serology is of no value in vaccinated animals

Treatment of viral conjunctivitis
- Topical antiviral treatment for FHV-1 is described under Cornea. Calicivirus is not sensitive to the antiviral drugs that are currently available.
- Nasal and ocular discharges should be removed by regular, gentle cleaning and topical antibiotic applied to control secondary bacterial infection. White petroleum jelly can be smeared below the eyes to prevent skin excoriation
- Nursing care (rehydration and good nutrition)
- Systemic broad-spectrum antibiotic will also be needed when upper respiratory tract involvement is present
- Tear replacement therapy (e.g. 0.2% polyacrylic acid; 0.2% w/w carbomer 940) will be required if KCS is present until tear production returns to an adequate level. Occasionally parotid duct transposition is needed in the long term

Bacterial
Feline chlamydiosis (Figure 4.13)
Chlamydophila felis (obligate intracellular bacterium)

Clinical signs
- The most important bacterial feline conjunctival pathogen
- Clinical signs may be observed in cats from four weeks of age onwards
- Initially unilateral conjunctivitis, several days later it becomes bilateral. Initially there is a serous discharge with obvious chemosis and conjunctival hyperaemia, later the discharge can become mucopurulent and other organisms may be isolated
- There is no corneal involvement, and no primary respiratory disease, although mild rhinitis may be present. In a proportion of cases both respiratory tract viruses and *Chlamydophila felis* will be isolated
- Lymphoid follicle formation is common in chronic cases

Diagnosis
- Conjunctival swab, cytobrush, or a Kimura spatula, are used to obtain samples from the ventral conjunctival sac for culture and indirect fluorescent antibody or PCR testing
- Diagnosis is confirmed by chlamydial isolation and by demonstration of intracytoplasmic inclusion bodies in the epithelial cells during the acute phase of the disease. Intracytoplasmic inclusion bodies can be difficult to differentiate from intracytoplasmic pigment granules
- Serology is of limited value in that a low antibody titre is not diagnostic of

chlamydiosis, whereas a high antibody titre may indicate, but does not confirm, infection. Titres may remain high for up to a year after infection

Treatment

- Treatment consists of systemic treatment with the tetracycline group of antibiotics, for example, doxycycline (5 mg/kg by mouth every 12 hours for 3–4 weeks) or a combination of amoxycillin/clavulanate (12.5–25 mg/kg every 8–12 hours for 3–4 weeks). The tetracycline group should not be used in pregnant queens or kittens.
- Topical tetracycline is no longer made commercially in the UK. It is not always well tolerated in the cat as it may provoke a rapid hypersensitivity response initially and, if its use continues, marginal blepharitis can develop.
- A proportion of previously-infected cats become chronic carriers and may be a possible source of infection for other cats (the organism can be isolated from the urogenital and gastrointestinal tracts), a situation which may pose problems in catteries, especially for breeding colonies. In this type of environment all the cats will require systemic amoxycillin/clavulanate or tetracycline or erythromycin or doxycycline for at least four weeks.

Feline mycoplasmosis

Mycoplasma felis, possibly in association with primary pathogens such as FHV-1 and *Chlamydophila felis*, may be associated with feline conjunctivitis. *Mycoplasma felis* alone is unlikely to be a primary pathogen and can be isolated from the conjunctival sac of normal cats.

Clinical signs

Blepharospasm, epiphora and conjunctival hyperaemia, but within 14 days the most striking finding is pallor of the conjunctiva with some thickening and chemosis and a typical pseudomembranous conjunctivitis.

Diagnosis

Confirmation of mycoplasmal conjunctivitis is difficult, as isolation requires specific mycoplasma culture media and the possibility of concurrent pathogens must also be investigated.

Treatment

- *Mycoplasma felis* is susceptible to tetracycline given topically for 5–7 days, but with the potential disadvantages already outlined above
- The clinical course is shortened to some five days in treated cases; without treatment the time course is some 30–60 days

Other bacteria

- Other bacteria identified (e.g. *Pasteurella* spp, *Staphylococcus* spp, *Streptococcus* spp, *Salmonella* spp, *Moraxella* spp) are of uncertain pathogenicity
- Bacterial conjunctivitis may occur secondary to other ocular disease (ocular, adnexal or orbital infection, keratoconjunctivitis sicca, dacryocystitis) and in cats that are stressed or immune compromised
- *Pasteurella multocida* may be transmitted in fight injuries

FELINE OPHTHALMOLOGY

ALLERGIC CONJUNCTIVITIS

Allergic conjunctivitis (and allergic blepharitis) is most frequently encountered as a response to topically applied drugs and, less commonly, as a reaction to insect venom. Long-term treatment with topical preparations (e.g. tetracycline) is sometimes associated with periocular pigment loss and marginal blepharitis.

Treatment
- The allergen should be avoided
- Topical antihistamines or corticosteroids can be given, but most cases have resolved completely by 12–48 hours after removal from the allergen

Other causes of conjunctivitis are rare in cats and similar to those already described for the dog

LIMBUS, EPISCLERA AND SCLERA

NEOPLASIA

Primary
This is a rare site for primary neoplasia. Limbal epibulbar melanoma (scleral shelf melanoma) is the most frequently encountered and, in most cases, and unusually amongst feline tumours, is both slow growing and benign.

Treatment
Sequential observation without intervention, or total resection, or partial resection with radiotherapy or cryotherapy. A graft may be required at the excision site and such cases are usually referred.

Secondary
Secondary neoplasia associated with the feline leukaemia–lymphoma complex are the most likely to be encountered. For example, scleral deposits of lymphoma can present as a red and often painful eye. Biopsy is diagnostic.

CORNEA

Developmental and early onset corneal problems include inherited *neurometabolic disease* (e.g. mucopolysaccharidosis, mannosidosis, gangliosidosis). Specific enzyme deficiencies lead to the widespread accumulation of abnormal products in tissues and in the cornea this manifests as pancorneal clouding (Figure 4.15(a,b)).

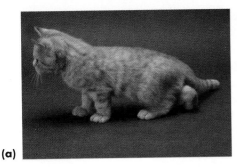

(a)

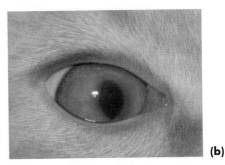

(b)

Figure 4.15 (a) Mucopolysaccharidosis in a 3-month old Domestic Shorthair. The kitten had facial dysmorphia (a broad flattened face) and disproportionately large paws. **(b)** The corneal clouding seen in the kitten in (a) was caused by pancorneal mucopolysaccharide accumulation.

Many of the acquired causes of corneal disease in the cat are similar to those found in the dog, although eyelid and cilia abnormalities as causes of ulcerative keratitis are uncommon in cats. Claw injuries are a common cause of feline ulcerative keratitis and bacterial infection is often introduced (Figures 4.16(a,b)). Damage to the feline lens following penetrating injury has been associated with the development of poorly differentiated, malignant, intraocular sarcomas up to several years later.

Feline herpes virus (FHV-1) is a primary corneal pathogen in the cat and it is important always to consider FHV-1 as a possible cause of feline ulcerative keratitis, in addition to other possible causes.

There is no primary pathogen in the dog and, in addition, corneal sequestrum and proliferative keratoconjunctivitis are feline conditions that have no direct parallel in the dog.

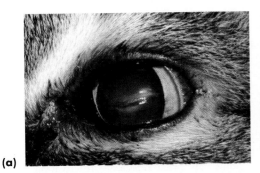

(a)

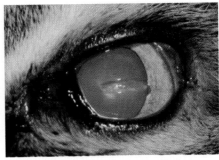

(b)

Figure 4.16(a,b)   Traumatic ulcerative keratitis in a Domestic Shorthair. The ulcer marks the site of a recent cat claw injury before (a) and after fluorescein application (b).

FELINE OPHTHALMOLOGY

ACQUIRED DISEASES OF THE FELINE CORNEA

Epithelial erosion

The cat appears to have a chronic type of refractory superficial erosion, which is similar to canine epithelial basement membrane dystrophy in presentation (see Section 3, pp 114–16, for description of typical clinical appearance) (Figure 4.17). In addition to the usual diagnostic work up (including tear production and adequacy of blink) it is worth checking for *feline herpes virus* (the commonest confirmed aetiological agent) and also the cat's FeLV and FIV status. In some cases there is also a history of topical or systemic corticosteroid use.

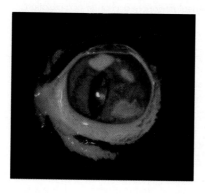

Figure 4.17 Epithelial erosion of the cornea in an adult Domestic Shorthair. The erosions have been stained with fluorescein and demonstrated using a cobalt blue light source, note that superficial vascularisation is also present.

Treatment

- If no predisposing cause can be found, the ulcer should be treated by removing redundant epithelium at the rim of the ulcer with saline-soaked cotton wool wound round the tips of Halstead's mosquito forceps
- The procedure can be performed under topical local anaesthesia and can be repeated after 10 days *only* if there has been no improvement, if the erosion persists despite treatment, consider referral
- A therapeutic soft contact lens can be used to provide protection and pain relief during healing (but avoid if tear production is abnormally low)
- If there is any suggestion of abnormal tear production, then topical tear replacement therapy should be given until tear production returns to normal, and for life if it does not

Herpetic keratitis
Aetiology and clinical signs

- Caused by feline herpes virus-1
- *Epithelial keratitis* occurs commonly during primary infection in young cats, but resolves spontaneously in most cases (Figure 4.18)
- Stromal keratitis (usually unilateral) in adult cats often represents reactivation of latent virus (see below); the prognosis is poor in these cases, because corneal complications are likely (Figure 4.19)

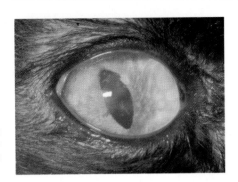

Figure 4.18 Acute herpetic keratitis in a Domestic Shorthair. The pathognomonic superficial dendritic lesions have been stained with fluorescein.

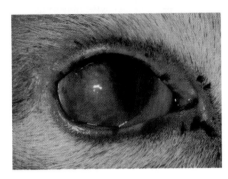

Figure 4.19 Chronic herpetic keratitis in a Domestic Shorthair. The lesions are predominantly stromal in the chronic phase. This cat was also FIV positive.

FELINE OPHTHALMOLOGY

Clinical findings
- Mild blepharospasm and lacrimation, or a serous ocular discharge, are common presentations in the initial stages
- The epithelial keratitis consists of discrete superficial punctate opacities in the early stages; later the pathognomonic linear branching (dendritic) ulcers may form and these can progress to produce an irregular and superficial geographical ulcer (Figure 4.18). These changes are the direct result of viral cytopathic effect on the corneal epithelium
- Chronic cases, with stromal involvement, are a consequence of a cell-mediated immune response
- Stromal keratitis is usually characterised by stromal oedema, superficial and deep vascularisation and cellular infiltration (Figure 4.19)
- A number of affected cats are FIV or FeLV positive, indicating that herpetic keratitis in these cases is an example of an essentially opportunist infection in an immunosuppressed host. The prognosis is poor in immunosuppressed animals

Diagnosis
Diagnosis is based on the clinical findings, which can be so diverse as to be unhelpful in chronic cases, and the detection of FHV-1 by viral isolation (insensitive in chronic cases) or FHV-1 DNA using PCR (more sensitive) from corneal samples.

Management

There is no simple and effective means of managing chronic disease. In practice, many cases *relapse* because of persistent conjunctival infection, or reactivation of a latent viral infection (in trigeminal ganglia). Reactivation of latent virus is triggered by many forms of stress (both local ocular and systemic), intercurrent disease and systemic corticosteroid administration. In view of the known association with FIV and FeLV, it is sensible to screen affected animals for the presence of these viruses.

Antiviral agents

Herpetic keratitis responds unpredictably to topical antiviral agents (e.g. idoxuridine, trifluorothymidine, acyclovir). Ideally, treatment should be given every 2–4 hours for at least six days, and then less frequently until the eye appears quiet. Acyclovir may also be given systemically (200 mg tid) but can cause bone marrow depression. All these agents, together with newer agents, such as ganciclovir (used to treat acute herpetic keratitis in humans), require evaluation in clinical trials to assess their efficacy against FHV-1.

Mechanical removal

Mechanical removal of affected corneal epithelium may assist in the treatment of epithelial keratitis, whereas *lamellar keratectomy* or even *penetrating keratoplasty* (corneal graft) may be of value in the treatment of stromal keratitis.

Immunotherapy

The use of one drop of intranasal vaccine to each eye, or oral human interferon alpha-$_2$ are being evaluated at present, as is *dietary therapy* with L-lysine (200 mg mixed with food on a daily basis, maximum 400 mg bid).

Corticosteroids

Topical corticosteroids may reduce post-herpetic scarring, but they should *only* be used in conjunction with antiviral agents in *chronic* cases as they will exacerbate *active* viral infection.

Corneal sequestrum

Aetiology

This is a condition of unknown cause, which has many descriptive names. It is unique to the cat and there is both a breed disposition (e.g. Colourpoint, Persian, Siamese, Birman, Himalayan) and a tendency for the condition to appear after previous corneal insult (e.g. trauma, herpetic keratitis), irrespective of breed (Figures 4.6 and 4.20).

Clinical findings

The condition is usually unilateral, although the other eye may be affected at a later date, and, both eyes may be involved at the same time in susceptible breeds. It is sensible to conduct a comprehensive examination, to exclude complicating factors, such as entropion, tear film abnormalities and infection, for the appearance of the lesion is often so striking that the necessity for complete examination is forgotten.

The lesion is of somewhat variable appearance, ranging from an ill-defined brown staining of the corneal stroma to a clearly-demarcated black plaque (sequestrum) which is raised above the level of the corneal epithelium (Figure 4.6). It is likely that the different appearances relate to the many causes and to different stages in the evolution of the opacity and that epithelial damage allows the pigment to deposit in the corneal stroma. The pigmented material contains melanin and it may derive from the preocular tear film and, in some cats, pigmented material also accumulates on and near the eyelid margins.

- A discrete zone of oedema sometimes surrounds the sequestrum and, apparently as a feature of chronicity, there may be obvious neovascularisation
- The sequestrum may extend as deeply as Descemet's membrane
- In most cases the corneal sequestrum is eventually sloughed, but this is a process that may take many months and, if ulceration or other problems are present, there may be long-term discomfort for the patient and risk of additional complications, such as corneal perforation

Management
This will depend on the extent and progression of the condition and the amount of discomfort that is present. In time, many of these lesions slough without complication and the cat may be treated with topical tear-replacement preparations or antibiotic ointment during this period if any discomfort is present.

A number of cases, however, will remain uncomfortable on conservative medical treatment and, in such cases, a therapeutic soft contact lens, or keratectomy combined with a conjunctival or free pedicle graft, gives good results. Superficial keratectomy greatly reduces the time course of the disease and potential surgical cases may be best referred.

After surgery, the patient is usually given a short course of topical antibiotic. Recurrence is unusual with careful assessment and treatment. In many respects, the management approach is similar to that adopted for ulcerative keratitis.

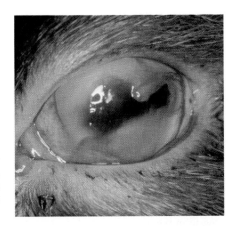

Figure 4.20 Corneal sequestrum as a complication of a traumatic ulcer in a Persian cat. The loose flap of lacerated cornea should have been removed at the time of the injury as this would have aided the healing process.

Eosinophilic (proliferative) keratoconjunctivitis
Aetiology
- The cause of this condition is unknown
- Some cats have a circulating eosinophilia, but many have only ocular involvement

- Ultraviolet light may be a predisposing factor, and the disease is strikingly similar to human vernal disease

Clinical findings (Figure 4.21)

- Usually unilateral initially, but without effective treatment it frequently progresses to affect both eyes
- The clinical appearance is of diffuse oedema, neovascularisation and plaque formation
- The dorsolateral corneal quadrant is most often affected
- The proliferative vascularised plaques are of bizarre and irregular form, frequently whitish in colour and sometimes resembling cottage cheese
- The eyelid margins of affected cats are often partly, and patchily, depigmented
- Adjacent conjunctiva is often inflamed, and the palpebral conjunctiva is invariably abnormal
- Ocular discomfort and a low-grade ocular discharge are usually present

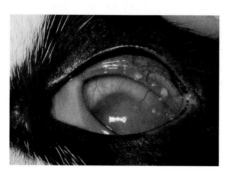

Figure 4.21 Eosinophilic keratoconjunctivitis in a Domestic Shorthair. Both eyes were involved. Note the superficial nature of the white deposits that are so characteristic of this disease, as well as the superficial corneal vascularisation.

Diagnosis

The clinical appearance is usually diagnostic, but the diagnosis can be confirmed by exfoliative corneal cytology.

Treatment

The condition responds to topical corticosteroid therapy and also to megestrol acetate given by mouth. All these drugs have potentially undesirable side effects. Megestrol acetate in particular may induce diabetes mellitus and should be used with great care.

Unfortunately, treatment usually achieves only remission rather than cure and this means that caution must be exercised in the long-term treatment of eosinophilic keratoconjunctivitis. In practice therefore, an initial short course of either topical corticosteroid (betamethasone, dexamethasone or prednisolone) or oral megestrol acetate is given and followed up with topical cyclosporin (once or twice daily) for long-term therapy.

UVEAL TRACT

The iris of young kittens is grey to slate blue in colour. In most adult cats the iris is yellow to gold in colour, but other variations include shades of green and blue. Occasionally, especially in oriental and white cats, each iris is of different colour, with one eye blue and the other yellow to green.

DIFFERENCES FROM THE DOG

- Less pigment in the iris of most cats, therefore normal vasculature and pathological changes such as neovascularisation and post-inflammatory darkening are easier to see
- Distinction between the iris collarette, ciliary zone and the pupillary zone of the normal iris is not always obvious, although when persistent pupillary membrane remnants are present, they arise most commonly from the collarette region, just as in the dog
- Iris vessels are relatively 'leaky' in kittens, but become less permeable with maturity, remaining, however, more permeable than those of the dog
- The dilated pupil is round, whereas the fully constricted pupil is a very narrow vertical slit
- The iris sphincter muscle has a scissor-like action dorsally and ventrally, which causes the vertical slit
- It is possible to perform a rudimentary examination of the iridocorneal (drainage) angle without using a gonioscopy lens, and the anterior chamber is relatively deep
- There is a high rate of aqueous production

FELINE OPHTHALMOLOGY

CONGENITAL AND EARLY ONSET DISORDERS OF THE FELINE UVEA

Sub-albinism
Partial or complete congenital deafness is not uncommon in white cats, especially when combined with a blue iris. There may also be ocular anomalies such as iris hypoplasia. Chédiak-Higashi syndrome is a rare type of partial oculocutaneous albinism, inherited as an autosomal recessive trait and the ocular abnormalities associated with the syndrome include cataracts and decreased pigmentation of the iris and fundus.

Anterior segment dysgenesis
Anterior segment dysgeneses are rare in cats. The commonest abnormality is persistence of the pupillary membrane, but it appears much less commonly in cats than in dogs.

UVEITIS

With the possible exception of uveitis resulting from acute traumatic injury, uveitis tends to be more insidious in cats than in dogs; therefore it is the *chronic* features that are most commonly seen. Many cases of uveitis in the cat are associated with systemic disease so it is easier to establish a specific aetiology, but consider referral if the cause cannot be established. It is worth noting that uveitis in cats rarely reaches the intensity of that seen in dogs, as chronic granulomatous types of uveitis account for a high proportion of cases.

Clinical signs of sub-acute/chronic feline uveitis
- No pain to mild discomfort, no inflammatory hyperaemia in most cases
- Usually no effect on vision, occasionally complications such as retinal detachment result in blindness
- Some or all of keratic precipitates, mutton fat deposits, hypopyon, fibrin and haemorrhage*
- Some or all of swollen iris, iris nodules, iris neovascularisation, pre-iridal fibrovascular membranes*
- Pupil responds normally to light unless synechiae are present*
- Synechiae distort pupil and result in an irregular shape*
- Intraocular pressure normal or low
- Snowflake opacities and retrolental snow banking may be seen when there is peripheral retinal vasculitis (*pars planitis* is the term used to describe the clinical appearance, but is actually an inaccurate description of the underlying pathology)
- Some or all of retinal vasculitis, perivascular exudates, chorioretinitis, retinal haemorrhage and retinal detachment
- Optic neuritis

Uveitis associated with infection
Systemic viral disease
Clinical signs
- It is often impossible to differentiate these conditions on clinical grounds when uveitis is the main presenting clinical sign.
- All the viruses may present with a low-grade anterior uveitis. In such cases there is a loss of iris detail and iris neovascularisation. Keratic precipitates may be obvious on the posterior cornea, especially ventrally. Frank hypopyon or cellular infiltration may be present in the ventral anterior chamber. Fibrin and haemorrhage may be present anterior to the lens and iris and may cause mechanical restriction of the pupil. Pupil mobility may also be affected by synechiae formation, so it is very common to find that the pupil shape is abnormal.
- The posterior segment should also be examined, as vasculitis and optic neuritis are possible presentations, occurring in conjunction with, or distinct from, anterior uveitis.

Feline infectious peritonitis (FIP) (Figures 4.22 and 4.23(a,b))
- This is a problem that is commoner in younger cats than older cats and is most common in pedigree cats kept in multicat households
- There is no specific diagnostic test, and it is known that enteric types of coronaviruses (FECV) may mutate to a more pathogenic type (FIPV). Interpretation of FIP serology is fraught with difficulty, as the tests detect antibody to any coronavirus, and while a high coronavirus antibody titre (>160) and hypergammaglobu-

---

* Readily identifiable key features

linaemia may be suggestive of FIP disease, an intermediate, low or even negative titre does not rule out infection
- Cats with FIP often demonstrate subtle neurological involvement and are often small for their age
- FIP infection is usually confirmed by histological examination, usually of post-mortem material

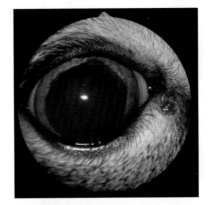

Figure 4.22 Anterior uveitis associated with feline infectious peritonitis. FIP is associated with typical perivascular pyogranulomatous inflammation and in this cat the aqueous is red-cell and fibrin rich and there is marked neovascularisation of the iris.

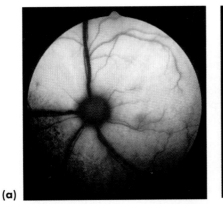

(a)

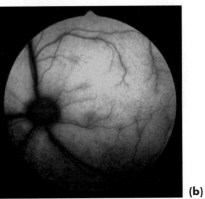

(b)

Figure 4.23(a,b) Posterior uveitis associated with feline infectious peritonitis in a Domestic Shorthair. White light (a) and blue light (b) photographs of the same area demonstrate the intense vasculitis and perivascular oedema. Both eyes were affected.

Feline leukaemia–lymphoma complex (FeLLC) (Figures 4.24 and 4.25)
- Cats of all ages may be infected by feline leukaemia virus (FeLV), although infection is commoner in young cats and is rare in cats over ten years of age
- The ophthalmic signs are usually a consequence of neoplastic involvement ± anaemia and thrombocytopenia
- Laboratory tests can provide confirmation of FeLV infection

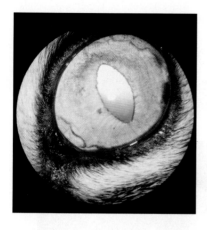

Figure 4.24 Hyphaema, originating from the major arterial circle, associated with the feline leukaemia–lymphoma complex in a Domestic Shorthair.

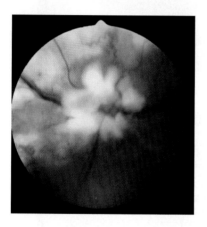

Figure 4.25 Neoplastic infiltration of the optic nerve (infiltrative optic neuropathy) and neovascularisation associated with the feline leukaemia–lymphoma complex in a Domestic Shorthair.

Feline immunodeficiency virus (FIV) (Figure 4.26(a,b))
- FIV occurs most often in adult, free ranging, non-pedigree cats and is more common in males than females
- A positive antibody test is diagnostic of FIV However, a significant proportion of FIV-infected cats have no detectable antibody, and therefore a negative antibody result does not preclude FIV infection

Treatment
Treatment of the uveitis associated with FeLV, FIV and FIP tends to be symptomatic and supportive, although there are chemotherapy protocols available to treat FeLV infection. Some cats with FIV and FeLV can be given a good quality of life for some years after the diagnosis has been made, but this is not usually the case for FIP, where any treatment tends to be palliative only.

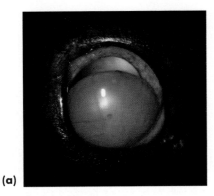
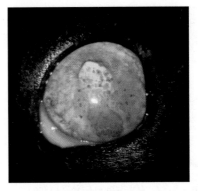

(a)   **(b)**

Figure 4.26(a,b) Chronic anterior uveitis in an FIV-positive Domestic Shorthair. Bilateral uveitis. Lens luxation has occurred in the right eye (a) and the lens has become secondarily cataractous. In the left eye (b), dark keratic precipitates (KPs) adherent to the ventral cornea indicate that the uveitis has been present for some time (KPs darken as they age). Lighter, fawn-coloured KPs indicate that the uveitis is still active. Both iridal surfaces show considerable new blood vessel formation. The anisocoria (inequality of pupil size) was due to the position of the luxated lens: the dorsal aspect was anterior and the ventral aspect occupied the pupillary aperture. Intraocular pressure (Mackay Marg) was 9 mm Hg in both eyes.

Bacterial infections

- *Generalised bacterial diseases* associated with uveitis are rare. Typical and atypical mycobacterial infections are rarely encountered, and ocular involvement is usually in the form of a granulomatous posterior uveitis. Combination treatment (e.g. oral clarithromycin at a dose rate of 10 mg/kg and rifampicin at a dose rate of 20 mg/kg) over a period of months may bring about resolution. Animals must be monitored carefully during treatment.
- *Local injury*, usually as a result of a bite or scratch, may result in direct intraocular inoculation of bacteria (e.g. *Pasteurella multocida*). This is a relatively common cause of uveitis which is amenable to symptomatic treatment for the uveitis and topical (e.g. chloramphenicol drops) and systemic administration of antibiotic (e.g. newer-generation penicillins).

Toxoplasmosis (Figures 4.27(a,b) and 4.28)

- *Toxoplasma gondii* is an intracellular coccidian parasite, and the domestic cat and other felidae are the only definitive hosts
- Clinical problems are most likely to be seen in debilitated or immunocompromised animals, and ocular features consist of retinitis, posterior uveitis, intermediate uveitis, anterior uveitis or panuveitis
- The zoonotic implications should be borne in mind, and it is important to discuss them with clients

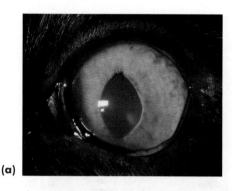

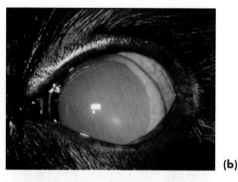

(a)   **(b)**

Figure 4.27 **(a)** Panuveitis in a Domestic Shorthair with toxoplasmosis. Keratic precipitates are present in the anterior chamber and the white 'snowbanking' behind the lens indicates inflammatory cells at this site. **(b)** The same eye as in (a) became glaucomatous some time later. Intraocular pressure measured with a Mackay Marg tonometer was 11 mm Hg in (a) and 49 mm Hg in (b).

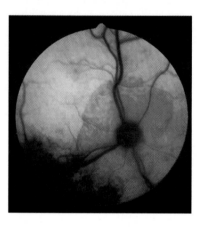

Figure 4.28 Posterior uveitis in a Domestic Shorthair with toxoplasmosis. Focal inflammatory lesions and peripapillary sub-retinal effusion with indications of retinal detachment and reattachment. Despite treatment, total detachment of the retina occurred in this eye.

Diagnosis
- Diagnosis of toxoplasmosis is based on ocular involvement and negative results for FeLV, FIV and FIP
- Detection of *T. gondii*-specific antibodies is helpful, and IgM titres >1:64 may be indicative of active infection
- Note that there is a strong association of toxoplasmosis with FIV-positive status

Systemic mycotic infections (Figure 4.29(a,b))
Systemic mycotic infections may occur in countries with suitable climatic conditions. Uveitis as a consequence of cryptococcosis is the commonest, although coccidiomycosis, blastomycosis, histoplasmosis and candidiasis have all been reported in cats. These problems are unlikely to be seen in the UK unless the animal has been imported or is immunosuppressed.

FELINE OPHTHALMOLOGY

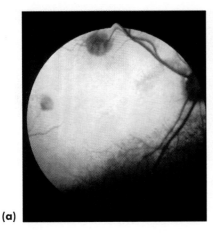 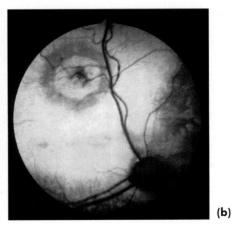

(a)   **(b)**

Figure 4.29   **(a)** Posterior uveitis associated with cryptococcosis in a Siamese cat. **(b)** The focal granulomatous lesions of active inflammation in (a) are less obvious than the same lesions when they have become inactive after the cat was treated with ketaconazole and 5-fluorocytosine.

Idiopathic uveitis (Figure 4.30)

- Idiopathic uveitis is of unknown cause, although an infectious origin is possible, and the problem may simply reflect the inadequate sensitivity of some diagnostic tests or the involvement of other organisms, such as feline herpes virus 1 and *Bartonella henselae*
- It tends to be commoner in older cats and responds poorly to treatment
- Idiopathic uveitis appears more likely to become complicated by epithelial erosion and secondary glaucoma ± lens luxation than other types, and because some of these complications could also relate to the long-term use of topical corticosteroids the benefits of treatment are equivocal
- Histopathology indicates lymphocytic and plasmacytic infiltration of the uveal tract

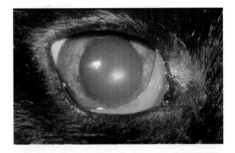

Figure 4.30   Idiopathic uveitis in a Domestic Shorthair. Note the keratic precipitates adherent to the ventral cornea and the dull metallic appearance of the iris.

Uveitis associated with trauma

Intraocular haemorrhage may be associated with blunt and penetrating trauma, and uveitis is a ubiquitous accompaniment (Figure 4.31(a,b)).

FELINE OPHTHALMOLOGY

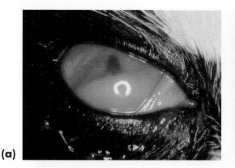
(a)

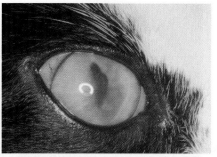
(b)

Figure 4.31 **(a)** Uveitis caused by a penetrating cat claw injury and complicated by intraocular infection. There was a delay of several days between the injury and the owner seeking veterinary help. **(b)** Note that the site of corneal penetration is not apparent until the hypopyon starts to resolve and that intensive use of mydriatics has failed to dilate the pupil because of extensive posterior synechiae coupled with continuing inflammation.

Differential diagnosis of common causes of intraocular haemorrhage in the cat

- Trauma
- Severe uveitis
- Systemic hypertensive disease
- Neoplasia
- Haematological problems such as severe anaemia, thrombocytopenia, vasculopathies, coagulopathies

Uveitis associated with lens damage
Direct lens trauma
Uveitis most commonly arises as a result of *direct lens trauma*, for example from a penetrating injury or gunshot wound (Figure 4.32). If the damage is not too severe it is often possible to control acute onset lens associated uveitis in cats, but the management of cases of this type is made more difficult because intraocular neoplasia can develop and is usually apparent about five years later.

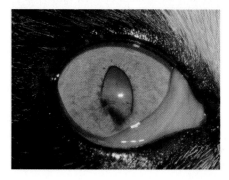

Figure 4.32 Domestic Shorthair with an old penetrating cat claw injury in which both corneal and lens penetration had occurred. The lens has become secondarily cataractous.

Blunt trauma

Blunt trauma is also a cause of lens associated uveitis. In milder injuries, when the eye survives the impact, cataract formation and chronic darkening of the iris may be the only chronic features, but the possibility of later sarcoma formation cannot be dismissed (see below).

Malignant intraocular sarcoma

Malignant intraocular sarcoma (Figure 4.33) seems to develop in feline eyes that have been subjected to major insult in the past (e.g. severe damage to the lens and uvea). The morphological features of these tumours indicate that some of them may be derived from lens epithelium. The tumours are malignant and both local and distant spread occur. Affected eyes are usually opaque and cartilage and bone may form within the tumour.

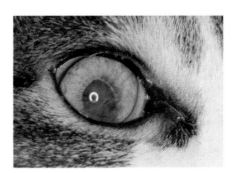

Figure 4.33 Malignant intraocular sarcoma in a Domestic Shorthair. The cat had received a penetrating injury to this eye some years earlier.

FELINE OPHTHALMOLOGY

Treatment

- The early consequences of lens trauma are managed as already described for the dog. Symptomatic treatment of accompanying uveitis is all that is required for mild injury, early advice and referral should be obtained for more serious insult. The owner should be alerted to the possibility of intraocular sarcoma.
- It is sensible to consider the early removal of blind traumatised eyes, rather than to risk subsequent neoplastic change. Histopathology of the enucleated globe is recommended.
- If there is any suspicion of intraocular sarcoma, ultrasonography of the eye, orbit and chest is indicated, as is examination of local lymph nodes. Thoracic radiography, or other diagnostic imaging techniques, may also be helpful. If the tumour is localised to the eye then globe removal and orbital exenteration should be performed.

Uveitis associated with neoplasia

Both primary and secondary neoplasia can involve the uveal tract and mimic uveitis and, in addition, neoplastic cells can elicit an inflammatory response.

UVEAL NEOPLASIA

Primary neoplasia

As in the dog, the commonest primary intraocular tumour is a *melanoma*, but although the histopathology is wide ranging, the tumour is usually more malignant in the cat than the dog with a greater potential for metastasis. The iris and ciliary body are more frequently affected than the choroid. There is a range of clinical presentations: sometimes the tumour involves a sector of iris, but often the iris is diffusely involved. Both pigmented and non-pigmented lesions occur, and there may also be hyphaema and intraocular inflammation. Consider referral if unsure of the diagnosis.

Treatment of discrete (nodular) melanomas
- If the growth pattern is slow then sector iridectomy or laser ablation may be an option, so specialist help should be sought
- If the growth pattern is fast then early enucleation, after ensuring that there has been no secondary spread, is the correct approach

Diffuse iris melanomas (Figure 4.34), with an initially benign behaviour pattern and superficial location, pose a real diagnostic challenge. In this type there is a change of iris colour (darkening and a velvety sheen) and extension into the iris stroma with subtle distortion of the pupil. Owners usually seek veterinary advice because of a change of iris colour or secondary glaucoma as a result of pigment-rich cells blocking the filtration angle. The clinical appearance is of benign melanosis initially, and the transformation to iris melanoma can take months or years, but the risk of metastasis increases with time, so early enucleation is usually the treatment of choice if progression is noted.

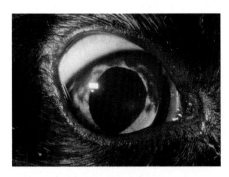

Figure 4.34 Diffuse iris melanoma in a Domestic Shorthair. The multiple patches of pigment have become slightly raised.

Other neoplasms

Tumours may also arise in other sites, such as the ciliary body (usually adenocarcinoma). The possibility of trauma-associated intraocular sarcoma, sometimes several years after the initial ocular trauma, should always be considered in cats.

Diagnosis
- Observation ± ultrasound or other imaging techniques

- The clinical presentation is various combinations of, for example, visible mass, uveitis, hyphaema, fundus changes, intraocular haemorrhage, retinal haemorrhage or detachment

Treatment
- If there is a chance of saving the eye and retaining vison then consider referral
- Early enucleation is the treatment of choice for the majority of primary feline uveal tumours, provided that there is no sign of distant metastasis

Secondary neoplasia
Lymphoma
Lymphoma associated with FeLV is the commonest secondary neoplasm affecting the feline eye and orbit and the uveal tract is commonly involved (Figure 4.35).

Clinical signs
- There is a range of clinical appearances and it is not always possible to differentiate lymphoma from other feline conditions on the basis of ocular appearance.
- General physical examination may locate abnormalities elsewhere in the body (e.g. intestinal and renal masses).
- Diagnosis is usually confirmed from a positive FeLV-antigen test, but some affected cats are FeLV negative. Tumour or bone marrow biopsies can be used to aid diagnosis in such cases.

Metastatic carcinoma
Metastatic carcinomas of the uveal tract should also be considered as causes of secondary uveal neoplasia. They arise from a number of primary sites (e.g. mammary gland) and the prognosis is grave.

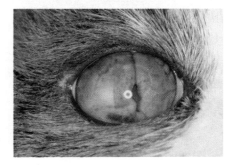

Figure 4.35 Lymphomatous infiltration of the iris in a Domestic Shorthair. Examination from the side indicated that the anterior chamber had been almost obliterated by the extent of the iris infiltration.

ANTERIOR CHAMBER AND AQUEOUS HUMOUR

Developmental defects can involve the anterior chamber (various types of anterior segment dysgenesis), but it is much commoner for anterior chamber abnormalities to be secondary to acquired disease in sites such as the uveal tract (e.g. uveitis) or

FELINE OPHTHALMOLOGY

generalised disease (e.g. dyslipoproteinaemias, multicentric lymphoma and systemic hypertensive disease).

Lipaemic aqueous

Transient *lipaemic aqueous* is encountered on occasions in apparently normal eyes, especially in young Burmese cats (Figure 4.36), and may be an ocular manifestation of familial primary hypertriglyceridaemia. It tends to become less common as the animal matures and the iris vessels become less leaky. Lipids and lipoproteins should always be analysed in cases with recurrent lipaemic aqueous and, if uveitis is a pre-disposing factor, it should be investigated and treated.

Differential diagnosis
• Hypopyon (usually post traumatic)
• Neoplastic infiltrates (most commonly lymphoma)

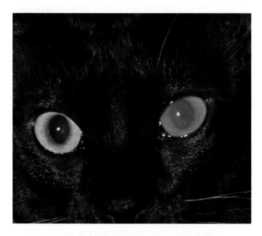

Figure   4.36 Unilateral lipaemic aqueous associated with hypertriglyceri-daemia in a young Burmese cat. The short-lasting phenomenon, which is self-limiting if the lipid levels return to normal, should be differentiated from genuine inflammation.

Hyphaema

Systemic hypertensive disease (this section, pp 223–225) is the commonest non-traumatic cause of hyphaema in the adult cat (Figure 4.37). Developmental causes (e.g. vascular anomalies) are exceptionally rare as a cause of hyphaema. Acquired disorders including coagulopathies, clotting disorders and hyperviscosity syndrome are also rare.

Differential diagnosis of hyphaema
• Systemic hypertensive disease
• Trauma (both blunt and penetrating)
• Neoplasia (e.g. associated with feline leukaemia)
• Uveitis (e.g. associated with feline infectious peritonitis)
• Haematogical problems

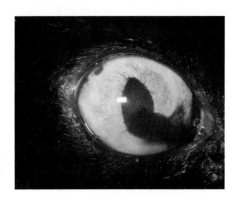

Figure 4.37 Hyphaema in an adult Domestic Shorthair caused by systemic hypertensive disease. The haemorrhage arises from the greater arterial circle.

GLAUCOMAS

Glaucoma (Figure 4.27(b)) in the cat is much less common than it is in the dog, partly because of the well-developed and deep drainage angle in this species. The feline drainage angle can be examined reasonably well by direct inspection. As in the dog, cases are best referred initially for specialist assessment.

Enlargement of the globe occurs more readily in cats than dogs, as the ocular coats stretch more easily. Glaucoma is often less painful, therefore, and vision is retained for longer than in dogs, because the retina is not subjected to such damaging pressure. However, exposure keratopathy is a likely complication of globe enlargement.

Most cases of glaucoma in cats are secondary to uveitis and neoplasia. Some may be associated with the chronic use of corticosteroids. Primary glaucoma is rare.

Clinical signs
- Less obvious than those encountered in dogs, the onset is frequently insidious
- Pain, redness, corneal oedema and Haab's striae are often absent or mild
- Dilated pupil, globe enlargement or a visual defect are first noticed
- Sometimes the underlying cause (e.g. inflammation or tumour) is obvious

Management
- If an underlying cause, such as uveitis, is identified, it should be treated (but idiopathic uveitis responds poorly). If there is pupil block because of adhesions (posterior synechiae), atropine is used in an attempt to dilate the pupil and break down the adhesions – but this is the only indication for the use of a mydriatic in glaucoma therapy.
- Cats do not tolerate oral medical treatment for glaucoma as well as do dogs (dichlorphenamide 0.5–2 mg/kg reduces IOP for four hours; acetazolamide 10 mg/kg reduces IOP for five hours). Inappetence is common and careful monitoring is required, so it is better to avoid their use.
- Topical carbonic anhydrase inhibitors (dorzolamide and brinzolamide) have no obvious systemic side effects and so they are both useful as the first line of therapy in cases with moderately elevated intraocular pressure.
- Surgical drainage procedures can be used, but are rarely employed because of the secondary nature of most cases.

- Enucleation is the preferred option for blind unsightly eyes with raised intraocular pressure.

LENS

The cat has a large lens (Figure 4.1(a)), of remarkable transparency in most individuals. Senile nuclear sclerosis does occur in old cats, but is much less obvious than it is in dogs. Congenital disorders are rare, and conditions such as microphakia, aphakia and congenital cataract are usually seen only in conjunction with other congenital ocular defects such as microphthalmos and persistent pupillary membrane.

CATARACT

Hereditary

Most types of cataract are rare in cats. Those reported as of possible inherited origin (British Blue and Himalayan) have been present from an early age and assumed to be congenital.

Traumatic

Trauma is a common cause of feline cataract and may be a consequence of blunt or, more usually, penetrating trauma. Cataracts may form some time after the initiating injury. The putative association of lens penetration with intraocular sarcoma must be remembered.

Post-inflammatory

Uveitis may be associated with secondary cataract. Cataract formation is usually associated with posterior synechiae and chronic inflammatory changes.

Lens luxation

Luxated lenses in cats invariably become cataractous if they are left *in situ*.

Glaucoma

Glaucoma with cataract formation is uncommon, but may sometimes be seen in chronic cases.

Metabolic and nutritional

Diabetic cataracts are less common and seem to progress more slowly in cats than dogs (Figure 4.38). Nutritional cataracts (e.g. associated with hand rearing on milk substitutes) are rare.

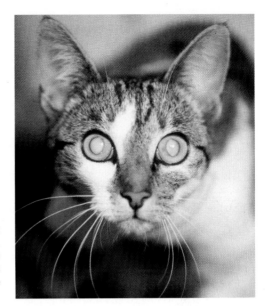

Figure 4.38 Bilateral cataracts in a Domestic Shorthair with diabetes mellitus. Diabetic cataract is commoner in dogs than cats, nevertheless in both species is probably the commonest cause of acute onset bilateral cataract.

LENS LUXATION

Lens luxation may follow chronic uveal inflammation (Figure 4.26(a)), trauma or be secondary to globe enlargement associated with chronic glaucoma. It may also be seen in old cats without any antecedent history, possibly as a form of primary lens luxation resulting from zonular degeneration. Chronic uveitis is the commonest cause, but note that lens luxation can itself provoke a mild uveitis. Lens luxation does not cause the severe problems seen in the dog and affected animals do not constitute ocular emergencies.

Diagnosis
- The diagnosis is usually straightforward, as the lens is large and easily visualised and secondary cataract is common
- As the eye is not particularly painful, it is generally easier to examine than a canine eye with lens luxation
- It is important to determine if uveitis is present and to measure the intraocular pressure, as these parameters may help in deciding treatment priorities

Treatment
- Treatment depends on the cause, the effect on vision and the amount of discomfort
- Lens luxation in the cat does not necessarily result in glaucoma, indeed the IOP may be reduced when lens luxation is secondary to uveitis, and management of the uveitis then takes priority
- Surgery for lens luxation carries an excellent prognosis in the right hands, provided that other factors have also been taken into account

FELINE OPHTHALMOLOGY

VITREOUS

Congenital disease of the feline vitreous is very rare, and acquired problems, as in other species, are usually a consequence of extension from neighbouring structures (e.g. snowflake opacities in *pars planitis*; intravitreal haemorrhage because of bleeding from retinal vessels in systemic hypertensive disease).

OCULAR FUNDUS

ANATOMY

The feline globe is well adapted to vision under dim lighting conditions (relatively large eye, large diameter cornea, large lens, rod-dominated retina and a highly efficient tapetum). Because the tapetum is highly reflective and the normal pupil constricts readily to a vertical slit, fundus examination should be performed with very low levels of illumination.

The fundus shows fewer variations of appearance than the normal canine fundus (Figures 4.1(b), 4.39(a,b) and 4.40(a,b)). The optic disc or optic nerve head (ONH) is circular and is located in the tapetal fundus when a tapetum is present. The retinal vessels often hook over the edge. It is not unusual to see a rim of pigment or other colour surrounding the disc: the latter variant may appear reflective and is known as *conus*.

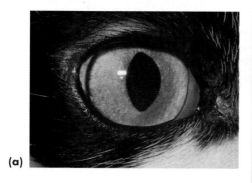
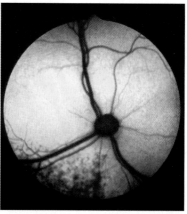

(a)

(b)

Figure 4.39(a,b) Normal iris (a) and ocular fundus (b) in a Domestic Shorthair. The optic nerve head is located in the tapetal fundus and is unmyelinated, so that the retinal vessels hook over its edge. The normal tapetal fundus is more reflective than that of the dog and herbivores, so the light intensity must be kept as low as possible if subtle fundus lesions are not to be missed.

The shape, size and colour of the optic disc show much less variation in cats than dogs. In dogs, most of the variations are related to the degree of myelination, whereas in cats, myelination does not usually extend beyond the *lamina cribrosa* and is rarely observed in the retinal nerve-fibre layer. The physiological pit is often obvious and the ONH appears slightly 'cupped' in most cats, a detail more readily appreciated using the slit beam option on a direct ophthalmoscope.

Different fundus appearances are largely related to the amount of pigment present and the presence or absence of a tapetum. The tapetum develops postnatally and its colour varies between yellow to green, sometimes blue. Sub-albinotic eyes are usually atapetal (Figure 4.40(a)).

The retinal blood supply is holangiotic. The usual pattern of retinal vessels consists of three major cilioretinal arterioles and a similar pattern of veins, the veins being of greater diameter and slightly darker than the arterioles. In the commonest fundus appearance, choroidal vessels, which perforate the tapetum to supply the choriocapillaris, may be viewed end on against the tapetal background. In colour-dilute cats where the fundus lacks pigment, or those in which there is no tapetum, considerably greater detail of the choroidal vasculature is apparent (Figure 4.40(b)).

The *area centralis* (equivalent of human *macula*) is located dorsolateral to the optic disc and is usually obvious because of the lack of blood vessels in the region. The *area centralis* contains the highest concentration of cones in the retina; even so, the feline fundus is rod dominated.

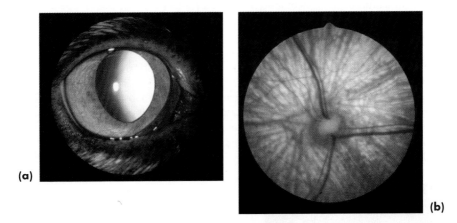

(a)

(b)

Figure 4.40(a,b) Normal sub-albinotic iris (a) and fundus (b) in a blue-eyed Domestic Shorthair.

CONDITIONS OF THE OCULAR FUNDUS

Neurometabolic diseases (lysosomal storage disorders)
- Although the enzyme defect is present from birth in these unusual lysosomal storage disorders, the progressive clinical signs appear later because of the accumulation of substrate in many cells throughout the body. In the retina, retinal ganglion cells and the retinal pigment epithelium are involved. There are more reports of ocular involvement with lysosomal storage diseases in cats than dogs.
- Retinal involvement has been reported in GM_1-gangliosidosis, α-mannosidosis, mucopolysaccharidosis (type VI) and mucolipidosis (type II).

- It is often difficult or impossible to identify the subtle fundus changes (e.g. multiple focal spots) because of accumulation of substrate in the corneal cells, which produces corneal cloudiness.

Retinal dysplasia
- Uncommon in cats and usually associated with perinatal viral infection (e.g. natural infection with feline panleucopenia virus and experimental infection with feline leukaemia virus)
- In addition to impaired retinal development, the development of cerebral and cerebellar tissues may also be affected and the commonest neurological signs relate to cerebellar hypoplasia with feline panleucopaemia virus infection

Inherited progressive retinal atrophy (PRA)
- An autosomal-dominant rod–cone dysplasia observable ophthalmoscopically at 8–12 weeks of age exists in a closed colony of Abyssinian cats at the Animal Health Trust in the UK. There is also an autosomal recessive type of rod-cone degeneration observable ophthalmoscopically at 1.5–2 years in this breed
- The British Shorthair and Siamese are other breeds in which inherited PRA might occur
- The ophthalmoscopic signs of inherited PRA are a bilateral increase in tapetal reflectivity, vascular attenuation and a poor PLR; the changes are symmetrical
- PRA is much less common in cats than dogs and, as in dogs, there is no treatment

Nutritional retinopathies
Taurine deficiency retinopathy
Taurine deficiency produces a retinal degeneration that is most obvious in the *area centralis* in the early stages, hence the description of feline central retinal degeneration (Figure 4.41). Progression of the condition results in a band-shaped lesion dorsal to the optic disc and eventually there is generalised retinal degeneration and irreversible blindness.

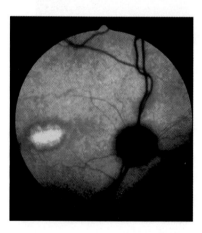

Figure 4.41 Taurine deficiency retinopathy photographed in blue light. Note the somewhat granular hyperreflective zone in the region of the *area centralis* in this Domestic Shorthair.

Taurine deficiency retinopathy is not uncommon. It may be a consequence of inadequate intake or faulty absorption and metabolism, and it is possible to produce this condition in some cats by feeding unusual diets, for example, exclusively dog food, which lacks taurine. This is because taurine is an essential amino acid for cats, whereas dogs can synthesise their own.

Treatment involves taurine supplementation (the daily requirement for an adult cat is 10 mg/kg body weight).

Thiamine deficiency retinopathy

- Thiamine deficiency is unusual and may be a consequence of feeding diets deficient in thiamine (e.g. heat-processed commercial cat foods) or containing thiaminases (e.g. raw fish)
- Clinical signs include anorexia and neurological signs (mydriasis with normal vision, ataxia, ventroflexion of the head and neck)
- Fundus examination may reveal retinal haemorrhage, papilloedema, peripapillary oedema and neovascularisation
- Coma and death result if the condition remains untreated
- Treatment involves thiamine (50–75 mg per dose every eight hours) to reverse the deficit, and corticosteroids to reduce the oedema; both may be given intravenously

Infections
Viral infection
Feline infectious peritonitis (FIP)
Fundus changes are associated with vasculitis, pyogranulomatous inflammation or hyperviscosity because of increased protein levels.

Feline leukaemia–lymphoma complex (FeLLC)
Fundus changes are usually a consequence of neoplastic involvement ± anaemia and thrombocytopaenia.

Feline immunodeficiency virus (FIV)
Fundus changes are probably related to concurrent toxoplasmosis.

Bacterial infection
Mycobacteria
Mycobacterial infections may be associated with chorioretinitis and retinal detachment.

Sepsis
Sepsis can produce multifocal inflammatory lesions by haematogenous spread.

Parasitic infection
Toxoplasmosis
The parasite may invade the retina and choroid, but the inflammation it produces is not distinctive and concurrent infection (e.g. FIV) is possible.

Ophthalmomyiasis interna
Dipteran larvae may gain access to the eye and produce highly-characteristic criss-crossing tracks in the fundus.

FELINE OPHTHALMOLOGY

Systemic mycotic infection

Fundus changes are usually the result of haematogenous spread and consist of sub-retinal and intraretinal pyogranulomas.

Neoplastia

- Primary tumours include astrocytoma and meningioma
- Metastatic tumours include lymphoma, squamous cell carcinoma, adenocarcinoma and haemangiosarcoma
- Ophthalmoscopic findings include neoplastic infiltration, retinal detachment, retinal haemorrhage and retinal degeneration
- Ischaemic degenerative changes, including pigmentary disturbance, have been associated with angioinvasive tumours such as primary bronchogenic carcinoma

Trauma

Blunt trauma

- Retinal detachment may be associated with blunt trauma. Although the retina may reattach spontaneously, degenerative changes will mark the site of the original detachment
- Intraocular haemorrhage, including hyphaema, may also be associated with trauma

Penetrating trauma

- Intraocular haemorrhage is the commonest complication
- Prognosis depends upon the site and extent of the injury
- Damage to the lens ± uveal tract may be complicated by malignant intraocular sarcoma formation, sometimes years after the initial injury

Toxic changes

- Acute retinal degeneration/necrosis may follow the administration of substances toxic to the feline retina
- Parenteral *enrofloxacin* (and possibly other quinolone antibiotics) has been associated with an apparently idiosyncratic adverse reaction. Affected cats become acutely blind, with widely-dilated non-responsive pupils, often within hours of treatment (Figures 2.24 and 4.42)
- Bilateral diffuse retinal degeneration is apparent within a few days of drug administration
- The outer retina, particularly the photoreceptor layer, is damaged
- There is no specific treatment, but there may be a degree of recovery if the association is recognised and the drug stopped immediately
- If this antibiotic is selected for use in cats the dose rate should not exceed 5 mg/kg every 24 hours

FELINE OPHTHALMOLOGY

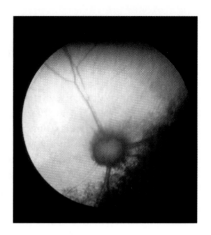

Figure 4.42 Enrofloxacin-associated retinal degeneration in a Domestic Shorthair. The cat went acutely blind overnight (Figure 2.24, Section 2, p. 58) and bilateral retinal degeneration was apparent within a week of the cat receiving the drug.

Systemic hypertensive disease

Both primary and secondary systemic hypertension occurs in cats and is certainly the commonest reason for fundus abnormality in older cats. The eye is a sensitive and readily-examined target organ, and ophthalmoscopic examination of both eyes must be performed in any adult cat that presents with haemorrhage in the anterior chamber.

Hypertensive fundus changes and their progression (Figures 4.43–4.45)

- The hypertension-induced damage to the choroidal, retinal and optic nerve head vasculature (mainly the result of ischaemia followed by degeneration) allows serum and even whole blood to escape
- Leakage may first be apparent as focal, hazy areas associated with choroidal vessels, mainly arterioles, which are viewed end on as the 'stars of Winslow'. These vessels are most easily viewed in the tapetal fundus as they pierce the tapetum en route to the choriocapillaris
- The histology of the normal tapetal retina and choroid is illustrated at the head of this section, and a choroidal vessel perforating the tapetum can clearly be seen (Figure 4.1(a))
- Leakage at this site allows subretinal fluid to accumulate. Subretinal fluid accumulation results in focal bullous retinal detachment
- In the early stages partial retinal detachment may be followed by reattachment in some patients, producing pathognomonic, often localised, branching linear folds, but eventually total detachment will occur if the condition is not recognised
- The retinal vessels become grossly abnormal (variable diameter, notably narrow segments ± aneurysmal dilatations)
- Arterioles are most severely affected
- Haemorrhage from choroidal and retinal vessels can produce marked intraocular haemorrhage and, in some cases, there will also be haemorrhage from iris vessels and hyphaema
- The optic nerve head may become oedematous (papilloedema)
- Retinal detachment and intraocular haemorrhage are the complicating factors most likely to be encountered
- End-stage fundus changes comprise panretinal degeneration and optic atrophy, and,

although such animals are irreversibly blind, they can still have a good quality of life if the systemic hypertension is treated
• The differential diagnosis of feline panretinal degeneration is summarised later

Diagnosis

It is important to recognise systemic hypertension as early as possible, ideally when the choroidal vessels appear 'fuzzy' and there is early mild subretinal fluid accumulation. Vision will be severely compromised or lost once retinal detachment has occurred, as retinal degeneration starts within hours of detachment in the cat. All cats of eight years of age and older should undergo regular screening (including examination of the ocular fundus and blood-pressure measurement) to detect early systemic hypertensive changes.
• History (e.g. to identify secondary associations such as renal failure and hyperthyroidism) and clinical signs
• Systemic arterial blood pressure (if there are no facilities for accurate measurement such as Döppler flow oscillometry, then the cat should be referred)
• Relevant laboratory tests

Management

• Emergency treatment of systemic hypertensive crises may include titrated dosage of sodium nitroprusside and can only be attempted when specialist facilities for continuous monitoring of blood pressure are available. This is unlikely to be available in all but a limited number of referral centres.
• The cause of the systemic hypertension must be investigated to establish whether it is primary or secondary to other conditions such as chronic renal failure or hyperthyroidism.
• Patients can be given good quality of life on medical treatment (usually a low-sodium diet and oral medication). The drugs used most commonly are ACE inhibitors, such as benazepril (0.25 mg/kg each day), or calcium channel blockers, such as amlodipine besylate (0.625 mg total dose every 24 hours). These drugs may be given alone, or if either drug alone is insufficient, they may be given together.
• Treatment aims to keep the mean systolic blood pressure below 180 mm Hg and ideally approximately 160 mm Hg.

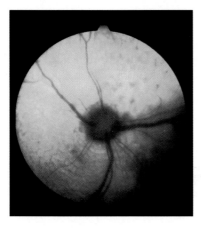

Figure 4.43 Systemic hypertensive disease in a Domestic Shorthair. The earliest fundus signs are consistent with leakage from abnormal choroidal vessels to produce a serous subretinal effusion and subtle areas of retinal detachment. Similar leakage from retinal vessels produces intraretinal oedema. The combination of subretinal effusion, intraretinal oedema and regions of retinal detachment, creates a false impression of variation of retinal-vessel calibre. Mean systolic blood pressure was 245 mm Hg at the time of the photograph.

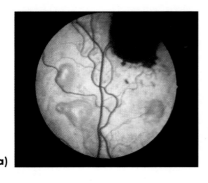 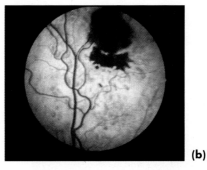

(a)   (b)

FELINE OPHTHALMOLOGY

Figure 4.44 **(a)** Systemic hypertensive disease in a Domestic Shorthair. In this fairly severe case there are true variations of retinal-vessel calibre. Preretinal haemorrhage is apparent dorsally. Multiple bullous detachments are present as a consequence of subretinal effusion. Mean systolic blood pressure was 280 mm Hg at the time of the photograph. **(b)** Within a week of initiating treatment to reduce the systemic blood pressure the retina has re-attached and the large preretinal haemorrhage has begun to resorb. Mean systolic blood pressure was 210 mm Hg at the time of the photograph.

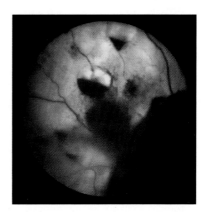

Figure 4.45 Systemic hypertensive disease in a Domestic Shorthair. In this blind and severely-affected cat there is extensive intraocular haemorrhage and retinal detachment. The two distinct blood-containing bullae, at approximately 11 and 12 o'clock, indicate haemorrhage from ruptured aneurysms. The more extensive haemorrhage, from 4 o'clock to 8 o'clock, is associated with extensive retinal detachment. The optic nerve head of this eye was obscured by the haemorrhage, but papilloedema was present in the other eye. Mean systolic blood pressure was 360 mm Hg at the time of the photograph.

End-stage retinal degeneration and its differential diagnosis
(Figure 4.46)
Congenital and developmental conditions
- Feline panleucopenia virus infection in foetus

Acquired conditions
- Inherited progressive retinal atrophy
- Taurine deficiency retinopathy
- Post-inflammatory chorioretinopathy
- Retinotoxicity
- End-stage glaucoma
- End-stage systemic hypertension

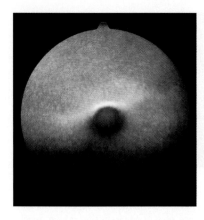

Figure 4.46 Panretinal degeneration and optic atrophy. The cause was unknown in this cat, the condition was bilateral and severe vascular attenuation and intense tapetal hyperreflectivity are notable features.

Haematological disorders associated with retinal haemorrhage
- *Anaemia*, especially when profound, may be associated with haemorrhage and is also a cause of bullous detachments. Retinal vessels (and choroidal vessels if visible) will be pale
- *Coagulopathies* and *vasculopathies*
- *Myeloproliferative* and *myelodysplastic* disorders
- Platelet defects such as *thrombocytopaenia*

Hyperviscosity syndromes
Vessels, especially retinal veins and venules, appear engorged and tortuous. If cyanosis is also present their colour will reflect this, as will the colour of the visible mucous membranes.
- Raised *plasma proteins* (e.g. FIP)
- Increased *red cells* (polycythaemia)
- Increased *white cells* (leukaemia)

Lipaemia retinalis (Figure 4.47)
- Chylomicron-rich blood (circulating triacylglycerides exceed 25 mmol/l) imparts a tomato-soup to creamy appearance to the blood column in retinal vessels
- *Lipaemia retinalis* can be caused by inherited primary chylomicronaemia and chylomicronaemia secondary to disease (e.g. diabetes mellitus)

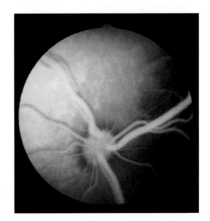

Figure 4.47 *Lipaemia retinalis* in a kitten with chylomicronaemia (serum triacylglycerides 41.6mmol/l). This four week-old kitten was also anaemic because of a heavy flea burden.

NEURO-OPHTHALMOLOGY

Most complex neurological problems in cats require referral for comprehensive investigation.

Feline dysautonomia

This is an autonomic polygangliopathy and any ocular involvement will be bilateral. The commonest ocular feature is widely-dilated non-responsive pupils and there may also be prominent third eyelids and reduced tear production. Generalised signs include depression, anorexia, weight loss, dry mucous membranes, megoesophagus, intermittent regurgitation, constipation, ileus, urinary retention and bradycardia.

Management
- Patients require long-term nursing and avoidance of stress
- Complete recovery may not occur and relapses are possible

Anisocoria

Anisocoria is common in cats and may be of CNS (e.g. inflammation or neoplasia) or ocular origin (e.g. Horner's syndrome).

Temporary Horner's syndrome is common after bulla osteotomy and may also be seen after aural administration of ototoxic agents (Figure 4.48).

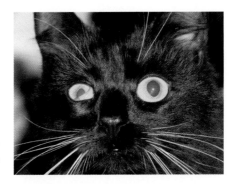

Figure 4.48 Horner's syndrome (right eye) in a young cat, which developed after the ears were cleaned with detergent solution.

FELINE OPHTHALMOLOGY

SECTION 5
RABBIT OPHTHALMOLOGY

INTRODUCTION

The normal eye is illustrated in Figure 5.1(a,b). As is to be expected of a prey species, the rabbit has prominent laterally-placed eyes with large uniocular fields on each side and very small binocular fields in front and behind. The rabbit fundus is described below (this section, pp 237–8).

Applied anatomy features of note are:

- Communication between the right and left orbits
- The presence of an orbital venous sinus – this makes enucleation hazardous and it is safer to perform transconjunctival enucleation or eviscerate the globe
- Lacrimal and accessory lacrimal glands
- The third eyelid has a superficial nictitans gland and a deep Harderian gland that is closely invested by the orbital venous sinus
- A single ventromedially-placed lacrimal punctum and a rather tortuous nasolacrimal duct; the nasolacrimal duct is largely encased in bone and passes close to the roots of both the molar and incisor teeth before terminating within the nasal vestibule

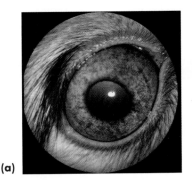 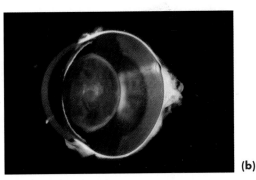

(a)   (b)

Figure 5.1 **(a)** Normal rabbit eye. **(b)** Normal gross rabbit globe (with acknowledgements to J.R.B. Mould).

Points to note about clinical disease in the rabbit

- Husbandry, environment and stress factors are of critical importance.
- Infectious organisms, notably *Staphylococcus* spp and *Pasteurella multocida* may be of relevance in orbital cellulitis, orbital abscess, blepharitis, blepharoconjunctivitis, conjunctivitis, dacryocystitis, uveitis and endophthalmitis.

The common ocular and adnexal conditions of the rabbit and those that are important to recognise because of the serious implications of misdiagnosis are summarised in Box 5.1.

RABBIT OPHTHALMOLOGY

RABBIT OPHTHALMOLOGY

Box 5.1 Common and important rabbit ocular and adnexal conditions

- Traumatic damage (especially cornea)
- Congenital defects such as colobomas of the retina, choroid and optic nerve head (and, less commonly, other ocular tissues such as the lens)
- Orbital infection
- Globe prolapse
- Ocular lipid infiltration and deposition linked with high fat (usually high cholesterol) diets
- Blepharoconjunctivitis and conjunctivitis (e.g. myxomatosis, rabbit syphilis, bacterial infections)
- Dacryocystitis
- Ulcerative keratitis
- Lens-induced uveitis and cataracts associated with *E. cuniculi*
- Neoplasia, most commonly squamous cell carcinoma affecting the eyelids
- Glaucoma

ORBIT

Traumatic globe prolapse

The prominent nature of the globe means that it is relatively easy to displace it from the orbit. Prognosis for retention of vision after the globe has been restored to the orbit is guarded.

Orbital abscess and orbital cellulitis

Orbital infection is common in rabbits, and may be associated with septicaemia or dental disease (Figure 5.2). Diagnosis is as for other species, and the common presentation is exophthalmos and third eyelid prominence. Most cases are unilateral.

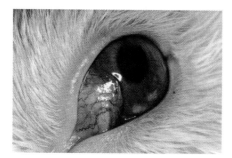

Figure 5.2 Orbital abscess (prominent and hyperaemic third eyelid) and iris abscessation (two caseous plaques) as the ocular manifestations of disseminated infection. At post mortem, multiple abscesses were present and *Staphylococcus aureus* was cultured.

Differential diagnosis
- Whilst bilateral exophthalmos may be a consequence of disseminated infection (e.g. pyaemia and septicaemia) it is more likely to reflect the jugular engorgement that may accompany cardiothoracic disease, including neoplasia (e.g. lymphoma and thymoma).
- Prolapse of the nictitans gland or the Harderian gland of the third eyelid should be distinguished from third eyelid prominence due to a space occupying lesion of the orbit.

Treatment
- Attend to any dental problems
- Drainage is difficult, even if orbital exenteration is performed, because of poor access and the tenacious nature of the pus
- Systemic antibiotics effective against *Staphylococcus* spp and *Pasteurella multocida* are indicated – instillation of gentamicin after evacuation may help

EYELIDS AND CONJUNCTIVA

Conjunctival overgrowth
The cause of this condition is unknown and it may be either congenital or acquired (Figure 5.3). As with symblepharon surgery, there is a tendency for the condition to recur following simple resection, so referral for more complex procedures, such as the Arlt technique, should be considered.

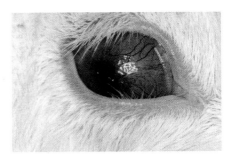

Figure 5.3 Unilateral conjunctival over-growth in a young rabbit, presumed to be congenital in this case.

Conjunctivitis
- Blepharoedema and blepharoconjunctivitis may be caused by *myxomatosis* (myxovirus). The severe, white, ocular discharge is probably a feature of secondary bacterial infection. Although most commonly seen in wild rabbits, it may also be seen in domestic pets and animals at risk are best vaccinated to provide protection.
- *Treponema cuniculi* (rabbit syphilis) also presents with blepharoconjunctivitis and blepharitis and is transmitted to the neonate by genital infection in the dam.
- Conjunctivitis can be secondary to environmental factors (e.g. dust from poor-quality hay).
- Secondary bacterial infections (e.g. *Staphylococcus aureus* and *Pasteurella* spp) are also causes of conjunctivitis.

Neoplasia

Squamous cell carcinoma is the most common eyelid tumour to be encountered, and is usually treated surgically ± cryotherapy.

LACRIMAL SYSTEM

Normal tear production shows marked breed variation, and zero Schirmer I tear test readings can be recorded in apparently normal eyes. Average Schirmer I tear test values are about 5 mm/minute. When unilateral ocular surface disease is thought to be associated with tear film abnormalities, careful comparison of both eyes, including Schirmer tear testing, is essential.

Dacryocystitis
Aetiology

- Dacryocystitis is common and is usually a consequence of dental disease causing obstruction of the nasolacrimal duct and secondary bacterial infection
- *Staphylococcus* spp and *Pasteurella* spp are important isolates from rabbits with epiphora or frank dacryocystitis, but other bacteria (e.g. *Bordetella* spp, *Moraxella* spp, *Neisseria* spp and *Streptococcus* spp) may also contribute
- Predisposing factors include poor husbandry (e.g. dietary imbalance, poor ventilation, ammonia build up)

Clinical signs

- The rabbit is unusual in that drainage of tears takes place through a single large punctum located in the ventromedial fornix, and a profuse white ocular discharge can be seen to originate from the lacrimal punctum (Figure 5.4(a,b))
- Conjunctivitis and, less commonly, corneal ulceration or a corneal abscess, may also be present

Management

- Address any underlying husbandry problems
- Take samples for culture and sensitivity
- For mildly-affected cases, topical chloramphenicol drops are applied directly into the lacrimal punctum after careful cleaning
- For more serious cases, the lacrimal punctum is cannulated with a 22- or 23-gauge catheter or similar, and gentle irrigation with sterile water used to restore patency, followed by application of aqueous antibiotic solution (e.g. chloramphenicol or fusidic acid, or a combination of fusidic acid and gentamicin drops)
- The catheter can be reinserted for each treatment or left *in situ*, but the latter is not always well tolerated and the catheter needs to be fixed in place
- In the later stages of dental disease, parenteral treatment with antibiotics, e.g. cephalexin given by subcutaneous injection at a dose rate of 20 mg/kg for 5–10 days, may be required
- Treatment may need to be repeated at regular intervals, especially if the dental disease progresses

Prognosis

The prognosis is guarded to poor, depending on the extent of any underlying dental disease and the adequacy of the husbandry.

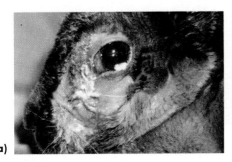

(a)

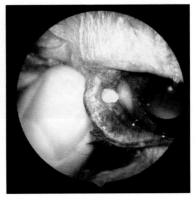

(b)

Figure 5.4 **(a)** Dacryocystitis, with extensive periocular changes, including a copious ocular discharge. **(b)** A closer view of the ventral conjunctival sac shows pus emerging from the single lacrimal punctum and secondary corneal involvement.

CORNEA

Keratitis

Ulcerative keratitis is not uncommon and is often the result of trauma from fibrous bedding or feed. There also appears to be a form of recurrent epithelial erosion.

Lipid deposition

Corneal lipid deposition will occur readily if fat-rich foods are fed by well meaning, but misguided, owners. The rabbit, as an obligate herbivore, is particularly susceptible to the adverse effects of high circulating cholesterol. Normal circulating levels of total cholesterol are usually less than 3 mmol/l; on a high cholesterol diet the levels often exceed 25 mmol/l. Accelerated atherosclerosis develops if these abnormal levels are maintained, and there is widespread infiltration and deposition of lipid in the tissues, including those of the eye (Figure 5.5(a,b)).

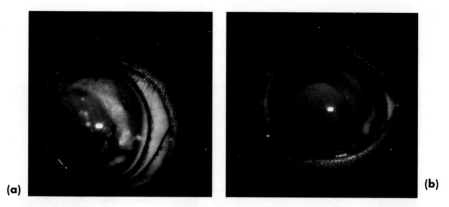

(a)   **(b)**

Figure 5.5 **(a)** Bilateral ocular lipid deposition as a result of a diet that included butter and cheese. In the right eye lipid can be visualised in the cornea, iris, ciliary body and lens. **(b)** The left eye is not so heavily infiltrated (with acknowledgement to S.D. Carrington).

UVEAL TRACT

Uveitis

Uveitis may be a consequence of disseminated infection or the result of lens infection by the ubiquitous microsporidium parasite *Encephalitozoon cuniculi* (Figures 5.6(a,b)). Intralenticular *Encephalitozoon cuniculi* (probably acquired *in utero* from an infected dam) causes eventual lens rupture (usually the anterior lens capsule) and release of lens material with consequent phacoclastic uveitis.

Encephalitozoonosis can be treated by phacoemulsification to remove the lens contents, and agents such as oral albendazole (15–30 mg/kg daily) or fenbendazole (10–20 mg/kg daily) over 2–4 weeks, may eliminate infection.

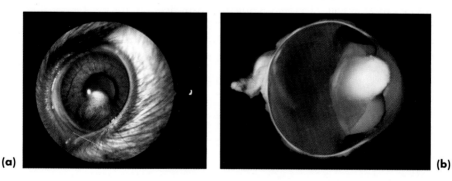

(a)   **(b)**

Figure 5.6 **(a)** Phacoclastic uveitis secondary to intralenticular *Encephalitozoon cuniculi*. **(b)** Gross globe from another rabbit with this condition to illustrate the lens rupture (with acknowledgements to J. R. B. Mould).

LENS

Cataract
Aetiology
- Intralenticular *E. cuniculi*
- Trauma
- Inherited cataract
- Posterior capsular lens opacities may be observed in conjunction with persistent hyperplastic primary vitreous

GLAUCOMAS

Glaucoma
Congenital glaucoma (buphthalmos) is known to be inherited (recessive) in the New Zealand White rabbit, but is also seen in other breeds. It develops in early life (1–3 months of age) and is associated with pectinate ligament dysplasia.

Clinical signs
- Most typically corneal oedema and globe enlargement (Figure 5.7)
- Severe cupping of the optic disc is an easily-recognisable feature, but early cupping is not easy to diagnose because of the depth and extent of the normal physiological pit

Treatment
Treatment may not be necessary as the condition is not painful, and the intraocular pressure often returns to normal when degenerative changes in the ciliary body cause a reduction in aqueous production.

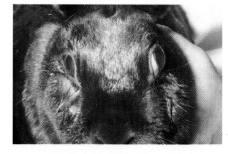

Figure 5.7 Unilateral glaucoma affecting the left eye. Note the globe enlargement and lack of pain.

FUNDUS

Anatomy
The rabbit has a merangiotic (i.e. a partially-vascularised) retina and the retinal blood vessels are confined to a horizontal zone on either side of the optic nerve head (ONH). The horizontally-located vessels consist of a major temporal (lateral) and nasal (medial) veins and usually several arterioles. No tapetum is present in the rabbit fundus.

The ONH has such a deep physiological cup that the surface and bottom of the pit cannot be viewed in focus together using a direct ophthalmoscope. This normal recession also makes it difficult to diagnose early pathological cupping in glaucoma cases. The optic cup may occupy up to half the diameter of the ONH.

In the pigmented rabbit, obvious myelinated nerve fibres, the medullary rays, are present beneath the retinal blood vessels, and additional myelinated nerve fibres are often present ventral to the ONH (Figure 5.8(a)). The ONH is located dorsal to the horizontal midline of the eye and the *area centralis* is in the form of a broad horizontal band located ventral to the ONH. There is a greyish crescent immediately ventral to the ONH, which is usually more obvious in albinos (Figure 5.8(b)).

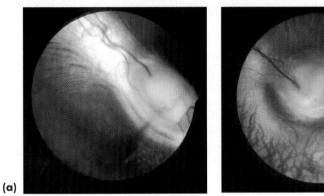 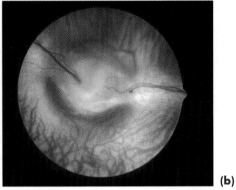

(a)   (b)

Figure 5.8 **(a)** Rabbit fundus. In this pigmented rabbit, there are obvious myelinated nerve fibres present beneath the horizontally located retinal blood vessels and ventral to the ONH. **(b)** In the albino rabbit fundus, there is an obvious greyish crescent immediately ventral to the ONH. In both fundi note that there is no tapetum and the physiological pit is deep and extensive.

Congenital abnormalities of the rabbit fundus

Colobomatous defects of the optic nerve, retina and choroid are commonest in microphthalmic eyes and usually of no clinical relevance.

Acquired abnormalities of the rabbit fundus

Active chorioretinitis and inactive chorioretinopathy are seen occasionally, but are uncommon. Other changes observed include pigmentary disturbance and retinal atrophy. The aetiology of acquired fundus lesions is poorly understood in rabbits.

FARM ANIMAL OPHTHALMOLOGY

INTRODUCTION

Neonatal animals and small farm animals are remarkably easy to examine, but larger farm animals will require good handling facilities (e.g. halter and cattle crush). Chemical restraint may be required in adult cattle in addition to physical restraint, especially when ocular pain is present. Any neuro-ophthalmological tests required should be performed before sedatives are administered.

ANATOMY

The eyes are laterally placed, especially in sheep, goats and cattle, so the binocular visual field is small and the uniocular visual fields extensive. The orbit is enclosed and the orbital floor is incomplete; there is substantial orbital fat in cattle.

An upper and lower lacrimal punctum is the usual arrangement for tear drainage in farm animal species. In the *pig*, however, a single upper punctum is usually all that is present. In *cattle*, the nasal ostium is obvious. Supernumerary openings are sometimes present in the nasolacrimal duct, but do not necessarily give rise to any clinical problems.

In *ruminants*, the pupil is horizontally oval and *granula iridica* (*corpora nigra*) are located on the dorsal and ventral pupillary borders. Heterochromia of the iris is common and related to iris pigmentation and coat colour. True albinos have a white to pink iris; with greater amounts of pigment the iris appears blue, grey or brown, the latter being the commonest adult colour. In *pigs*, the pupil is circular when dilated and a subtle horizontal oval at rest. *Granula iridica* are absent.

A patent hyaloid artery is a common finding in young *ruminants*, whereas in adults the site of the original attachment of the hyaloid artery at the optic nerve head is marked by prominent glial tissue known as Bergmeister's papilla. Details of normal fundus variations are outlined later (this section, pp 261–262).

HANDLING AND EXAMINATION

Sedation and analgesia
- Intramuscular injection of xylazine (approximately 0.05 mg/kg) provides excellent sedation in cattle some 25 minutes after administration. Note that xylazine should not be used in the last trimester of bovine pregnancy.
- In pigs, azaperone administered by deep intramuscular injection at a dose rate of 1–2 mg/kg will provide effective sedation some 20 minutes after administration.
- An auriculopalpebral nerve block can be given, if required, once the animal is sedated. In cattle, some 10–15 ml of lignocaine 2% is injected beneath the fascia at approximately the highest point of the dorsal border of the zygomatic arch and in front of the base of the ear.
- Application of topical local anaesthetic will be needed if the eye is painful, as the auriculopalpebral nerve block is motor and not sensory.

FARM ANIMAL OPHTHALMOLOGY

FARM ANIMAL OPHTHALMOLOGY

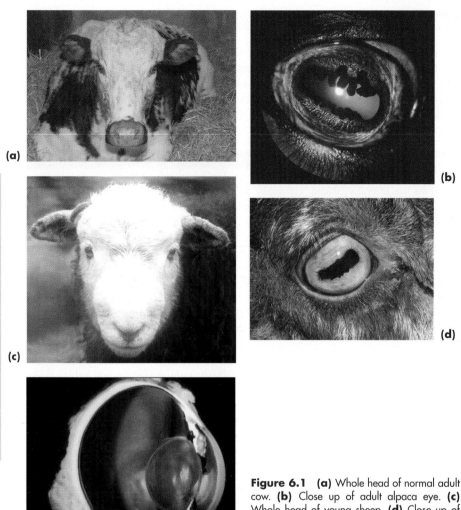

Figure 6.1 **(a)** Whole head of normal adult cow. **(b)** Close up of adult alpaca eye. **(c)** Whole head of young sheep. **(d)** Close up of the eye of an adult sheep. **(e)** Cross-section of the globe of a normal sheep (with acknowledgements to J.R.B Mould for illustration of the globe).

History and ophthalmic examination

As with other species, careful history-taking is essential and should include details of previous or present drug therapy, nutrition, including feed supplements, and the animal's normal environment. Any potential exposure to poisons or toxins should be investigated. The animal should be observed unrestrained in its normal environment initially and note taken of its body condition, size for age, posture and coordination.

Examination of the eyes and their adnexa follows the usual protocol. Assessment of ocular abnormalities are rendered simpler if normal species variations are recognised and understood (Figure 6.1a–e).

- The complete bony orbital rim should be palpated as part of ocular examination
- The direction of the well developed upper eyelid lashes should be noted, to aid identification of exophthalmos or enophthalmos
- Constriction of the pupil in response to a bright light stimulus is slower than that of the dog and cat

Common and important farm animal ocular and adnexal conditions

The common farm animal ocular and adnexal conditions and those that are important to recognise because of the serious implications of misdiagnosis are summarised in Box 6.1.

Some of these conditions are important because of the financial implications of disease, particularly so when there is herd or flock involvement. Unfortunately, the harsh economics of many commercial enterprises means that management decisions are frequently made on purely economic grounds, but veterinary surgeons must also be aware of the welfare implications of such decisions.

Nutritional deficiencies – and excesses – including those of trace elements, are commoner in production animals than other domestic species, and ocular manifestations are one aspect of such variations. They may be seen in progeny born of affected mothers and in animals that become affected later in life. It is important to ask about husbandry practices in any investigation of production animal disease, especially when a number of animals are affected. Flock and herd problems tend to be of infectious, nutritional, toxic or environmental origin. Hereditary factors may also be of importance when groups of animals are affected.

FARM ANIMAL OPHTHALMOLOGY

Box 6.1   Common and important farm animal ocular and adnexal conditions

- Ocular and adnexal trauma in most farm animal species, pigs seem least likely to suffer traumatic damage.
- Neoplasia, particularly squamous cell carcinoma and lymphoma (all farm animal species, particularly cattle).
- Multiple ocular defects associated with nutrition, toxins and teratogens (e.g. bovine virus diarrhoea in cattle).
- Entropion (lambs) and a variety of eyelid defects in some breeds of overweight pet pig (e.g. Vietnamese pot bellied pig).
- Infectious keratoconjunctivitis (cattle, sheep and goats).
- Cataract (congenital nuclear cataract in cattle is commonest).
- Uveitis from a variety of causes (in all farm animal species).
- Blindness from a variety of nutritional (e.g. hypovitaminosis A, in cattle and piglets), toxic (e.g. lead in all farm animal species, bracken in sheep), metabolic (e.g. pregnancy toxaemia in sheep and ketosis in cattle) and generalised diseases.

CONGENITAL AND EARLY-ONSET DEVELOPMENTAL CONDITIONS

Ocular congenital and early-onset defects have been recorded in all farm animal species. The most important economically are entropion in *lambs*, some forms of cataract in *cattle* and defects associated with teratogens, of which the most notable is bovine virus diarrhoea.

Other neonatal diseases of infectious origin in *ruminants* (e.g. blue tongue virus and *Listeria monocytogenes*) may also present with ocular manifestations.

Rare developmental conditions that are not discussed further include lysosomal storage diseases (e.g. ceroid lipofuscinosis, globoid cell leukodystrophy, gangliosidosis, mannosidosis) in *ruminants*.

Globe abnormalities – anophthalmos, cystic eye and microphthalmos
(Figures 6.2 and 6.3)
- Rare, but described in *all* farm animals
- The cause is often impossible to determine, but infectious, toxic, nutritional, environmental and inherited factors should be considered
- May be unilateral or bilateral, occurring as isolated ocular defects or in conjunction with defects elsewhere (e.g. muscular dystrophy and hydrocephalus in Hereford *cattle* and blue tongue virus, usually in *sheep*)

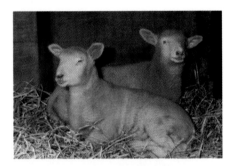

Figure 6.2 Bilateral cystic eyes in twins. The cause was unknown.

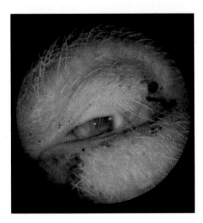

Figure 6.3 Microphthalmos in a piglet due to maternal vitamin A deficiency. The other piglets in the litter were also affected.

Bovine virus diarrhoea (BVD) and ocular abnormality

- The pestivirus which causes the bovine virus diarrhoea–mucosal disease complex (BVD-MD) has a worldwide distribution.
- Persistently-infected *cattle* are the major source of transmission, as they shed large amounts of virus throughout life, but acutely-infected cattle are also an important source of BVD-MD virus transmission.
- The developing foetus can be infected transplacentally in either acutely-infected or persistently-infected cattle.
- BVD virus is a common cause of ocular insult to the developing eye and produces a range of defects in *calves* when the mother is infected (Figure 6.4(a,b)). The ocular manifestations depend upon the age at which the foetus is infected, with the developing eye being most susceptible to infection at about 150 days of gestation. Persistent infection occurs when there is *in utero* exposure of the foetus to BVD virus earlier than at 125 days of gestation.
- The teratogenic insult coincides with immune-system development, so that there is also an inflammatory response to infection. Many of the fundus changes observed in young calves are a consequence of inflammation and post-necrotic scarring (e.g. retinal degeneration after *in utero* chorioretinitis and optic atrophy after *in utero* optic neuritis).
- Acute BVD virus infections may result in immunosuppression.
- BVD should always be considered as a likely diagnosis for any congenital ocular lesion in cattle (e.g. blindness, nystagmus, microphthalmos, corneal lesions, persistent pupillary membrane, cataracts, retinal dysplasia, retinal degeneration, optic atrophy).
- As the foetus is infected during the final stages of nervous-system development, affected calves may also have hydrocephalus, hypomyelinogenesis and cerebellar hypoplasia and consequent gross ataxia. Other likely changes include skeletal defects, hypotrichosis and retarded growth.
- Pre-colostral serum samples from calves are diagnostic when they show titres to BVD virus.

FARM ANIMAL OPHTHALMOLOGY

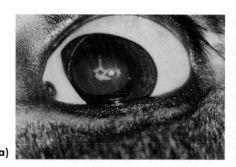

(a)

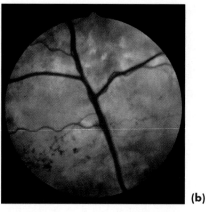

(b)

Figure 6.4 (a) Multiple ocular anomalies in a calf, associated with the teratogenic effects of BVD-MD. Both eyes were affected. The left eye (pictured here) is microphthalmic (note the large amount of exposed 'white' of the eye and slight prominence of the third eyelid). Persistent pupillary membrane remnants are present and there is a dense focal cataract where they are in contact with the anterior lens capsule. **(b)** The fundi of both eyes were also abnormal. That of the right eye is illustrated and shows marked attenuation of the retinal vessels and retinal hyperreflectivity.

Progressive exophthalmos and strabismus

In *cattle*, particularly, there are a number of rare abnormalities, some with a genetic basis, that are associated with progressive exophthalmos and strabismus (both convergent squint – *esotropia* – and divergent squint – *exotropia*). There is no treatment and animals will effectively become blind if the strabismus is severe enough.

Dermoid

Dermoids occur in all species, and in *farm animals* can arise from various sites (cornea, conjunctiva and eyelids) as isolated ocular defects, or in association with other diseases (e.g. BVD).

Eyelid coloboma

Colobomatous defects of the eyelid (usually upper eyelid) may be inherited in Jacob and Manx *sheep* and is seen most often in those with four horns (Figure 6.5(a)).

Treatment

The eyelid should be reconstructed to avoid exposure keratopathy, most simply by freshening the edges of the defect with a deep V-shaped incision (Figure 6.5(b)). The full-thickness wound created is closed with a single layer of sutures, commencing at the eyelid margin, using a figure of eight suture or a simple interrupted suture pattern.

FARM ANIMAL OPHTHALMOLOGY

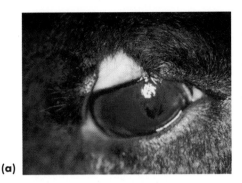 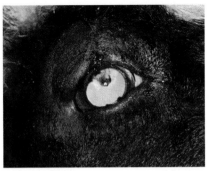

(a) **(b)**

Figure 6.5 (a) Upper eyelid coloboma in a Jacob sheep. Note the exposure keratopathy and frank vascular and pigmentary keratitis in the area of cornea devoid of eyelid protection. **(b)** Appearance following repair utilising a deep, full-thickness, V-shaped incision and primary closure with 4-0 silk. The keratitis soon resolved following surgery and retroillumination highlights a number of corneal ghost vessels.

Entropion

Entropion may be inherited as a polygenic trait in certain breeds of *sheep*, usually affecting the lower eyelid of one or both eyes from birth or soon afterwards, although it is often not detected until the lamb shows signs of ocular pain as a consequence of keratitis. Untreated severe cases usually progress to corneal ulceration with additional secondary spastic entropion. Bilaterally affected animals can go blind, if the condition goes undiagnosed, due to complications such as corneal granulation tissue, corneal perforation and endophthalmitis. Blind lambs may die of starvation.

- In some Piebald *sheep*, the upper eyelid is notched and ectropion is present at the notch with entropion to either side
- Entropion can be inherited in miniature *pigs*. The upper eyelids of neonatal animals are affected, and treatment is not usually needed
- Anatomical entropion is also seen in breeds such as the Vietnamese pot-bellied pig and these cases may require surgical correction (usually Hotz-Celsus technique) and strict weight control
- Previous injury is a common reason for secondary (cicatricial) entropion in all species

Management of entropion in sheep

Lambs with entropion should not form part of the future breeding flock, and rams that produce affected lambs should not be kept for breeding. For primary entropion in lambs there are many treatment techniques available. The method to select is the one that is simple, cost effective and curative. Dry the eyelids carefully first whichever treatment option is selected.

Manual eversion

Manual eversion can work in mild cases and may need to be combined with manual pinching.

- After drying the eyelids, a fold of lower-eyelid skin, close to the eyelid margin and sufficient to correct the entropion, is taken between finger and thumb and pressed briefly and firmly

- Lambs appear unconcerned by this manoeuvre
- This squeezing technique can be repeated in several other sites parallel to the eyelid margin
- The mild swelling that this provokes is often sufficient to break the vicious cycle of lower eyelid inversion
- The shepherd can carry out this technique

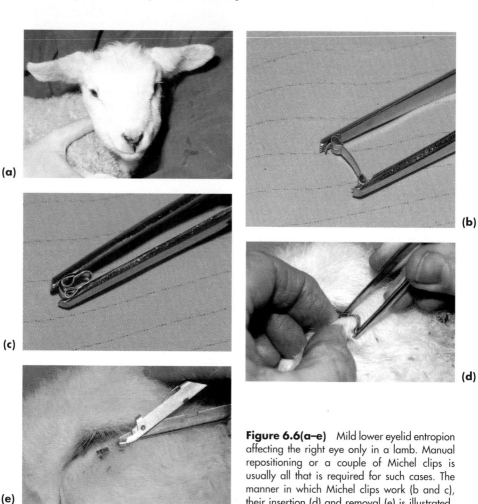

(a)

(b)

(c)

(d)

(e)

Figure 6.6(a–e) Mild lower eyelid entropion affecting the right eye only in a lamb. Manual repositioning or a couple of Michel clips is usually all that is required for such cases. The manner in which Michel clips work (b and c), their insertion (d) and removal (e) is illustrated.

Michel clips

Some 2–4 Michel clips (e.g. 14 × 3 mm size) can be inserted approximately 3–5 mm below and parallel to the eyelid margin, in order to evert the eyelid (Figure 6.6(b,c,d,e).

- A fold of skin is tented up between thumb and forefinger, or, occasionally, with tissue forceps in very small lambs, and the clips inserted with Michel forceps
- This method is probably the quickest and arguably the most economical for those cases that do not respond to simple eyelid drying and eversion ± squeezing

- The clips are usually left *in situ*, as the majority fall out naturally within a week or so; they can also be removed, if necessary, using the clip remover provided

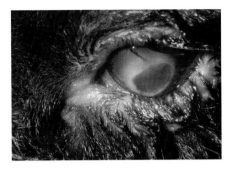

Figure 6.7 Severe lower eyelid entropion. The whole of the lower eyelid is involved and secondary corneal damage has occurred. Michel clips are the quickest means of restoring normal eyelid congruity in such cases.

Retention sutures

It is relatively easy to insert 2–4 temporary retention sutures (e.g. vertical mattress sutures) through the intact skin of the affected eyelid to evert the eyelid margin in the same position and manner outlined for Michel clips, but it is difficult to maintain cleanliness if large numbers are involved. One large horizontal mattress suture is a quicker, but less aesthetically pleasing, alternative.

Adhesive

Various types of impact adhesive applied to the skin to create the effect achieved by Michel clips or skin sutures can also be effective, but it is obvious that such adhesives must be applied with precision and the technique is more time consuming.

Injection into the eyelid

Many veterinary surgeons favour the use of antibiotic preparations or, occasionally, air, injected into the eyelid, most easily via the palpebral conjunctiva. It is difficult to maintain cleanliness if many lambs are involved, and it is slower, and therefore potentially less cost effective, than Michel clips.

A one-inch, 18–20 gauge needle is inserted through the lateral aspect of the palpebral conjunctiva of the lower eyelid and pushed medially. Antibiotic (1 ml) or air is injected as the needle is slowly withdrawn. The use of liquid paraffin is not recommended as it provokes a persistent granulomatous response.

Surgery

Non-responsive congenital entropion and acquired types of entropion may require the standard skin–muscle resection techniques already described in Sections 2 and 3, or other blepharoplastic surgery according to cause, extent, use and value of the animal.

Cataract

- Congenital cataracts are commonest in *cattle*, but have also been reported in *sheep* and *goats*
- Congenital cataracts may be associated with BVD infection in *calves* (usually cortical)
- Congenital, bilateral, progressive cataracts, possibly hereditary, in Holstein–Friesian, Hereford and Jersey *cattle*

Optic nerve coloboma
Typical colobomas of the papillary and peripapillary region are inherited and common in Charolais *cattle*.

GLOBE AND ORBIT

Exophthalmos
- In all farm animal species, exophthalmos may be a consequence of a space-occupying lesion in the orbit or periorbita. Acquired exophthalmos should be differentiated from the progressive developmental exophthalmos described earlier.
- Examples of possible causes include tooth abscess, maxillary cysts, sinusitis (sinusitis can be a complication of dehorning), granulomatous infections, pituitary abscess, neoplasia (squamous cell carcinoma and lymphoma).

Orbital neoplasia
- Investigations include careful examination to determine whether the mass is of primary (e.g. squamous cell carcinoma) or secondary (e.g. lymphoma) origin.
- Lymphoma is the commonest secondary tumour in farm animals, particularly *cattle*, and the orbit is the predilection site (Figure 6.8). Chemosis may be part of the presentation (probably because of impeded venous drainage from the orbit) and gross conjunctival thickening is a consequence of neoplastic infiltration.

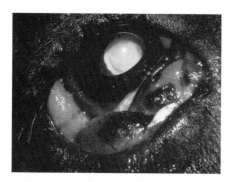

Figure 6.8 Orbital lymphoma in a Friesian cow. A grass seed is adherent to the desiccated, tumour-infiltrated, palpebral conjunctiva. This animal also has bilateral nuclear cataracts.

EYELIDS

Causes of third eyelid (nictitating membrane) prominence
- Orbital, para-orbital or retro-orbital space-occupying lesions
- Inflammation (e.g. solar-induced) of the conjunctiva of the third eyelid
- Pain
- Neoplasia, most commonly squamous cell carcinoma (treat by local resection or third eyelid removal) or lymphoma (not usually treated, affected animals are sent for slaughter)
- *Phthisis bulbi*
- Tetanus is associated with bilateral involvement, usually as a rapid and intermittent protrusion

Upper and lower eyelid neoplasia

Squamous cell carcinoma (eyelids, conjunctiva, limbus, cornea) is the commonest primary neoplasm of *cattle*, especially Hereford cattle in countries with a high incidence of sunlight (Figure 6.9(a,b)). Affected animals are at least four years of age, usually seven to nine years. It is rarer, but still the commonest eyelid tumour, in *sheep*. Solar-induced inflammation may precede neoplastic changes in those animals that are 'at risk' because they lack protective pigment.

Papillomas are sometimes encountered in young *cattle* and *sheep*. They are of viral origin and may disappear with age. Although trauma can be associated with spread, papillomas are usually self-limiting, so treatment is not normally required.

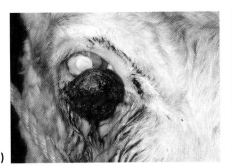

(a)

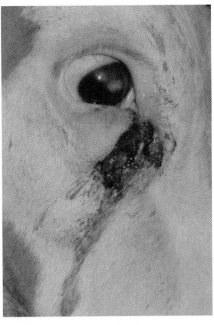

(b)

FARM ANIMAL OPHTHALMOLOGY

Figure 6.9 (a) Periocular squamous cell carcinoma (SCC) in a Hereford cow. SCC in this region may be of rapid and invasive growth and the history is often a good guide to prognosis. In this case, the prognosis was adjudged to be poor because of the rapid growth of the tumour (from commencement to presentation in approximately 15 days). This animal was pregnant, but because the tumour was causing corneal damage and pain it was felt necessary to intervene on welfare grounds. The tumour was debulked under local infiltration anaesthesia. **(b)** The corneal damage healed rapidly, but tumour regrowth occurred within a month.

Management

Squamous cell carcinoma (SCC) can usually be treated by local radiotherapy or surgical debulking, combined with cryotherapy or radiotherapy (see Section 7, pp 294–306). Complex cases may require referral. Occasionally, highly-malignant squamous cell carcinomas, especially those involving the periocular skin, with a rapid growth pattern and potential for spread are seen in cattle. The growth rate, size and position of the lesion, as well as the value of the animal, will determine the correct approach.

FARM ANIMAL OPHTHALMOLOGY

LACRIMAL SYSTEM

Investigative procedures are as for small animals, except that in cattle the nasal ostium is usually visible and accessible and so is used in preference to the lacrimal puncta for cannulation and retrograde irrigation. Normal STT I in *cattle* is at least 20–30 mm per minute.

Problems of tear production and drainage are very rare. In the very unlikely event of KCS, parotid duct transposition should not be contemplated in ruminants as they secrete saliva continuously.

CONJUNCTIVA

Conjunctivitis
Causes include allergies, viruses (infectious bovine rhinotracheitis), bacteria (*Moraxella bovis*) and parasites (*Thelazia* spp).

Infectious bovine rhinotracheitis (IBR)
- The main ocular manifestation of IBR in *cattle* is conjunctivitis, which may be unilateral or bilateral
- Conjunctival form of IBR can occur as a herd disease with or without respiratory infection
- Typified by excessive lacrimation initially, progressing to copious mucopurulent discharge
- Affected cattle do not usually exhibit blepharospasm or photophobia, but chemosis and conjunctival hyperaemia ± petechiation can be marked
- Multiple, small, focal, white plaques may develop on the conjunctiva within two weeks of the onset of clinical signs; Peripheral corneal involvement is rare
- Most cases resolve in 2–3 weeks and do not require treatment, although topical antibiotic can be given to prevent secondary bacterial infection

Differential diagnosis of IBR and other causes of keratoconjunctivitis
- Classical IBR can be distinguished from *infections bovine keratoconjunctivitis* (IBKC) by the lack of central corneal involvement, however, both conditions can occur concurrently with more severe and extensive ocular manifestations.
- IBR is easily differentiated from *malignant catarrhal fever* in which severe anterior uveitis is the predominant early ocular sign, and generalised vasculitis contributes substantially to the clinical presentation.
- *Listeriosis* may be associated with keratoconjunctivitis in ruminants and is usually readily distinguished from other causes because of the accompanying neorological signs.

Infectious bovine keratoconjunctivitis (IBKC) (New Forest Eye)
IBKC (New Forest Eye or pink eye) affects *cattle* and is the most important ocular cause of suffering and economic loss in this species.

Aetiology
- *Moraxella bovis* (a Gram-ve bacillus) is the pathogen most commonly isolated from clinical cases

- Piliated strains are associated with clinical disease, as they can adhere to the corneal surface
- Haemolytic strains are more likely to be isolated from clinical cases
- Pathogenic strains of *Moraxella bovis* are able to invade an intact cornea, although the mechanism whereby this is achieved is unknown
- Some strains of *M. bovis* may release factors that encourage the detachment of epithelial cells and there may even be a direct cytotoxic effect on corneal epithelial cells

Pathogenesis

- The condition is commonest in young animals at pasture in summer, but in susceptible herds cattle of any age and under a wide variety of management systems can be affected
- The infection is highly contagious and is spread by direct contact, ocular and nasal discharges and mechanical factors such as flies (e.g. *Musca autumnalis*, *Musca domestica*, *Stomoxys calcitrans*)
- Flies cause local mechanical irritation, and the organism may survive on their legs for several days. *M. autumnalis* is the most important insect vector
- Stocking density is an important factor in the spread of disease
- Incidence varies from year to year, but spread within a group is very rapid and morbidity can be as high as 80%
- Although some recovered animals develop protective immunity, subclinical carriers are a problem. In such cases *M. bovis* can be isolated from ocular and nasal discharges throughout the year
- In some herds the infection becomes endemic

Other factors that may contribute to the pathogenesis of disease

- Environmental factors, such as flies, dust, ultraviolet radiation, geographical location, season and climate
- Systemic factors, such as breed, age, immune status and the effects of stress
- Concurrent pathogens (e.g. infectious bovine rhinotracheitis virus and possibly *Mycoplasma* spp)
- Vaccination with modified, live IBR virus will also place animals at greater risk of IBKC, and the ocular signs in affected animals are more severe
- Local ocular factors, such as superficial trauma and the amount of ocular pigment may also be of relevance

Clinical signs

- Affected animals are commonly inappetent and dull
- Usually one eye is affected initially, but infection will often spread to the other eye so that ocular signs may be unilateral or bilateral
- Typically there are pain, blepharospasm, photophobia and excessive lacrimation
- A serous or mucopurulent discharge develops later in the time course of disease
- Conjunctivitis (hyperaemia and chemosis) and keratitis (tiny superficial vesicles and corneal oedema) are relatively early clinical features; there are sometimes also eyelid oedema and blepharitis
- A greyish-white, centrally-located corneal opacity develops, usually within 2–4 days of the initial signs of discomfort, followed by corneal necrosis (white or yellow in appearance) and central corneal ulceration (Figure 6.10(a))

FARM ANIMAL OPHTHALMOLOGY

- Ulcerative changes may be confined to one eye
- The extent and depth of corneal vascularisation depends upon the age of the lesion and the extent of corneal involvement
- Despite the spectacular appearance, the cornea heals with minimal scarring in most cases over some 2–3 weeks, but when there has been stromal involvement and more serious ulceration, dense axial corneal scarring can persist (Figure 6.10(b))
- Unusual sequelae, usually as a complication of globe rupture, include blindness, endophthalmitis, panophthalmitis and even death, because of ascending infection to the central nervous system
- The time course and extent of ocular involvement is variable, for example the condition can follow a more protracted and severe course (some 2–3 months) in younger animals
- Some cattle become carriers and show no clinical signs, or there may be intermittent or more persistent excessive lacrimation in such animals
- Reasonable protective immunity follows infection

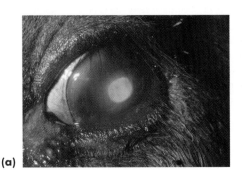 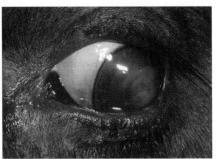

(a)   (b)

Figure 6.10 **(a)** Infectious bovine keratoconjunctivitis in a Friesian heifer. Some 30% of the herd were affected at the time of examination. Note the cellular infiltration of the central cornea (associated with corneal necrosis). There is also mild conjunctival hyperaemia, perilimbal oedema, fine corneal neovascularisation and peripheral cellular infiltration. **(b)** Within a few days of treatment, corneal healing is progressing well.

Preventative measures
It is impossible to eliminate the organism, so most measures seek to prevent clinical disease.
- Cull carrier animals
- Regular inspection of animals and their immediate isolation in the event of identification of disease is crucial
- Stringent measures should be taken to control flies
- Adequate feed space should be provided
- Other factors such as the reduction of stress (e.g. avoidance of long journeys) may reduce the potential for disease transmission
- Vaccination is not yet an effective means of preventing clinical disease

Management
Affected animals should be isolated to limit spread and shade should be provided.

Topical treatment

Topical benzathine cloxacillin ointment or cephalonium ointment both give effective therapeutic levels for 24–48 hours, and one or other is the treatment of choice in the UK. One or two treatments are effective. Other effective topical antibiotics include tetracyclines, gentamicin and first-generation cephalosporins.

Subconjunctival injections

Subconjunctival injections are painful for the animal and difficult to administer in the correct site (beneath the bulbar conjunctiva) in a clean fashion to multiple animals. The uptake of antibiotic, and therefore the therapeutic levels achieved, are quite variable, although tear-film concentrations of antibiotic may be adequate. Injections beneath the conjunctiva of the eyelids may not achieve therapeutic levels, as the blood flow tends to be away from the eye. Bulbar subconjunctival procaine penicillin given once daily for three days has been claimed to be an effective treatment for dairy cattle.

Parenteral treatment

Parenterally administered antibiotics are also effective, but the potential disadvantage of this route is the meat and milk withdrawal period. In commercial beef animals not close to slaughter, intramuscular long-acting tetracycline (20 mg/kg, two doses, 72 hours apart) is probably the drug of choice. In dairy herds, procaine penicillin is more likely to be used as the milk withdrawal time for this drug is only three days. The withdrawal period provisions may not apply to non-commercial enterprises.

Other

In severe cases corneal protection (e.g. temporary tarsorrhaphy) should be provided. Enucleation is rarely required.

Infectious ovine keratoconjunctivitis (IOKC)

IOKC (pink eye) occurs in sheep and goats throughout the world and affects animals of all ages, although adults are usually the most severely affected. *Mycoplasma* spp (most frequent isolate) and *Chlamydophila* spp (next most frequent isolate) are thought to be primary pathogens. Other bacteria may be involved, but it is likely that they play a secondary role.

Aetiology

- *Mycoplasma* spp (*M. conjunctivae* var *ovis* and *M. mycoides* var *capri*)
- *Chlamydophila* (formerly *Chlamydia*) spp (*C. psittaci* group)
- Aerobic bacteria (*Branhamella ovis*, *Escherichia coli* and *Staphylococcus aureus*).

Pathogenesis

- Infection is usually introduced into a flock by mildly-infected or carrier animals
- Spread within the flock is more likely when the animals are in close proximity (e.g. when gathered, housed, penned, fed or transported)
- Outbreaks occur at all times of year, but are usually seen in winter and early spring in the UK because of the increased crowding associated with, for example, supplementary feeding and lambing
- Ultraviolet light may be an exacerbating factor, as cases tend to be more severely affected during the summer

- Post-infection immunity after chlamydophiliosis is poor, and some animals can become infected repeatedly; immunity after mycoplasmosis seems to be rather better
- Carriers can pose a problem as both *Mycoplasma* and *Chlamydophila* can be isolated from the eyes after apparent recovery. Mycoplasma organisms show greater persistence and some previously-infected animals can provide a source of infection the following year
- Relapse can occur after *Mycoplasma* and *Chlamydophila* infection in both naturally-recovered and treated animals

Ocular signs

The ocular signs are similar, irrespective of the causal agent. Resolution can occur after any of the stages outlined and treatment tends to diminish the severity of the clinical signs and shorten the time-course of disease (Figures 6.11(a,b,c) and 6.12(a,b)).
- Initially there are pain, blepharospasm, increased lacrimation and conjunctival hyperaemia, first in one eye and then, within a few days, in both eyes
- Corneal oedema develops and new blood vessels enter the cornea from the limbus; vascularisation is usually first apparent in the dorsal cornea and both superficial and deep vessels can be distinguished.
- The ocular discharge becomes more serous
- The serous discharge becomes more purulent, cellular infiltration and microabscesses may become apparent in the cornea and corneal ulceration can develop
- Conjunctival lymphoid follicular hyperplasia is common in established infection.
- Frank corneal abscessation ± hypopyon and iritis may be found in some severe cases.
- Complications are rare and include blindness, permanent corneal opacities and scarring, endophthalmitis and *phthisis bulbi*

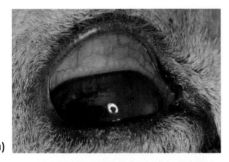

(a)

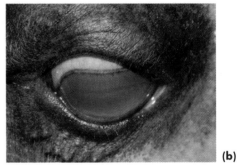

(b)

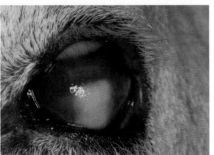

(c)

Figure 6.11(a–c) Infectious ovine kerato-conjunctivitis affecting a high proportion of a flock of crossbred ewes at the time of examination. Three are illustrated. In (a), the predominant findings on ophthalmic examination were conjunctival hyperaemia and perilimbal corneal oedema with some vascularisation, particularly dorsally. In (b), peripheral corneal vascularisation is prominent and in (c) there is also marked cellular infiltration of the cornea.

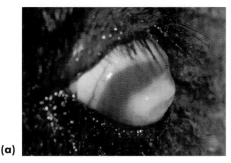
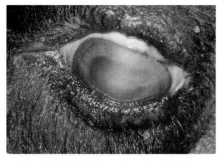

(a)   **(b)**

Figure 6.12 **(a)** Infectious ovine keratoconjunctivitis associated with frank corneal abscessation. There is also a change of corneal profile. **(b)** Temporary tarsorrhaphy was performed and corneal healing was progressing well when the tarsorrhaphy was taken down ten days later.

Diagnosis

Diagnosis is based on clinical signs and laboratory samples, which should be taken early in the course of disease. Only samples taken from the conjunctival sac are listed.

- Swabs and scrapes should be taken into mycoplasma transport medium, chlamydial and viral transport medium and Stuart's transport medium for bacteriology
- Culture of *Mycoplasma* requires special media, whereas culture of *Chlamydophila* is slightly easier and culture of other bacteria is straight forward
- Experimental work identifying these organisms by polymerase chain reaction (PCR) offers the possibility of rapid and specific diagnosis
- Giemsa staining can be used to detect *Mycoplasma* and *Chlamydophila* in smears and scrapes, but it is easy to confuse intracytoplasmic inclusion bodies and melanin granules, so fluorescent antibody tests with specific antisera are more accurate.

Treatment

- Affected animals should be isolated to limit the spread of disease, and treated affected animals should be separated from untreated ones
- If the problem is severe and widespread, the whole flock should be treated
- Although in many cases the ocular signs associated with *Mycoplasma* and *Chlamydophila* are self-limiting, it is usual to shorten the time course of disease by treating affected animals and to consider prophylactic treatment for others at risk
- Adults and weaned stock can be treated with a single intramuscular injection of long-acting oxytetracycline (10–20 mg/kg body weight). The higher dose can be used prophylactically at 48–72 hour intervals
- Local treatment poses difficulties, as topical ophthalmic tetracycline ointment is no longer available. Topical powders (contain local anaesthetic) or intramammary preparations (contain corticosteroids) do not provide suitable alternative choices and there are no ideal antibiotics for subconjunctival use
- Recovery usually starts within 3–4 days and is complete within a week *with* treatment and rather longer than this *without* treatment
- Although medical treatment produces a good clinical response within days, it does not eliminate either *M. conjunctivae* or *Chlamydophila*

FARM ANIMAL OPHTHALMOLOGY

CORNEA

For IBKC in *cattle* and IOKC in *sheep* and *goats* see pp 252–257. Ulcerative keratitis is usually of infectious or traumatic origin (Figure 6.13).

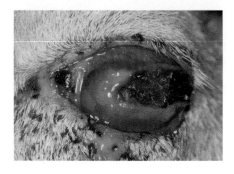

Figure 6.13 Severe keratitis in a ram following chronic traumatic damage from the animal's own misdirected horn. The horn had grown too close to the eye and was removed prior to photography.

UVEAL TRACT

Neonatal uveitis
Neonatal uveitis (Figure 6.14) may be associated with, for example, umbilical infection (navel-ill), pneumonia and septicaemia in all farm animals.

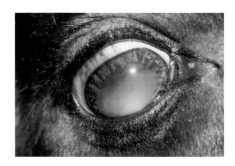

Figure 6.14 Neonatal uveitis associated with navel-ill in a calf. Mild hypopyon is the most obvious feature and the eye is reasonably comfortable. Although topical symptomatic treatment for uveitis is usually given, the systemic treatment of the underlying cause is the most important aspect of management in resolution of the ocular signs.

Acquired uveitis
Uveitis may be associated with trauma, severe keratoconjunctivitis and keratitis, toxins, immune-mediated and generalised disease, including neoplasia (e.g. lymphoma). As in other species, the uveitis is termed idiopathic when a precise aetiology cannot be determined.

Malignant catarrhal fever
- Malignant catarrhal fever is a high mortality, low morbidity, pansystemic vasculopathy of ruminants caused by a herpes virus
- The virus affects all epithelial surfaces as well as vascular endothelium
- Pyrexia, generalised lymphadenopathy, oral erosions, mucopurulent nasal discharge, diarrhoea, lameness and encephalitis are possible systemic features in *cattle*

- Ocular manifestations include keratoconjunctivitis, uveitis and dense corneal oedema (Figure 6.15(a,b,c))
- Treatment of severely-affected animals is not usually attempted, as it is not particularly successful
- Animals with severe disease usually die; those with mild disease may survive

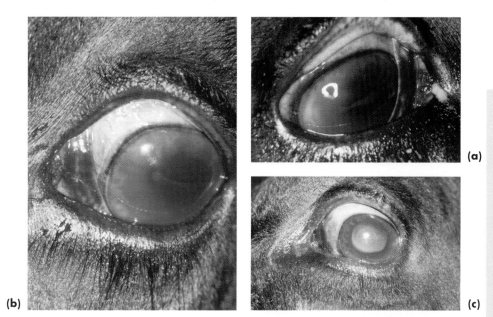

(a)

(b)

(c)

Figure 6.15 (a,b) Uveitis associated with malignant catarrhal fever in a Friesian steer. Note the intense pupillary constriction and loss of iris detail (right [a] and left [b] eyes). Corneal changes include peripheral cellular infiltration and vascularisation as well as mild corneal oedema. When viewed from the side the anterior chamber was relatively shallow because of the swollen, inflamed iris. **(c)** The left eye is shown after topical treatment with atropine and prednisolone acetate, which produced considerable symptomatic relief.

Listeriosis
- The feeding of silage (especially big bale) has been associated with uveitis (usually unilateral presentation) in *cattle* and *sheep*
- Affected animals should be taken off silage
- In neonates, listeriosis is most likely to be associated with encephalitis or septicaemia and infection is acquired from the mother's milk
- Note that when listeriosis affects the nervous system of *ruminants* (notably cattle, sheep and goats), the ocular manifestations include nystagmus, blindness, facial paresis or paralysis (upper eyelid ptosis) and strabismus (usually medial and on the same side as involvement of the abducens nucleus)

Thromboembolic meningoencephalitis
- Infectious thromboembolic meningoencephalitis (TEME) is a septicaemia caused by the Gram-ve bacterium *Haemophilus somnus* in young *cattle* (commonest at less than one year of age)

- Of economic significance in the USA and Canada, but is apparently rare in the UK
- Ocular manifestations include conjunctivitis, retinitis (thrombosis of retinal vessels) and chorioretinitis
- Anterior segment involvement is less common

Other infectious causes of uveitis
- *Toxoplasmosis* can be a cause of uveitis and retinitis in *sheep*
- Uveitis may be associated with *leptospirosis* and bovine *tuberculosis* in *cattle*
- Uveitis may also be seen as part of the clinical presentation in adult animals with *septic foci and septicaemia* (e.g. mastitis, metritis, traumatic reticuloperitonitis and reticulopericarditis)

Signs of acute anterior uveitis
- Pain, blepharospasm, lacrimation (anterior segment triad)
- Photophobia
- Hypotony, corneal vascularisation, corneal oedema, anterior chamber infiltration, miosis, loss of iris detail and early synechiae formation

Signs of chronic anterior uveitis
Synechiae, darkening of iris, fixed, irregular pupil, iris rests, cataract, hydrophthalmos, and, sometimes, *phthisis bulbi* (Figure 6.16).

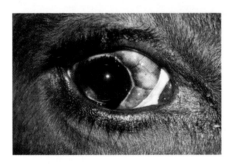

Figure 6.16 *Phthisis bulbi* following post-traumatic uveitis in a cow. Note that there is also prolapse of orbital fat.

Symptomatic treatment of anterior uveitis
- Topical corticosteroids, but avoid if corneal ulceration is present
- Topical mydriatics (1–4% atropine sulphate)
- Topical antibiotic (e.g. tetracycline)
- Intravenous or intramuscular long-acting tetracycline is useful as a first-choice antibiotic in silage-associated types, and may be effective in halting the development of uveitis if given early

LENS

Cataract
- Secondary to teratogens (e.g. BVD-MD virus), ill-defined insult (e.g. environmental factors), anterior uveitis and trauma
- Nutritional cataracts have been reported following use of the feed additive hygromycin B in *pigs*

OCULAR FUNDUS

ANATOMY

The *optic nerve head* is often myelinated and of variable shape and size in farm animals, and may be heavily pigmented in *sheep*. It is usually located within the non-tapetal fundus.

The *retinal blood supply* is holangiotic. The 3–4 primary retinal vessels are large and very distinct, and it is not unusual to find that the dorsal arteriole and venule spiral around each other. The small choroidal vessels (mainly capillaries) that perforate the tapetum en route for the choriocapillaris can be viewed ophthalmoscopically as distinct dark dots – the stars of Winslow.

The *tapetum* of *herbivores*, yellow, green or blue in colour, is formed from collagen (*tapetum fibrosum*) and this forms an effective barrier, so that in herbivores generally it is often easier to identify fundus pathology by examining the non-tapetal fundus. *Pigs* do not have a tapetum, and the fundus is a uniform light grey to red-brown colour in most pigs and of pinker appearance when less pigment is present.

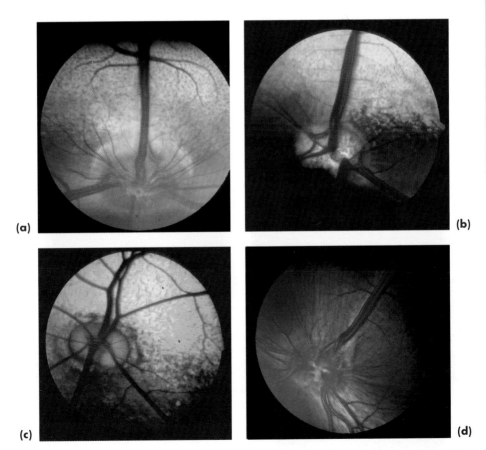

(a)   (b)   (c)   (d)

Figure 6.17(a–d) Normal bovine fundus (a), ovine fundus (b), caprine fundus (c) and camelid fundus (d).

FARM ANIMAL OPHTHALMOLOGY

ACQUIRED DISEASES INVOLVING THE FUNDUS

Infectious disease
- Tuberculosis (*Mycobacterium bovis*), malignant catarrhal fever, infectious thromboembolic meningoencephalitis – TEME (*Haemophilus somnus*), in cattle
- Blue tongue virus, Borna disease and scrapie in sheep
- Teschen disease and Aujeszky's disease in *pigs*

Nutritional and toxic disease
- *Hypovitaminosis A* (mainly *cattle*, *sheep* and *goats*)
  - Occurs because there is no access to pasture and deficiencies in compounded rations
  - In *cattle* associated with poor dark adaptation initially, then night blindness, then complete blindness if unrecognised (Figure 6.18(a,b,c))
  - There is raised intracranial pressure, stenosis of the optic canals, papilloedema and, eventually, retinal degeneration and optic atrophy
  - There may also be decreased corneal sensitivity as well as more generalised signs such as unsteadiness, diarrhoea, convulsions and fading hair colour
- *Bright blindness*, a retinopathy from consumption of bracken (*Pteridium aquilina*), in *sheep*
- *Rafoxanide* toxicity in *sheep* and *goats* (optic nerve damage)
- *Arsanilic acid* toxicity in *pigs* (demyelination and axonal degeneration of optic nerve and optic tract)

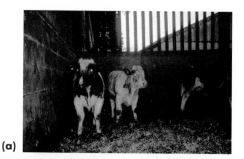

(a)

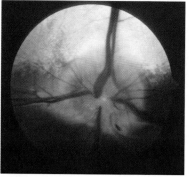

(b)

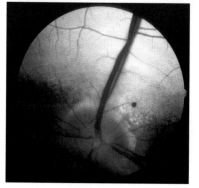

(c)

Figure 6.18 **(a)** Hypovitaminosis A in young bulls as a consequence of improper compounding of their rations. Note the widely-dilated pupils (photographed under daylight conditions in a covered yard). **(b)** Fundus examination revealed abnormalities in most of the group. Here there is a degree of papilloedema, peripapillary haemorrhage and subtle attenuation of the retinal vessels. **(c)** The vascular attenuation is more obvious here, and there is a degree of optic atrophy and a small haemorrhage between 1 and 2 o'clock.

SOME CAUSES OF CORTICAL BLINDNESS IN FARM ANIMALS

- Lead poisoning – most farm animals
- Thiamine deficiency (polioencephalomalacia or cerebrocortical necrosis) – most farm animals
- Ketosis in *cattle*
- Pregnancy toxaemia in *sheep*
- Hydatid disease (*Coenurus cerebralis*) in *sheep*
- Sodium toxicosis (salt poisoning) and water deprivation in *ruminants*
- Meningoencephalitis and encephalitis from any cause (e.g. TEME in *cattle*, listeriosis in *cattle*, *sheep* and *goats*, toxoplasmosis in *sheep*, sarcocystosis in *cattle*, *sheep* and *goats*)

SECTION 7
EQUINE OPHTHALMOLOGY

EQUINE OPHTHALMOLOGY

INTRODUCTION

The horse has laterally-placed eyes with large, panoramic, uniocular visual fields and small binocular visual fields (Figures 7.1(a–c) and 7.2(a,b)). As in all species with laterally placed eyes, there is a high percentage of crossover (some 85%) at the optic chiasma. The lateral positioning of the eyes enables the horse to have extensive panoramic vision, and the large eye, coupled with a large retinal surface area, produces a relative image size some 50% greater than that of the human eye. Visual acuity is less than that of humans, but greater than that of the dog and cat.

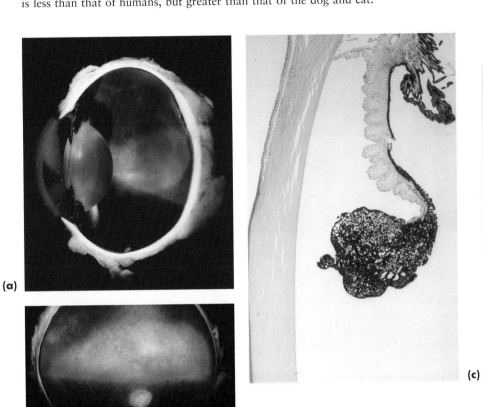

(a)

(b)

(c)

EQUINE OPHTHALMOLOGY

Figure 7.1(a–c) Normal gross equine globe (a); fundus (b); cornea and dorsal iris and *granula iridica* (c) (with acknowledgements to J. R. B. Mould).

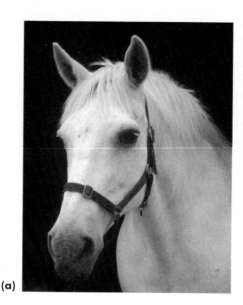

(a)

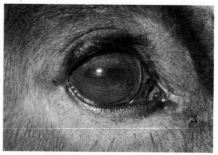

(b)

Figure 7.2 **(a)** Whole head of normal horse. **(b)** External eye of normal horse.

ANATOMY

- The supraorbital fossa and direction of the well-developed eyelashes on the upper eyelid should always be inspected as part of ocular examination. The supraorbital fossa should also be palpated.
- Obvious indentations, the dorsal and ventral orbital sulci, are apparent close to and parallel to the eyelid margins. A rounded prominence, the *lacrimal caruncle*, located in the medial canthus proximal to the third eyelid is an obvious feature of many horses; it may be pigmented or non-pigmented and usually bears fine hairs.
- The nasal palpebral aperture and cornea are wider medially than laterally and the pupil is horizontally oval.
- The grey lines that are such a striking feature of the medial and lateral cornea in some horses mark the insertion of the pectinate ligaments into the termination of the cornea at Descemet's membrane. The pectinate ligaments and entrance to the drainage angle can be directly observed in these regions.
- The commonest iris colour is dark brown, although heterochromia of the whole iris, or a sector of the iris, are common (this section, pp 294–295) and persistent pupillary membrane remnants are a very common finding (this section, p. 294). Colour dilution is associated with blue, cream or tan iris colour and there is usually focal or diffuse lack of stromal pigment as well as a relatively under-developed iris.
- The *granula iridica* are better developed on the dorsal pupillary border.
- Although the pupillary light response to a penlight is often somewhat slow and incomplete, the pupil responds briskly and completely when exposed to bright sunlight.

EQUINE OPHTHALMOLOGY

- The equine lens is large and may demonstrate a number of non-progressive minor aberrations. The lens suture lines are usually apparent: the anterior suture lines are usually in the shape of an upright Y, whereas the posterior suture lines may be in the form of an inverted Y or of stellate or sawhorse configuration. The tips of the suture lines sometimes have a somewhat feathered appearance. It is very common to be able to visualise the nuclear–cortical interface.
- As the eye is relatively large, some details of vitreal structure, such as the fibrillar condensations, are often quite clearly defined. For example, the anterior hyaloid face is readily visualised with a slit lamp and appears as an irregular, grey, veil-like structure just posterior to the posterior lens capsule. Hyaloid remnants persist to some four months of age in most foals.
- The fundus has a number of features of note – the retinal blood supply is paurangiotic, the optic nerve head is located within the non-tapetal fundus and two regions of higher visual acuity (approximating to the human macula) have been identified.

EXAMINATION

ASSESSMENT

The initial assessment is important and should include details of the horse's age, breed, coat colour and sex, plus family history and any previous illnesses, together with details of their treatment. The animal's lifestyle, management, performance and behaviour should also be recorded.

The nature of the present problem should be established, especially in relation to the clinical signs observed, including the rapidity of onset and whether there have been similar problems in the past. Any treatment that the animal has received should be documented, as should the response to treatment.

Ophthalmic examination is usually carried out in a loose box from which light has been excluded. Any stray light entering may complicate interpretation as the light reflects on the cornea and lens.

Proper handling is essential and a twitch is occasionally required. Sedation and analgesia will be needed on occasions, particularly if the eye is painful, but in most cases routine ophthalmic examination is performed without chemical restraint. Local nerve blocks, if needed, should be administered after systemic sedation has been given, although motor nerve blocks may be unnecessary after effective sedation.

Note that if the significance of any ophthalmic finding at a pre-purchase examination is not apparent, then referral should be considered.

SEDATION AND ANALGESIA

The drugs (Table 7.1) are given by slow intravenous injection, and additional, smaller doses can be given if deeper sedation is required. The horse should be left undisturbed to allow these drugs to take effect before proceeding to the next stage. Young foals should not be given injectable sedatives and analgesics.

EQUINE OPHTHALMOLOGY

Table 7.1 Sedation for ophthalmic examination

Purpose	Drug	Dosage
Sedation	Detomidine	up to 10 mcg/kg
	Romifidine	up to 50 mcg/kg
Profound sedation	Detomidine or romifidine	
	+ systemic analgesic, e.g. butorphanol	0.02–0.05 mg/kg

mcg = micrograms   mg = milligrams

LOCAL ANAESTHESIA

Topical anaesthesia (Figure 7.3)
- As an aid to examination of a painful eye and for diagnostic techniques such as corneal culture, conjunctival biopsy and cannulation of the lacrimal puncta or nasal ostium.
- Topical local anaesthetic can be administered directly from the single use ampoule or using a 1 ml hypodermic syringe to which the hub of a 23-gauge needle, from which the needle has been broken off, has been fitted.
- Proxymetacaine hydrochloride 0.5% drops are most commonly used to desensitise the ocular surface, and this agent produces excellent short-term analgesia of rapid onset.
- Amethocaine hydrochloride (tetracaine hydrochloride), 0.5% and 1%, provides an alternative when more profound anaesthesia is needed.

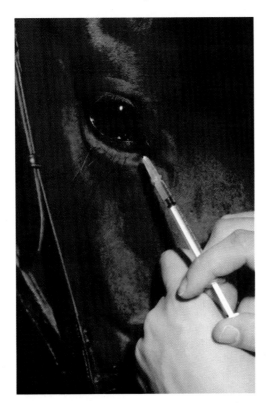

Figure 7.3 Application of topical anaesthesia using a 1 ml hypodermic syringe and 23-gauge needle hub with the needle broken off (with acknowledgements to R. C. Lowe).

EQUINE OPHTHALMOLOGY

Local infiltration anaesthesia

- Local infiltration of the eyelid is needed prior to placing a subpalpebral medication device (this section, pp 272–274)
- Local infiltration is also used prior to skin suture placement in the conscious horse
- Lignocaine hydrochloride (lidocaine hydrochloride) 1% or 2%, with adrenaline, and mepivacaine hydrochloride 2% are effective

Auriculopalpebral nerve block

- This motor-nerve block is of value when blepharospasm makes examination difficult and if there is any possibility that full-thickness rupture of the globe may be present. The auriculopalpebral nerve is a branch of the facial nerve.
- The sensory supply to the eye (ophthalmic division of the trigeminal nerve) is not affected by this block which is why topical local anaesthetic may also be required if there is ocular pain.
- The palpebral branch of the auriculopalpebral nerve can be blocked as it crosses the dorsal border of the zygomatic arch, immediately medial and slightly anterior to the highest point of the zygomatic arch and approximately halfway between the eye and the ear. A 5/8-inch 22- to 25-gauge needle and 2–3 ml of prilocaine hydrochloride 1% or mepivacaine hydrochloride 2% are used for this block.
- Alternatively, the auriculopalpebral nerve can be blocked just caudal to the ramus of the mandible, approximately one inch below its highest point (Figure 7.4). A one inch 22–23 gauge needle and 5–7 ml of prilocaine hydrochloride 1% or mepivacaine hydrochloride 2% are used for this block.

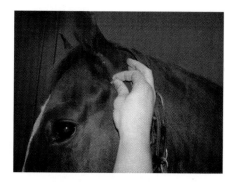

Figure 7.4 Administration of an auriculopalpebral nerve block (with acknowledgements to R. C. Lowe).

Supraorbital nerve block

- The supraorbital or frontal nerve is a branch of the ophthalmic division of the trigeminal nerve and supplies sensory innervation to the medial two thirds of the upper eyelid. The supraorbital foramen is located on the orbital rim in the supraorbital process of the frontal bone dorsal to the medial canthus of the eye.
- The supraorbital nerve block anaesthetises the upper eyelid and makes ophthalmic examination easier, as the animal cannot feel the manipulations of the eyelid.
- The nerve is blocked by injecting 3–5 ml of prilocaine hydrochloride 1% or mepivacaine hydrochloride 2% using a 5/8-inch 22- to 25-gauge needle placed in the region of the supraorbital foramen to a depth of no more than a quarter of an inch. There is no need to place the needle through the foramen as the globe is located not far beneath.

- Some motor paralysis of the facial nerve may also be produced, as there are palpebral branches at this site.
- The supraorbital block is useful for reducing blepharospasm and prior to minor eyelid surgery, including eyelid biopsies.

PRE-PURCHASE AND INSURANCE EXAMINATION

At examinations for purchase and insurance purposes, findings that may be difficult for non-specialists to interpret include opacities of the ocular media, especially those involving the cornea, lens or vitreous, iris variations including those affecting the *granula iridica* and normal and pathological alterations in the appearance of the ocular fundus. Many of the findings are normal variants – indeed this type of examination is usually conducted on the assumption that the eye will be normal. There is no doubt that, as in other species, examination of as many normal animals as possible is the best way of gaining confidence in interpreting the findings.

The intended use of the animal is obviously of relevance when purchase and insurance examination is carried out: for example, what is expected of an animal used for quiet hacking places quite different demands on the eye than those that would be required of a three-day eventer. It is always sensible to categorise changes identified at these examinations as anomalies or abnormalities of no clinical significance, abnormalities of minor clinical significance and abnormalities of major clinical significance.

Abnormalities of major clinical significance include:
- Any abnormality that may become, or already is, painful
- Any abnormality that affects, or may affect, vision
- Any abnormality that is progressive, chronic or recurrent
- Any abnormality that cannot be cured by a course of medical treatment or by surgical correction

LAVAGE DEVICES

Highly-strung animals, particularly those in pain, can be difficult or impossible to treat with topical medication applied directly to the eye and it is sensible to consider inserting some form of indwelling medication device at the initiation of treatment. These devices can be inserted in the sedated conscious horse following infiltration with local anaesthetic, or at the end of any surgical procedure under general anaesthesia.

Subpalpebral lavage devices
Two types are available: single entry and double entry. The single-entry type consists of delivery tubing at the end of which is a small central hole surrounded by a footplate. Inserting this type is associated with fewer complications for the occasional user than the double entry type and its insertion is described below (Figure 7.5(a–d)).

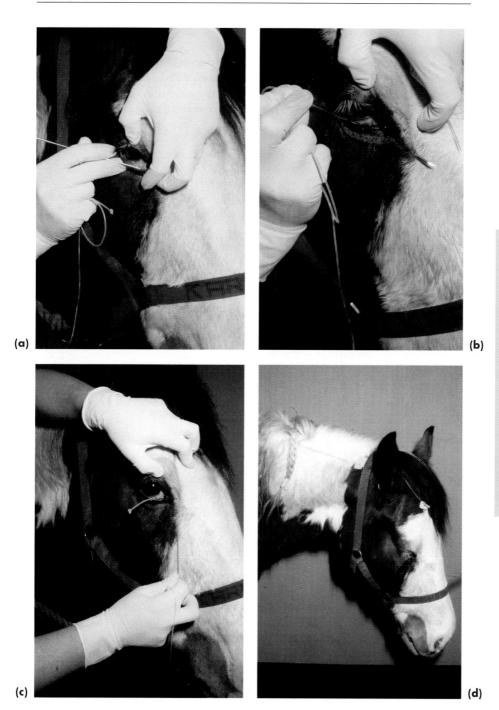

(a)

(b)

(c)

(d)

Figure 7.5(a–d) Insertion of a single-entry subpalpebral lavage device via the ventromedial approach (with acknowledgements to R. C. Lowe).

- In the conscious animal, topical anaesthetic is applied to the cornea and local anaesthetic is infiltrated at the site where the trochar (or needle) will exit.
- The trochar is placed as deeply as possible in the dorsal or ventral conjunctival sac at almost 90 degrees to the eyelid margin and then pushed decisively to emerge through the skin (Figure 7.5(a,b)). This is slightly more difficult to achieve when using a ventral approach, but it is probably the position of choice, because the location of the third eyelid makes inadvertent corneal damage from the footplate less likely (Figure 7.5(c)).
- The tubing is then threaded through the trochar, after which the trochar is removed and the tubing is adjusted so that the footplate rests snugly against the conjunctiva.
- The tubing is retained in place with skin sutures or cyanoacrylate adhesive, applied to 'butterflies' made from zinc oxide tape wrapped around the tubing. The first suture is placed close to the eyelid, the second one closer to the midline between the eyes and a third, if required, close to the ear. It is usually convenient to lead the tubing between the ears, or to some other point where it may be attached to the head collar (Figure 7.5(d)).
- Topical solutions are injected into the system and flushed through with air. If multiple solutions are used in therapy, at least five minutes should be allowed to elapse between different drugs.
- These devices should be checked regularly as a number of complications can occur, including local haemorrhage when they are inserted and simple blockage during use.
- Eyelid swelling and corneal damage can result if they are improperly located, or become displaced from their original position.

Indwelling nasolacrimal cannula (Figure 2.20, p. 53)

A commercial cannula is available, which is inserted into the nasolacrimal duct via the nasal ostium after applying local anaesthetic drops to the lower lacrimal punctum and local anaesthetic spray or gel to the nasal ostium. Indwelling nasolacrimal cannulae and catheters may be used as a means of delivering drugs or other preparations to the eye, or to the nasolacrimal drainage system, or as a means of retaining patency within the nasolacrimal drainage system. The volume of lavage solution used in this system is greater than that required for subpalpebral devices, although if air is used to drive the bolus of drug the difference is insignificant.

- The indwelling cannula is passed into the nasal ostium via a stab incision over the cranial aspect of the false nostril and fed up the nasolacrimal duct until the moulded collar abuts against the ostium
- Non-absorbable sutures are used to retain the cannula in place at this point
- The remainder of the tubing is led up between the ears and kept in place as already described for the subpalpebral lavage device

OCULAR AND ADNEXAL CONDITIONS

The common equine ocular and adnexal conditions and those that are important to recognise because of the serious implications of misdiagnosis are summarised in Box 7.1.

> **Box 7.1** Common and important equine ocular and adnexal conditions
>
> - Ocular and adnexal trauma
> - Entropion (foals)
> - Non-ulcerative and ulcerative keratitis, including melting ulcers
> - Uveitis from a variety of causes; the immune-mediated aspects are of particular significance
> - Neoplasia, particularly periocular sarcoids and ocular and adnexal squamous cell carcinoma. Less common, but clinically significant, tumours include uveal melanoma and lymphoma
> - Differentiation of normal variants and pathological changes affecting the cornea, iris, lens, vitreous and fundus
> - Space-occupying orbital and paraorbital neoplastic and non-neoplastic lesions are uncommon, but important in terms of differential diagnosis and prognosis

GLOBE AND ORBIT

PHTHISIS BULBI

The commonest sequel to severe ocular damage in horses is *phthisis bulbi* – a small, shrunken, blind, painless globe (Figure 7.6). It should be distinguished from a congenitally small eye (e.g. microphthalmos).

No treatment is required, unless there is an unacceptable amount of ocular discharge, which may, in turn, attract flies and lead to chronic infection. In such cases the eye should be removed.

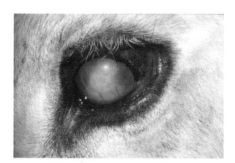

Figure 7.6 *Phthisis bulbi* following severe intraocular inflammation.

ORBITAL, RETRO-ORBITAL AND PARAORBITAL LESIONS

Exophthalmos
- The depression of the supraorbital fossa may be obliterated, and there may be

swelling in this region. It is comparison of each side that is most revealing. This is an early and important sign in many cases
- Exophthalmos is a frequent finding ± an associated strabismus
- The third eyelid may become prominent
- Note, also, the direction of the eyelashes – they may be more horizontal than usual when exophthalmos develops

Aetiology and diagnosis
- Neoplastic, inflammatory, cystic (hydatid disease) and other space-occupying lesions within the orbit (retrobulbar) and outside the orbit (paranasal, retro-orbital and paraorbital). For example, both ethmoidal haematoma and carcinoma involving the ethmoidal labyrinth can produce exophthalmos as the ethmoidal labyrinth is anatomically close to the orbit (Figure 7.7).
- Extraorbital lesions are a commoner cause of exophthalmos in horses than intra-orbital lesions
- Radiology, ultrasonography, sinus trephination and endoscopy (including of the guttural pouch) can help in differentiation, and such cases are often best referred for comprehensive investigation

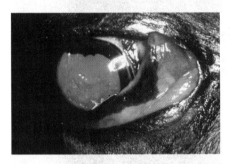

Figure 7.7 Exophthalmos and third-eyelid prominence because of an ethmoidal carcinoma. Note that the pupil is widely dilated as a result of chronic compressive optic neuropathy – optic atrophy was apparent on ophthalmic examination.

EYELIDS

THIRD EYELID (NICTITATING MEMBRANE)

Prominence – summary
- Orbital, retro-orbital and paraorbital space-occupying lesions
- Prolapse of the extraorbital fat pad (*corpus adiposum extraorbitale*)
- Inflammation of the third eyelid (including solar-induced inflammation in non-pigmented lids)
- Neoplasia of the third eyelid, most commonly SCC or lymphoma
- Tetanus: in all species there is bilateral prominence of the third eyelid in this disease, but it is more likely to be seen in herbivores than carnivores.
- Horner's syndrome is *rare* in horses. Ptosis is usually the most obvious feature, and the third eyelid is often *not* prominent. Increased skin temperature and sweating

may also be observed and give a useful insight into the location of the damage to the neurological pathway.

Neoplasia (Figures 7.8(a,b) and 7.9(a,b,c))

See also under Conjunctiva and Upper and Lower Eyelids (this section pp 285–287 and pp 278–281). Commonest tumour is squamous cell carcinoma (SCC) of the third eyelid and this condition (and pre-cancerous solar-induced inflammation) should *always* be considered in animals with an unexplained ocular discharge. Animals in which the eyelids and caruncle are poorly pigmented are most at risk.

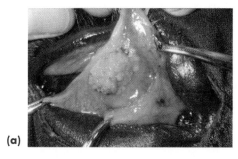
(a)

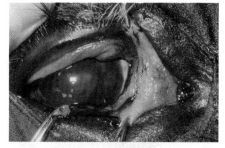
(b)

Figure 7.8 **(a)** Squamous cell carcinoma of the third eyelid in a Thoroughbred. The third eyelid has been protruded prior to excisional surgery of the tumour and part of the third eyelid. **(b)** The immediate postoperative appearance of the eye in (a). The third eyelid conjunctiva was closed with a continuous buried suture of 5-0 polyglactin 910.

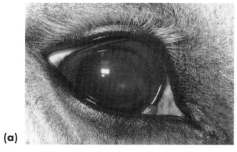
(a)

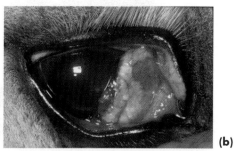
(b)

Figure 7.9(a–c) Squamous cell carcinoma of the third eyelid in a Shire X Thoroughbred. Appearance at rest (a) and after manual protrusion of the third eyelid (b). The third eyelid was resected at its base and there were no problems relating to either squamous cell carcinoma or loss of the third eyelid during a six-year follow up (c).

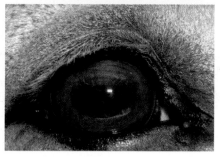
(c)

EQUINE OPHTHALMOLOGY

Diagnosis
- Affects non-pigmented or poorly pigmented third eyelids ± caruncle and the appearance is usually characteristic (e.g. plaque-like or follicular)
- The full extent of the tumour should be assessed by protruding the third eyelid
- Exfoliative cytology from impression smears can be helpful to aid diagnosis prior to surgery, but it is best to submit excised tissue for histopathology to confirm the diagnosis

Treatment
- Local resection of the third eyelid with a full-thickness wedge excision of the tumour and a wide margin of normal tissue, or complete removal of the third eyelid at its base if the tumour is more extensive
- Whichever technique is needed, the wound should be closed with a continuous buried suture of absorbable material (e.g. 5-0 to 6-0 polyglactin 910) because of the possibility of extraorbital fat herniation and because it produces a better postoperative and long-term appearance
- Additional forms of therapy are not usually required at this site, but would follow the lines outlined under upper and lower eyelids as set out below

UPPER AND LOWER EYELIDS

Entropion (Figure 7.10(a,b,c))
- May be perinatal or acquired
- Sick foals are at risk of the early onset type, which is bilateral
- Previous injury the commonest reason for acquired unilateral (cicatricial) entropion

Diagnosis
The appearance is characteristic and the history may be helpful.

Treatment
- Perinatal entropion in foals may correct spontaneously in the first few weeks of life and mild cases require no treatment other than management of any underlying disease (usually including rehydration), careful drying of the eyelids and manual correction of the entropion.
- For congenital entropion that is producing pain and corneal damage, temporary retention ('tacking') sutures (5-0 silk or polyglactin 910 vertical mattress or horizontal mattress) through the skin of the affected eyelid, close to the eyelid margin, are usually sufficient to evert the eyelid (Figure 7.10(c)).
- Non-responsive perinatal (and acquired) entropion may require standard skin –muscle resection techniques, or cosmetic surgery, according to cause and extent.

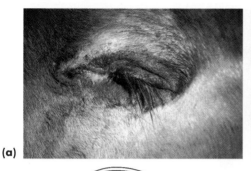
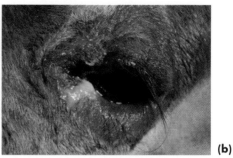

(a)
(b)

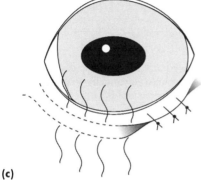

(c)

Figure 7.10 **(a)** Entropion (bilateral) in a foal. The whole of the lower eyelid is involved. **(b)** There is a spastic component because of low-grade corneal trauma, but the entropion persisted after topical local anaesthesia. **(c)** Temporary tacking sutures were used to rectify the problem.

Neoplasia

- *Periocular papilloma* of viral origin may be encountered in young horses and most gradually disappear over a period of months, so no treatment is required
- *Sarcoid* is the commonest periocular and eyelid tumour of horses and donkeys in the UK. Sarcoids may be single or multiple (Figure 7.11)
- *Squamous cell carcinoma* (adnexa and eyelids) is also common and this tumour may also involve the conjunctiva, limbus and cornea (Figure 7.12(a,b))
- *Melanoma* is a common tumour of grey horses, and the eyelids and caruncle are possible sites
- Less common primary eyelid tumours include adenoma, adenocarcinoma, angioma, angiosarcoma, basal cell carcinoma, fibroma, fibrosarcoma, haemangiosarcoma and mast cell tumour
- Both isolated and metastatic *lymphoma* may involve the eyelids

Diagnosis

- Clinical appearance of the lesion
- Biopsy should be submitted for confirmatory histopathology

Differential diagnosis

- Tumours should be differentiated from inflammation (e.g. granulomas associated with habronemiasis)
- Infiltrative conjunctival tumours should be differentiated from very rare conditions like amyloidosis
- Differentiation may only be possible after an adequate biopsy has been obtained

EQUINE OPHTHALMOLOGY

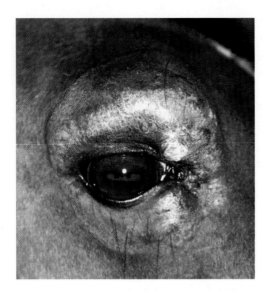

Figure 7.11 Periocular sarcoid. This was treated successfully using intralesional injections of BCG.

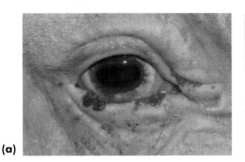

(a)

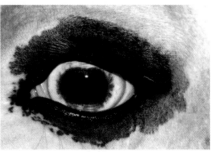

(b)

Figure 7.12 **(a)** Squamous cell carcinoma (SCC) of the lower eyelid. Note the lack of upper and lower eyelid pigment. **(b)** The other eye had normally pigmented upper and lower eyelids and no pathology. In both eyes, the third eyelid lacked pigment and it is important to assess this region carefully for any signs of solar-induced inflammatory change or SCC.

Treatment
Periocular sarcoids
- Periocular sarcoids are usually treated with intralesional injections of BCG in general practice
- Usually 1 ml of intradermal BCG is injected into each lesion, and the treatment is repeated in 2–3 weeks
- Usually two treatments are sufficient, but occasionally three are required
- Intralesional cisplatin and radiotherapy are alternative forms of treatment
- Surgery should *not* be used, as the recurrence rate (80%) is unacceptably high

Squamous cell carcinoma

- Standard treatments for SCC of the upper and lower eyelids include surgical excision, chemotherapy (e.g. intralesional cisplatin), radiotherapy (e.g. iridium 192), immunotherapy (e.g. BCG) or cryotherapy.
- For cryotherapy, liquid nitrogen is the cryogen of choice and a double freeze–thaw cycle is used. The temperature should be lowered to –25°C throughout the affected tissue, and the ice ball should extend 2 mm into healthy tissue.

Melanomas

Melanomas are usually surgically excised or treated using cryotherapy (as outlined for SCC). Cryotherapy can be used alone or after prior surgical debulking of the mass.

Other types of neoplasia

Most other tumours are surgically removed, as already described in the general and canine section. Advice should be sought if the management strategy is unclear, and a proportion of cases will require referral.

LACRIMAL SYSTEM

TEAR FILM PRODUCTION AND DISTRIBUTION PROBLEMS

The trigeminal nerve (Vth cranial nerve) provides the sensory supply to the eye and both sensory and autonomic nerve fibres to the lacrimal gland. The ophthalmic division of the Vth cranial nerve supplies the afferent arm of the trigeminal–lacrimal reflex pathway and the facial nerve (VIIth cranial nerve) supplies the efferent arm.

Damage to the motor fibres of the facial nerve may result in an inadequate blink and poor tear film distribution. Exposure keratopathy is the likely consequence.

Keratoconjunctivitis sicca (KCS)
Aetiology
- Trauma associated with fractures of the stylohyoid bone or mandible is the commonest cause of damage to the parasympathetic fibres that run in the superficial petrosal nerve to supply the lacrimal gland
- Guttural-pouch pathology, middle ear disease and vestibular disease may also be associated with keratoconjunctivitis sicca
- Damage to the lacrimal gland itself (e.g. toxic, eosinophilic and chronic dacryoadenitis) can affect lacrimal-gland function so that keratoconjunctivitis sicca results

Clinical signs of KCS (Figure 7.13)
- Ocular discomfort or more obvious pain
- Blepharospasm, but without any signs of excessive lacrimation
- Lacklustre cornea – the corneal light reflex is disrupted. Subtle epithelial defects or frank ulceration may be present, as well as fine neovascularisation
- There is often rather sparse ocular discharge and any accompanying conjunctivitis is mild

EQUINE OPHTHALMOLOGY

Diagnosis
- History and clinical signs
- Mean normal STT I in the horse is approximately 13 mm ± 9 mm/minute. Consistent values of 10 mm/minute or less should be regarded as indicative of KCS, especially in conjunction with relevant clinical signs

Treatment
- KCS is usually treated with topical ocular lubricants (e.g. polyvinyl alcohol or carbomers such as polyacrylic acid)
- *Neurogenic* dry eye is the commonest type of KCS encountered in the horse, but there has been no clinical evaluation of the efficacy of parasympathomimetics such as pilocarpine (topical or oral)
- *Immune-mediated* KCS has not been identified as a specific entity in the horse, so it is unlikely that immunosuppressive drugs, such an important mode of treatment in the dog, would achieve a great deal

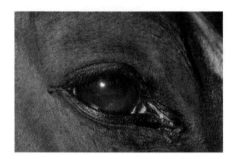

Figure 7.13 Unilateral keratoconjunctivitis sicca following head trauma. The Schirmer tear test reading was 6 mm wetting/minute in the affected eye and 14 mm wetting/minute in the fellow eye.

TEAR-FILM DRAINAGE PROBLEMS

These problems are not uncommon, and they can be congenital or acquired. Investigative procedures are as for small animals, with the important difference that in horses the nasal ostium is visible and accessible and so can be used instead of the lacrimal puncta for cannulation and retrograde irrigation. Some drainage problems are quite complex and affected animals will be best referred.

Congenital dysgenesis
Dysgenesis (abnormal development), including atresia (absence) of the nasal ostium and varying portions of the rostral (nasal or distal) nasolacrimal duct, is the commonest abnormality of the lacrimal system encountered in foals.

Clinical diagnosis
- Veterinary advice is usually sought when the animal is quite young; the problem is usually unilateral

- Clinical examination reveals no sign of a nasal ostium and considerable epiphora, or a mucopurulent discharge, may be present at the medial canthus and on the side of the face (Figure 7.14(a))
- If the nasal ostium is absent it is likely that surgery will be required, therefore the additional investigations are usually performed under general anaesthesia so that surgery can follow immediately

Additional investigations
- Congenital dysgenesis cases are often referred, following the initial clinical examination, for additional investigations and treatment
- A sterile catheter (e.g. feline urinary catheter) can be passed via the upper lacrimal punctum and down the nasolacrimal duct to establish the degree of abnormality
- Dacryocystorhinography may also be required to establish the extent of any dysgenesis (Figure 7.14(b)). Note that it is not uncommon to encounter diverticula, both patent and impatent, at the rostral (nasal) end of the nasolacrimal duct in some horses

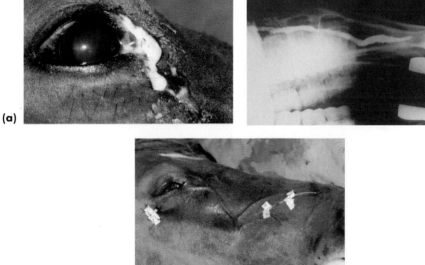

(a)

(b)

(c)

Figure 7.14 (a) Congenital dysgenesis of the rostral (distal) nasolacrimal drainage system. External inspection indicated that there was no sign of a nasal ostium. **(b)** Dacryocystorhinography was used to confirm that the terminal portion of the rostral nasolacrimal duct was absent. **(c)** Patency was established by passing a catheter to the site of obstruction, incising the mucosa overlying the tip of the catheter, delivering the catheter through the incision and retaining it *in situ* for about three weeks to ensure permanent canalisation.

Treatment
- The end of a catheter that has been passed from the upper punctum down the

EQUINE OPHTHALMOLOGY

nasolacrimal duct is palpated and a cruciate incision made over the tip, the four flaps of tissue are then excised, so creating a nasal punctum
- The proximal end of the catheter will be retained with more comfort for the patient if it is placed as for subpalpebral lavage devices; the rostral end can be routed to the skin via the false nostril as described previously for indwelling nasal cannulae
- The catheter is left *in situ* for 2–3 weeks and is kept in place by sutures or superglue through 'butterflies' made from sticking plaster (Figure 7.14(c))

Acquired drainage problems – trauma, infection, inflammation and neoplasia

Stenosis or occlusion of the lacrimal drainage system may be a complication of inflammatory, infectious, neoplastic or traumatic disease processes within the drainage system or external to it (Figure 7.15(a,b)). Granulomatous reactions (parasitic and fungal) should always be considered as a cause of obstruction in horses and donkeys. Cases of traumatic injury to the lacrimal drainage apparatus are usually complex and referral should be considered.

EQUINE OPHTHALMOLOGY

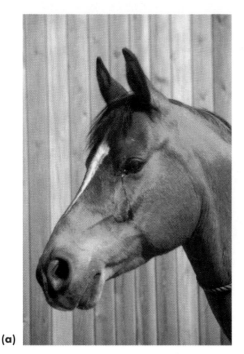

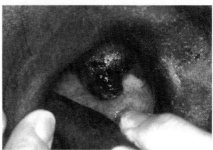

(b)

Figure 7.15 (a) Acquired obstruction of nasolacrimal drainage because of a mast cell tumour occluding the nasal ostium. **(b)** Diagnosis was made by external inspection, and removal of the mast cell tumour solved the problem.

(a)

Aetiology
- Internal reasons for obstruction of the nasolacrimal duct include dacryocystitis (inflammation of the lacrimal sac and duct), neoplasia, parasites (*Habronema* spp and *Thelazia* spp), foreign bodies and other traumatic causes

- External reasons for obstruction of the nasolacrimal duct include trauma, neoplasia, rhinitis, sinusitis and upper-arcade dental disease

Clinical signs of acquired drainage problems
- Epiphora or some form of ocular discharge
- Identifiable cause of obstruction by direct inspection (lacrimal puncta or nasal ostium) or by indirect inference (e.g. dental disease, sinusitis)

Clinical signs of habronemiasis
- Usually a rapid onset of swelling, which is both painful and pruritic. The lesion is usually raised and ulcerated, or of caseous plaque-like appearance (Figure 7.16)
- In addition to causing lacrimal drainage obstruction and secondary dacryocystitis, habronemiasis may also be associated with granulomas of the eyelids and conjunctiva, especially in the region of the medial canthus
- The diagnosis is confirmed by biopsy

Treatment of parasitic causes of dacryocystitis
A single dose of oral ivermectin (0.2 mg/kg) is usually effective.

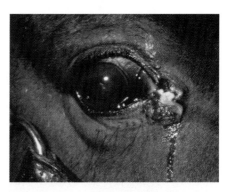

Figure 7.16 Habronemiasis as a cause of acquired obstruction of nasolacrimal drainage.

EQUINE OPHTHALMOLOGY

CONJUNCTIVA

Conjunctivitis
Aetiology
Causes of conjunctivitis include foreign debris (e.g. dust), allergies (e.g. fly spray and drugs), parasites (e.g. *Habronema* spp, *Thelazia* spp and *Onchocerca* spp), viruses (e.g. equine viral arteritis, equine herpes virus and adenovirus), bacteria (almost exclusively secondary pathogens) and mycoses in tropical countries (e.g. blastomycosis) (Figure 7.17).

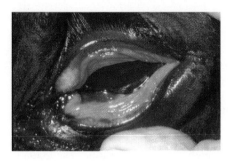

Figure 7.17 Acute allergic conjunctivitis in a Hanoverian. Acute blepharoconjunctivitis is often a painful condition in horses, as is apparent here.

Treatment
- Treatment of conjunctivitis depends upon establishing and eliminating the cause
- Environmental factors are the commonest causes (physical, chemical and allergic)
- As horses live in a relatively contaminated environment, growth of organisms from conjunctival swabs is common, but they may not be pathogenic, so expert assistance may be required if the clinical significance of any isolates is unclear

Neoplasia involving the bulbar conjunctiva
- Squamous cell carcinoma is the commonest and may be confirmed by histopathology (Figure 7.18)
- Other tumours are uncommon and include papilloma, haemangioma, haemangiosarcoma, melanoma and lymphoma
- The extent of the tumour, and any indications of local or distant spread, should be established before contemplating removal

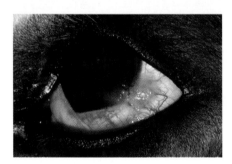

Figure 7.18 Squamous cell carcinoma involving the conjunctiva, limbus and cornea.

Differential diagnosis
Tumours that involve the conjunctiva (bulbar, palpebral or nictitating) should be differentiated from amyloidosis, which is very rare.

Treatment
- For SCC involving the conjunctiva of the lids, see under Eyelids (this section pp 276–281)
- For SCC involving the bulbar conjunctiva, limbus and cornea, keratectomy and conjunctivectomy can be used to debulk or excise the tumour

- Surgery can be combined with radiotherapy (e.g. beta irradiation with a strontium 90 applicator) or radiotherapy can be used on its own
- The presence of unrecognised micrometastases can complicate the management of these cases, as local ischaemia and limbal keratomalacia may result
- Referral should be considered for any case with corneal involvement (e.g. SCC and carcinoma *in situ*)
- Other tumours can usually be removed using wide-based excision, and, as with SCC, the diagnosis should be confirmed by histopathology

CORNEA

Non-specific corneal opacities
Band opacities
Band opacities (linear keratopathy), in the form of linear streaks crossing the cornea, are an occasional finding. They represent thin regions of Descemet's membrane and are most commonly associated with glaucoma ± globe enlargement, so the rest of the eye should be checked very carefully.

Corneal oedema
Corneal oedema is not uncommon in horses. It may be a primary 'dystrophic' condition, but is more likely to be a sequel to a variety of ocular insults (e.g. blunt trauma, keratitis, uveitis and glaucoma).

Keratitis
Keratitis accounts for a high proportion of all eye cases examined in equine practice – and donkeys and mules, as well as horses, are involved. There are a number of possible causes that include trauma (physical and chemical), infection, hypersensitivity, immune-mediated disease and neoplasia, and it is important to try to establish the aetiology if treatment is to be effective. On occasions it is impossible to establish the cause, so early specialist advice may be required to help with such cases.

When pain and blepharospasm are features of the clinical presentation, topical local anaesthesia, systemic sedation ± analgesia and an auriculopalpebral nerve block may be required for examination. If indicated, Schirmer I tear tests should be performed before local anaesthetic is applied and swabs and scrapes should be taken before agents such as fluorescein and rose bengal are applied. The insertion of an indwelling medication device after initial assessment may make subsequent management easier.

Non-ulcerative keratitis
Eosinophilic keratoconjunctivitis
Eosinophilic keratoconjunctivitis is an unusual form of limbal-based keratoconjunctivitis of possible immune-mediated origin. It bears comparison with human vernal disease, canine chronic superficial keratoconjunctivitis and feline proliferative keratoconjunctivitis. Horses present with conjunctival hyperaemia and chemosis, as well as characteristic superficial, white, corneolimbal plaques. There is usually some ocular discomfort with blepharospasm and lacrimation and, sometimes, a mucoid discharge.

Treatment consists of topical 0.1% lodoxamide four times daily. Alternatively, topical corticosteroids may be effective.

EQUINE OPHTHALMOLOGY

Keratouveitis

Keratouveitis is a rare limbal-based type of inflammation of unknown cause, also presumed to be immune-mediated, but the stromal infiltrate is more deeply situated and uveitis is also present.

Treatment consists of topical immunosuppressive agents (e.g. cyclosporin) and/or topical corticosteroids, together with mydriatic cycloplegics (atropine) used to effect. Systemic non-steroidal anti-inflammatories may also be indicated.

Differential diagnosis of limbus-based disease of the equine cornea

- Neoplastic – squamous cell carcinoma and related neoplasia (e.g. papilloma, including keratosis, intraepithelial carcinoma), isolated and metastatic lymphoma
- Non-neoplastic – this broad category includes inflammatory and degenerative causes, possible immune-mediated disease and parasitic disease
  - Stromal abscess, eosinophilic keratoconjunctivitis, keratouveitis
  - Limbal-based keratomalacia
  - Amyloidosis
  - Onchocerciasis

Ulcerative keratitis (Figure 2.20, Section 2, p. 53 and Figures 7.19–7.21)

- Ulcerative keratitis is common, and *all* corneal ulcers in horses should be viewed as potentially serious
- The blink rate should be assessed
- A Schirmer I tear test should be performed on most occasions and it may also be necessary to assess corneal sensitivity
- Topical local anaesthetic is applied before swabs and scrapes are taken
- *All* corneas should be stained with fluorescein to check for ulceration
- Subtle erosions may be easier to identify in the dark with a blue light source
- Refer early if there are problems. Many eyes are lost because of poor work-up and late referral
- The earlier sections on the general approach to corneal ulceration should also be consulted (Section 2, pp 51–52)

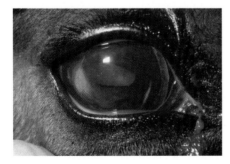

Figure 7.19 Equine ulcerative keratitis. Note the lateral position of the ulcer, which is in a region of relatively exposed cornea, beyond the range of third eyelid excursion. Investigations in cases of this type must include assessment of the production and distribution of the tear film.

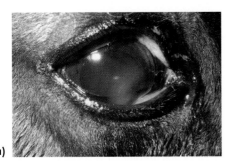
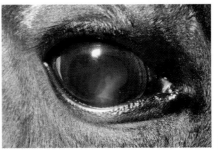

(a)   **(b)**

Figure 7.20 **(a)** Equine ulcerative keratitis, superficial medial ulcer. **(b)** Support for healing provided by therapeutic soft contact lens.

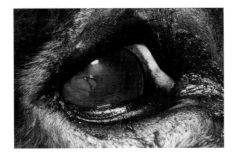

Figure 7.21 Superficial geographic ulceration in a donkey. It was thought that this presentation might indicate a viral aetiology, as acute-phase lesions of putative viral keratitis are likely to be superficial, with a range of possible appearances in affected animals (punctate, geographic). These superficial lesions take up fluorescein, but the staining is not always obvious and examination in the dark using a cobalt blue light is advised, or rose bengal can be used after fluorescein to pick up subtle staining. No virus was isolated from this case, or other donkeys similarly affected, using a variety of techniques.

Complications of equine ulcerative keratitis
- Progression – e.g. descemetocoele formation and corneal perforation
- Keratomalacia and liquefactive stromal necrosis (see Section 2, pp 52–54)
- Corneal stromal abscesses – most abscesses follow penetrating injury in which there is implantation of foreign material, usually organic in nature
- Bacterial or fungal infection may follow because the implanted material, which may also include infectious agents, is effectively walled off when neighbouring epithelial cells divide and migrate to cover the micropuncture site
- Once the foreign material is encapsulated, it is difficult for medical treatment to achieve therapeutically effective levels
- Endophthalmitis

Superficial 'indolent' ulcers
As in the dog and cat, superficial non-healing ulcers of unknown aetiology can occur and, in horses, ulcers of this type are often located laterally.

EQUINE OPHTHALMOLOGY

Clinical signs
- Usual anterior-segment triad associated with pain (blepharospasm, lacrimation and photophobia)
- Superficial, fluorescein-positive erosion, with epithelial loss only and a characteristic rim of non-attached epithelium
- No indication of inflammatory reaction or neovascularisation

Treatment
- Mechanical debridement is probably the treatment of choice
- Pain relief and support for healing can be provided by use of a therapeutic soft contact lens

Viral keratitis

Equine herpes virus (e.g. EHV 2) has long been suspected as a cause of equine keratitis, but, despite these suspicions, there is as yet no definitive proof that equine herpes virus, or indeed any other equine virus, is a primary corneal pathogen in clinical patients. The diagnosis is usually made by default, in so far as response to treatment, rather than actual virus isolation and serological findings, are taken as confirmatory.

In view of the doubts as to the pathogenicity of the ubiquitous herpes virus, it is important to make quite sure that no other potential causes are present, particularly as equine herpes virus has been isolated from normal eyes as well as those with disease.

Putative viral keratitis should be differentiated from other forms of ocular surface disease and corneal conditions.

Clinical signs
- Acute onset of, usually, unilateral pain, blepharospasm and lacrimation
- The clinical appearance is variable. The commonest presentation is multiple, punctate and, less commonly, faint linear, superficial corneal opacities. More extensive superficial geographic erosions, of similar or identical appearance to the superficial indolent ulceration described above, may also be encountered
- The focal lesions may stain with fluorescein 1%, but if they are fluorescein −ve then rose bengal 1% should be applied, and this is often retained after excess stain has been removed by gentle irrigation with sterile saline
- Neovascularisation and stromal involvement both seem to be more typical of chronicity and it is possible that immune-mediated mechanisms are of relevance in the pathogenesis

Differential diagnosis
- Ocular surface disease associated with production (quantity and quality) and distribution of the preocular tear film
- Corneal pathology associated with poor corneal sensitivity and exposure keratopathy
- Superficial indolent ulcers and other types of epithelial erosion
- Unsuitable topical treatment regimes for corneal disease (e.g. topical corticosteroids for fluorescein +ve lesions)

Treatment
- Treatment of acute cases consists of topical antiviral agents, such as trifluorothymidine

or acyclovir, every two hours for the first two days, then three to four times daily for approximately five days
- Antiviral agents are epitheliotoxic and should not therefore be used continuously for longer than 2–3 weeks

Bacterial keratitis
Bacterial keratitis may follow corneal injury or some other corneal insult, particularly when ulceration is present. Gram –ve organisms are the important pathogens. The intact cornea is resistant to bacteria.

Clinical signs
- Pain, blepharospasm and lacrimation initially
- The ocular discharge may become purulent and there may be marked conjunctival hyperaemia and chemosis
- Corneal oedema and frank ulceration may be present
- The cornea should be examined carefully for indications of penetrating injury or stromal abscess formation
- Anterior uveitis is a likely associated finding and hypopyon may also be present
- *Beware* those cases in which the appearance changes to one where the cornea becomes diffusely opaque or appears gelatinous or 'mushy', as this is typical of a *'melting' ulcer (liquefactive stromal necrosis)* (Figure 2.20) and demands immediate aggressive therapy if perforation and loss of the eye are to be avoided. Specialist help and referral should be sought early in such cases (see Section 2, pp 52–54)

Isolation of bacteria
It is important to take corneal scrapes and swabs (Gram staining, culture and sensitivity) at the onset of inflammation, because of the relatively contaminated environment and the possibility of liquefactive stromal necrosis.

Treatment
- The treatment of uncomplicated non-infected corneal ulcers where there has been epithelial loss consists of topical broad-spectrum antibiotic only applied four times a day (e.g. a triple preparation, such as Neosporin®, which contains gramicidin, neomycin sulphate, polymixin B sulphate)
- For deeper lesions, with stromal involvement, a lavage device should be inserted (this section pp 272–274)
- A commercially-available antibiotic preparation or fortified antibiotic solution, selected on the basis of cytology and confirmed by culture and sensitivity results, should be used
- The drops are applied topically every 15–30 minutes for the first six hours, then every 30–60 minutes for the next six hours, after which the frequency can be reduced, but not below four times daily, until the course of treatment is completed. The maximum duration of treatment should not exceed three weeks
- Gentamicin or tobramycin are effective against Gram +ve and Gram –ve rods. Cephazolin or tobramycin are effective against Gram +ve cocci. Fluoroquinolones, such as ciprofloxacin and ofloxacin, are effective against Gram –ve cocci

EQUINE OPHTHALMOLOGY

- When there is any possibility of a corneal 'melt' (e.g. Gram −ve organisms such as *Pseudomonas* or excessive numbers of inflammatory cells), debridement of necrotic tissue should be performed and an early decision taken with regard to providing support for healing (e.g. a conjunctival pedicle graft)
- Fortified antibiotic solutions should be selected for potential melting ulcers
- Empirical treatment with topical whole fresh serum, usually with 5–10% acetylcysteine, or other anticollagenases such as sodium EDTA, can also be used (the latter achieved most simply using large-animal EDTA vacutainers made up with 3 ml of sterile, isotonic, saline or false tears)
- Heparin (1000 IU/ml) suppresses the migration of polymorphonuclear leukocytes (PMNs) into the ulcer, and has direct anticollagenase activity
- Serum or anticollagenases should be used every 1–2 hours until the situation has been brought under control. It is important to emphasise that these preparations have not yet been subjected to rigorous scientific evaluation in the horse
- Uveitis accompanies deep keratitis, and the pupil should be dilated with topical atropine 1% to relieve the pain of ciliary spasm. Once the pupil has dilated, the drug need only be applied frequently enough to maintain dilation (usually once daily or less)
- Non-steroidal anti-inflammatories (orally or intravenously) may be used under careful supervision because they will relieve ocular pain and help to stabilise the blood–aqueous barrier when uveitis is also present
- If the suggested regime cannot be followed, then early referral often gives the best results

Mycotic keratitis

Despite the fact that yeasts and fungi are present in the horse's environment and can often be isolated from the normal conjunctival sac, mycotic keratitis is rare in temperate climates, so is unusual in the UK. Climate change is likely to increase the prevalence of fungal ocular disease, particularly so when the weather is hot and humid (Figure 7.22). Mycotic keratitis should be considered in all instances of non-healing ulcers and refractory interstitial (stromal) keratitis, especially when the history suggests trauma or foreign body implantation originally and treatment has included corticosteroid ± antibiotic use. Specialist advice may be helpful when mycotic keratitis is suspected.

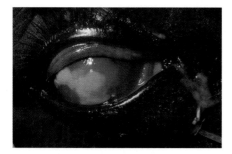

Figure 7.22 Mycotic keratitis associated with traumatic ulceration. Climatic conditions of heat and humidity at the time of the injury were such as to support rapid fungal growth. The diagnosis (*Aspergillus* spp) was confirmed by material from a deep corneal scrape.

Clinical features
- Pain, blepharospasm, lacrimation and photophobia
- A degree of uveitis is usually present, and hypopyon may also be a feature
- Opacities, usually whitish to yellowish in colour, can involve the ocular surface or superficial cornea as well as being subepithelial, stromal and at the level of Descemet's membrane
- Yeasts and fungi often demonstrate affinity for Descemet's membrane
- Stromal abscessation is a likely complication of deep implantation of fungal material (more so than after implantation of bacteria)
- Mycotic keratitis is usually a chronic problem in the UK, but when conditions are hot and humid it may present more acutely

Diagnosis
- Cytology and culture (corneal scrapes and swabs)
- Histopathology from keratectomy specimen

Management
- Keratectomy may be required to allow better access to the organisms located in the stroma and to obtain material for confirmation of diagnosis
- Antifungal preparations for the eye are not generally available in the UK, and are usually obtained on a per-case basis from hospital pharmacies
- Antifungal preparations for the treatment of non-ocular conditions such as vaginitis (e.g. miconazole 1%, clotrimazole 1%) are sometimes used
- When a deep, stromal, corneal abscess forms, the most effective treatment usually involves specialist techniques such as posterior lamellar keratoplasty, or even penetrating keratoplasty

Neoplastic keratitis
Primary corneal neoplasia is rare in most animals, but in horses may have *preneoplastic epithelial dysplasia* and *intraepithelial carcinoma in situ* as well as extension of *squamous cell carcinoma* from adjoining tissues (i.e. conjunctiva and limbus) (Figure 7.18).

Clinical features
- Superficial, white-to-pink corneal opacities
- The benign types (e.g. keratosis) are entirely superficial, usually originate in the lateral limbal region and do not involve the corneal stroma
- Squamous cell carcinoma infiltrating from adjoining tissues, most commonly the lateral limbus, is often of florid 'follicular' appearance and pinkish in colour
- Intraepithelial carcinoma *in situ* is usually whitish in colour, rather poorly defined and involves any region of the cornea

Management
- Specialist advice should be sought, as the most appropriate treatment is usually surgical excision followed by radiotherapy or cryotherapy
- It is important to perform histopathology to confirm the nature of the lesion

EQUINE OPHTHALMOLOGY

Trauma (see also Section 2)

Partial and full-thickness lacerations of the equine cornea are common, and early assessment and, usually, referral is required if a functional eye is to be retained. In most cases of perforation, aqueous loss and iris prolapse occur and the prolapsed iris frequently seals the wound. If the wound is left the iris becomes incarcerated and restoration of normal ocular anatomy is then difficult, if not impossible.

Immediate complications of corneal trauma include hyphaema, iris damage, lens luxation, loss of intraocular contents and collapse of the anterior chamber or the whole globe.

Delayed complications include corneal abscess, synechiae formation, intractable uveitis, secondary glaucoma, endophthalmitis and globe enlargement or *phthisis bulbi*. Partial or complete loss of vision can occur acutely or at a later date.

Diagnosis and management

- Diagnosis of corneal trauma is relatively easy, but calculating the true extent of any injuries requires such careful examination that topical local anaesthesia is mandatory and heavy sedation and analgesia *plus* auriculopalpebral (AP) block or, rarely, general anaesthesia, may be necessary
- An AP block ensures that there is no excessive pressure on the globe (e.g. from squeezing the eyelids shut) and, if the intraocular pressure is kept as low as possible, expulsion of intraocular contents through the wound is less likely
- The prognosis is much more guarded when intraocular haemorrhage is also present
- Superficial traumatic injury is managed as described previously (Section 2, pp 35–49)
- Early referral must be considered in most cases of extensive corneal trauma if the practice lacks facilities for intraocular surgery and expertise in this area

UVEAL TRACT

- The equine pupillary light response is slower than that of carnivores. In foals it is particularly weak for the first few days of life
- Whilst the pupillary aperture of adults is horizontally oval, that of foals is almost circular
- Pigmented *granula iridica (corpora nigra)* are a normal feature of the pupillary border in herbivores; in horses they are mainly located on the dorsal pupillary border (Figure 7.1(c))

Persistent pupillary membrane (PPM) (Figure 7.2(b))

Persistent pupillary membrane remnants are very common in horses, and are of no consequence unless related corneal opacity or cataract obstructs the visual axis.

Heterochromia (Figure 7.23)

- Heterochromia may involve a sector of the iris or the whole iris ('wall' eye or 'china' eye)
- Can occur in older horses
- Of no significance unless associated with uveal inflammation
- Sub-albinism is typified by a blue or grey iris and albinism by a pink or white iris
- Colour-dilute animals may be very photophobic

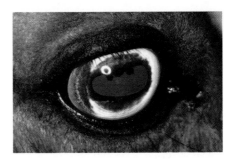

Figure 7.23 Heterochromia of the iris. A sector of the iris is normally pigmented and the majority of the iris is poorly pigmented. This is a normal variant.

Enlargement of the *granula iridica* (Figure 7.24(a,b))

Hyperplasia is quite common, and the enlarged *granula iridica* (which may also be cystic – see below) can be of considerable size without interfering with vision. Treatment is not usually necessary.

(a)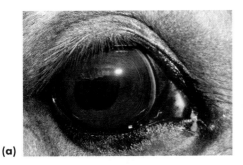

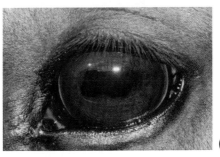 (b)

Figure 7.24(a,b) Enlargement of the *granula iridica*. This is a common finding and rarely of any functional significance. In this show jumper both eyes were affected (a–b), but without any discernible effects on vision.

Cystic anomalies (Figures 7.25–7.27)

Stromal 'cysts'

Stromal 'cysts' are associated with hypoplasia of the mid-dorsal portion of the iris in animals with pale irises (e.g. Welsh ponies) and very rarely in animals with a dark iris. The hypoplastic region bulges anteriorly, creating a 'cystic' appearance. No treatment is required.

Posterior pigment epithelium cysts and cysts of *granula iridica*

- Common
- Rarely, may enlarge to obstruct visual axis
- On the very rare occasions when vision is compromised or the horse's behaviour affected, evacuation of the cysts or laser ablation is effective
- Most cysts should be left alone

Iridociliary cysts can be associated with other ocular anomalies and glaucoma, especially in the Rocky Mountain horse.

EQUINE OPHTHALMOLOGY

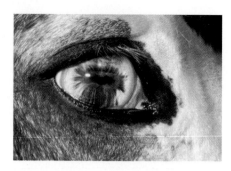

Figure 7.25 Bilateral hypoplasia of the iris and associated miosis in a colour-dilute horse. The right eye is illustrated.

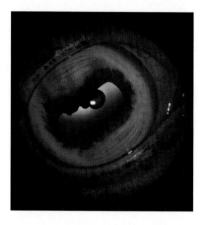

Figure 7.26 Uveal cysts arising from the *granula iridica*. Both cysts are round and smooth and can be transilluminated with a bright light.

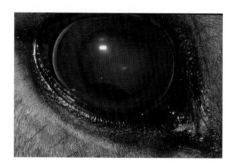

Figure 7.27 Pigmented uveal cyst in the ventral pupillary border. Cysts in this position appear more likely to cause horses to 'spook' than those positioned dorsally.

UVEITIS

Equine uveitis is an important and painful problem and is probably the single most common cause of blindness in this species. Prevalence may approach 25%. A proportion of cases (e.g. unknown aetiology, post-traumatic and unresponsive) may require referral.

EQUINE OPHTHALMOLOGY

Aetiology

In common with uveitis in other species there are a number of potential identifiable causes of *acute* equine uveitis. Triggering antigens include infectious agents such as *Leptospira* spp and non-infectious antigens (Table 7.2). Whatever the initiating event, the greatest concern is of immune-mediated *chronic* complications.

Table 7.2 Aetiology of equine uveitis

Aetiology of equine uveitis	Possible examples (most infectious causes are unproven)
Infectious agents	
	Viruses – Herpesvirus (EHV-1 and EHV-4), equine influenza virus
	Bacteria – *Leptospira interrogans* (number of serovars), *Rhodococcus equi*, *Escherichia coli*, *Streptococcus equi*
	Parasites –, *Toxoplasma gondii*[1], *Onchocerca cervicalis*[2], intestinal strongyles
Inflammation	
	Ulcerative and non-ulcerative keratitis
	Kerato-uveitis
Trauma	
	Blunt and penetrating trauma (including phacoclastic uveitis)
	Foreign bodies
	Surgery
	Physical and chemical injury
Immune-mediated	
	Delayed response to local or circulating antigens

[1] Serum and vitreous samples from animals with toxoplasmosis suggest that *T. gondii* is not implicated in ERU.

[2] *Onchocerca cervicalis* is probably not a primary initiator of uveitis.

Classical *equine recurrent uveitis* (ERU) consists of active episodes of uveitis followed by periods of quiescence. The disease is similar to immune-mediated recurrent uveitis in human patients. Acute, active ERU primarily involves the iris, ciliary body and choroid with concurrent involvement of the cornea, anterior chamber, lens, vitreous and retina (Figure 7.28(a,b)). After variable lengths of time, the quiescent, or chronic phase, is inevitably followed by further and increasingly severe episodes of acute uveitis. The severity of the clinical signs differs between cases and between attacks. It is possible to predict neither how long the quiescent period between attacks will last, nor how serious the next attack will be.

Although the precise aetiology of equine recurrent uveitis (ERU) is unknown and a specific triggering antigen has not been identified, it seems likely that a variety of circulating antigens (heteroantigens) or native ocular antigens (autoantigens) are involved, and the triggering antigens may well vary in different parts of the world. A T-cell-mediated autoimmune mechanism is the basis of the recurrent episodes of inflammation. T-lymphocytes are the predominant cell type to infiltrate the anterior uvea of horses with ERU and cell-mediated immunity to uveal antigens has been demonstrated in affected horses.

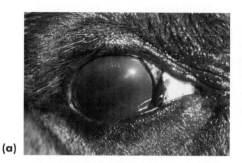 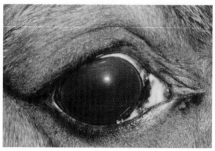

(a) **(b)**

Figure 7.28 **(a)** Acute equine uveitis as a consequence of a penetrating injury. The eye shows the classical signs of ocular pain. It is also reddened, aqueous flare is present and iris details are not apparent. The single most useful ocular sign of the acute iritis is intense pupillary constriction. Hyphaema marks the track of penetration and may indicate a retained foreign body. **(b)** The situation remains unclear, even after the haemorrhage had cleared. Note that application of combined topical atropine 4% and phenylephrine 10% has failed to dilate the pupil.

Diagnosis
Non-traumatic aetiology
- A careful and accurate case history should be taken, including any previous and current treatment. Thorough physical examination is required, and neurological function may also need to be assessed
- Examination of both eyes and their adnexa (orbital, paraorbital, eyelids and lacrimal system) must be meticulous, so that normal lighting and darkness will both be needed, as well as a penlight, some form of magnification, indirect and direct ophthalmoscopy
- Systemic sedation/analgesia and an auriculopalpebral nerve block may be necessary if the eye is painful, or if there is any doubt as to the integrity of the globe
- Relevant laboratory investigations (in most cases routine haematology, urea, enzymes, total protein, protein electrophoresis, faecal analysis for parasites and urinalysis)
- Serology (paired samples) should also be undertaken if a microbial cause is suspected, particularly for leptospirosal and viral antibodies
- If necessary, a conjunctival biopsy (e.g. in suspected onchocerciasis) and aqueous and vitreous paracentesis can be incorporated into the diagnostic work-up

Traumatic aetiology
- *Blunt trauma* is usually more damaging to the globe than penetrating injury, as the intraocular contents can be severely disrupted. Autoimmune uveitis may follow local release of potentially autoantigenic intracellular material when there is cellular damage. The prognosis after blunt injury is usually guarded to poor.

- *Penetrating trauma* is not uncommon in horses, and may involve entry via the cornea, limbus or sclera with or without direct injury to the iris and lens. Elective procedures such as corneal and intraocular surgery will also be associated with breakdown of the blood–aqueous barrier and consequent uveitis.
- Recurrent bouts of uveitis can follow traumatic injury, especially when uveal tissue is incarcerated in the wound, when there is leakage of lens material, when necrotic tissue is present, when haemorrhage persists, or when foreign bodies remain.
- Penetration of the lens can result in phacoclastic uveitis, which carries a poor prognosis, particularly if it is not recognised and treated aggressively in the early stages.
- The clinical signs of acute lens rupture include pain, blepharospasm excessive lacrimation, evidence of corneal penetration, aqueous flare, lens material in the anterior chamber, focal cataract and an intraocular pressure that is lower than normal.
- If uveitis cannot be controlled after traumatic injury, the eye may eventually become phthitic, a common sequel to serious ocular insult in the horse.
- Other findings in chronic trauma-related uveitis include corneal opacification, pigmentation and vascularisation, hypotony and blindness.

Key features of examination and diagnosis
- The examiner must ascertain that the globe is intact before the eyelids and globe are manipulated as part of the ocular examination.
- If aqueous leakage is a possibility, topical fluorescein (2%) should be used for Seidel's test – the escaping aqueous dilutes the fluorescein and causes it to fluoresce. This test is easier to interpret if the eye is examined in the dark with a blue light.
- If corneal ulceration is suspected, topical fluorescein (1%) should be used to check for uptake of the stain by the corneal stroma. The eye should be gently irrigated with sterile saline to remove excess fluorescein before checking for fluorescein uptake with a blue light in the dark.
- Ultrasonography may be needed to aid diagnosis if adequate intraocular examination cannot be performed.
- Radiography may be needed if there is any suggestion of orbital or periorbital damage.

Clinical features of acute equine uveitis (Figures 7.28(a,b) and 7.29(a,b))
- Pain, blepharospasm, lacrimation and genuine photophobia*
- Apparent enophthalmos – the painful eye is actively retracted, the third eyelid may be prominent and the upper eyelid lashes will be directed more downwards than normal
- Eyelid oedema may be present, as may chemosis
- Corneal oedema (especially near the limbus) and neovascularisation (an early response in horses)
- Eye may be reddened as a consequence of inflammatory hyperaemia (conjunctival and ciliary injection, particularly towards the limbus), but not necessarily so

* Readily identifiable key features

EQUINE OPHTHALMOLOGY

- Anterior chamber may appear shallower than normal because the iris is often swollen
- Plasmoid aqueous imparts a hazy appearance to the anterior chamber (a slit beam is the easiest way of detecting aqueous flare)
- Aqueous may be an abnormal colour (usually yellow, or green-tinged)
- Hyphaema is an occasional finding when non-traumatic uveitis is severe, but is a common finding in uveitis associated with trauma
- The pupil is miotic (constricted), often intensely so, and different lighting conditions do not usually have any effect on the intense constriction. It is helpful to compare the affected eye with an unaffected eye under the same lighting conditions to confirm this pathognomonic feature*
- Details of superficial iris structure are lost and the iris may appear thickened and dull in colour, mainly as a result of iris oedema and inflammatory hyperaemia
- Early posterior synechiae formation, abnormal pupil shape*
- Low intraocular pressure (hypotony)
- Inflammatory cells in vitreous (vitritis) – hazy appearance
- Vasculitis, perivascular oedema, focal or diffuse oedema (fundus details are indistinct), subretinal exudation, focal or diffuse chorioretinitis
- Optic neuritis and peripapillary oedema
- Vision may appear unaffected or show varying degrees of impairment. Some animals are blind

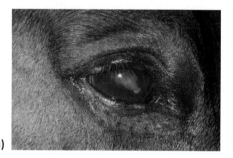 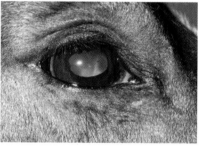

(a)   **(b)**

Figure 7.29 (a) Unilateral panuveitis of unknown cause. It is important always to examine the posterior segment in uveitis cases once topical treatment has achieved mydriasis, because inflammation may not be confined to the anterior segment. **(b)** In this case vitritis is present and inflammatory debris can be seen on the ventral pupil.

Additional clinical features of traumatic uveitis

- Indications of traumatic damage to the head, particularly periocular /periorbital/orbital – including soft tissue and bony damage e.g. eyelid lacerations and orbital fractures.
- Alterations of ocular appearance may include:
  - External signs of ocular penetration or splits in the ocular coats, aqueous loss, aqueous coagulation and iris prolapse

---

* Readily identifiable key features

  ○ Internal signs of damage to the anterior segment – hyphaema, irregular pupil, distortion of the iris, damage to the *granula iridica*, disruption of iridal pigment, change of anterior chamber depth, avulsion of the trabecular meshwork, anterior and posterior synechiae, lens opacities/cataract (often focal), perforation of the lens capsule, lens material in the anterior chamber

  ○ Internal signs of damage to the posterior segment – intraocular haemorrhage, disruption of vitreous, retinal oedema, retinal haemorrhage, retinal detachment, optic neuritis, extrusion of myelin in papillary and peripapillary region

Clinical features of chronic equine uveitis (Figures 7.30 and 7.31)

- Corneal neovascularisation
- Keratic precipitates (usually requires a slit lamp), hypopyon, hyphaema
- Focal or diffuse iris hypopigmentation and hyperpigmentation, loss of iris detail
- Marked darkening of the iris is the commonest chronic feature seen in the normal pigmented eye, but in animals with a pale iris the lack of pigment enables *rubeosis iridis* (neovascularisation of the iris) to be readily observed
- There is sometimes iris atrophy
- Alterations of iris colour are very common in chronic uveitis*
- Degeneration/absence of *granula iridica**
- Synechiae, usually posterior, but may be anterior synechiae when there has been previous corneal perforation*
- Pupillary seclusion (the adhesion of the whole pupillary circumference to the lens) and pupillary occlusion (opaque fibrous tissue crossing the pupil) are possible sequelae
- Immobile, or partially mobile, irregular pupil*
- Cell rests (pigment deposition on anterior lens capsule)*
- Cataract formation is a common complication, particularly in the presence of synechiae or cyclitic membranes (organized exudate behind the lens as a result of cyclitis) and such patients are unsuitable for cataract surgery
- Cataract may be incipient, immature, mature or hypermature, depending on chronicity*
- Lens subluxation/luxation
- There may be vitreal discolouration, opacities (floaters) and liquefaction (syneresis)
- Thickened vitreal membranes are quite common. Those of the posterior vitreous usually appear as grey striae radiating into the vitreous from the vicinity of the optic nerve head; unfortunately they may eventually cause traction detachments of the retina
- Retinal detachment is a possible complication of vitreal alterations, alternatively any subretinal and retinal oedema present during the acute inflammatory phase may contribute to subsequent retinal detachment
- Peripapillary chorioretinopathy, focal or diffuse inactive chorioretinopathy
- Optic atrophy
- Secondary glaucoma – intraocular pressure higher than normal, globe may enlarge
- Shrinkage of globe (*phthisis bulbi*) – intraocular pressure extremely low

EQUINE OPHTHALMOLOGY

---

* Readily identifiable key features

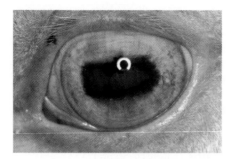

Figure 7.30 Subacute equine recurrent uveitis. In this colour-dilute eye it is possible to observe new blood vessels (*rubeosis iridis*) on the iris surface (*rubeosis iridis* is not usually apparent in darkly-pigmented eyes). In addition, the pupil is irregular, there is partial degeneration of the *granula iridica* and there are pigment deposits (iris rests) on the anterior lens capsule.

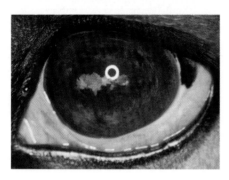

Figure 7.31 Chronic equine recurrent uveitis. The eye is quiet, but severely damaged by previous recurrent episodes. There is marked darkening of the iris, degeneration of the *granula iridica*, an irregular pupil, posterior synechiae, iris rests, secondary cataract and the eye is blind.

Management of uveitis

Complete resolution is achievable in some cases if early treatment is given the first time uveitis occurs and when the cause is readily identifiable (e.g. trauma). However, the prognosis in traumatic cases is guarded when there is extensive intraocular haemorrhage and/or disruption of the intraocular contents. The prognosis is also guarded when there have been previous episodes of inflammation, and the prognosis for restoration of normal visual function is very poor in chronic recurrent cases. Once vision is permanently lost, the only consideration is provision of adequate pain relief and this may be most readily achieved by removal of the globe.

The horse should be walked twice daily in dim light, and, in addition to the usual principles of animal management, vital signs should be monitored. It is important to be aware of any potential undesirable side effects of treatment.

- When uveitis is confirmed, house the affected animal in a dim, quiet and clean environment
- Dust and insects should be kept to a minimum (e.g. feed wet hay at ground level, avoid dusty bedding, control insects)
- Place a subpalpebral lavage device or similar at the time of the initial examination, preferably before sedation/analgesia and local nerve blocks have worn off
- Collect the requisite samples before treatment is started
- Any ocular discharge should be cleaned away before medication is applied
- Petroleum jelly should be applied to the face beneath the lower eyelid to avoid

scalding from excessive lacrimation and to protect from the effects of frequent medication
- Institute medical treatment promptly while investigations as to aetiology are in progress
- The response to treatment can often be gauged within an hour of commencing the combination of topical mydriatic cycloplegic and corticosteroid and systemic non-steroidal anti-inflammatory drugs
- The eye must be re-evaluated at regular intervals

Treatment
Topical
Mydriatics

A *mydriatic cycloplegic* (atropine sulphate 1–4%) should be applied with sufficient frequency to achieve and maintain mydriasis. This means that the drug is given intensively in the early stages of treatment, and once the pupil has responded it is only given as needed to maintain mydriasis (probably once daily). A directly-acting mydriatic such as phenylephrine hydrochloride 10% may be used in conjunction with atropine in an attempt to disrupt established synechiae.

If there is no pupil response to this two-drug combination within six hours of frequent applications, it is unlikely that successful mydriasis will be achieved. Treatment can be stopped when the eye is free of any signs of pain or inflammation. Owners should be advised that pupillary dilation may persist for up to four weeks after treatment has stopped.

Precautions – topical atropine may cause ileus and subsequent colic, especially in foals, and should only be used with sufficient frequency to maintain pupil dilation. If necessary, intestinal sounds can be monitored, but there is unlikely to be a problem if applications are not given more frequently than every six hours and atropine ointment is always an option in foals.

Corticosteroids

Topical prednisolone acetate 1% is the drug of choice, as it has excellent powers of intraocular penetration. It can be applied every 30 minutes for the first two hours and then every 2–4 hours for the next two days, tapering off to 3–4 times daily if the response is positive. The aim is to cease treatment approximately two weeks after clinical signs have resolved. Topical corticosteroids may be supplemented with less-frequent subconjunctival injections using 10–40 mg methylprednisolone acetate if frequent topical application is not possible.

Precautions – topical and subconjunctival corticosteroids are contraindicated when there is corneal ulceration or abrasion.

Non-steroidal anti-inflammatory drugs

Non-steroidal anti-inflammatory drugs (NSAIDs) are not as potent as corticosteroids and are more expensive. They may be added to a corticosteroid-based topical treatment regime in resistant cases. Ketorolac trometamol 0.5% and flurbiprofen sodium 0.03% every 6–12 hours are the drugs of choice.

Precautions NSAIDs should be used with caution and with regular reassessment when ulcerative keratitis is present.

EQUINE OPHTHALMOLOGY

Antibiotics

Topical antibiotics are only required if intensive and prolonged corticosteroid therapy encourages opportunistic bacteria.

Systemic
Non-steroidal anti-inflammatory drugs

Non-steroidal anti-inflammatory agents such as flunixin meglumine have proved of value as part of non-specific uveitis treatment. Initially flunixin meglumine can be given intravenously at a dose rate of 1 mg/kg body weight every 12 hours for 3–5 days. Flunixin meglumine can also be given at the same dose rate orally and intramuscularly. Ketoprofen can be used as an alternative to flunixin meglumine at a dose rate of 2 mg/kg every 24 hours for 3–5 days.

Follow-up treatment is given at the minimum effective dosage and can be effected with intravenous or oral dosage of flunixin meglumine (0.25–0.5 mg/kg twice daily) or other prostaglandin inhibitors like phenylbutazone (3–5 mg/kg twice daily). In cases that relapse, prolonged oral administration of acetylsalicylic acid (aspirin) at a dose rate of 15 mg/kg may be helpful, but it is not usually selected for acute cases.

Precautions – NSAIDs can produce gastrointestinal ulceration and haemorrhage and renal damage. These effects can be potentiated by concurrent use of corticosteroids.

Corticosteroids

Steroidal anti-inflammatory drugs can be used as well as, or instead of, the non-steroidal type, always providing that their use is not contraindicated. If both types of drug are given simultaneously there is an increased risk of gastrointestinal haemorrhage. Prednisolone is the drug of choice at a dose rate of 0.5–1.0 mg/kg per day for 5–7 days reducing thereafter. Dexamethasone (intramuscular dose rate of 10–40 mg/day) is more likely to be associated with undesirable side effects. Corticosteroids should be administered with caution in animals predisposed to laminitis.

Precautions Systemic corticosteroids can cause immunosuppression, laminitis and iatrogenic Cushing's syndrome. They should be used with appropriate cover if infection is present and with considerable care, or not at all, if corneal ulceration is present.

Antibiotics

If a specific cause for the uveitis is identified, then therapy can be targeted pharmacologically (e.g. parenteral penicillin-streptomycin may be selected if *Leptospira* titres are rising).

New therapeutic options under investigation
Cyclosporin

Cyclosporin is a non-cytotoxic immunosuppressive cyclic peptide that blocks the transcription of the cytokine interleukin-2 (IL-2) and therefore decreases the responsiveness of T-cells to inflammatory stimuli. The drug may therefore be of value in blocking the non-specific activation of T-cells in recurrent episodes of ERU.

Topical cyclosporin is hydrophobic and so does not penetrate the eye well enough to achieve effective intraocular levels. Intravitreal implantation of a sustained-release cyclosporin delivery device has been assessed in horses with experimentally-induced

ERU and naturally occurring ERU and the duration and severity of inflammation decreased significantly.

Subconjunctival delivery systems for cyclosporin are being evaluated, so as to avoid the necessity for intraocular microsurgery.

Pars plana vitrectomy

Pars plana vitrectomy has been used to obtain diagnostic material and remove vitreal debris (and leptospires in some cases). The technique is claimed to improve vision and delay progression of disease in affected horses and it is hypothesised that it works by removing the uveitis-induced 'immunological memory' in the vitreous, thereby reducing adverse interaction between the vitreous and the uveal tract. The results obtained have shown some variation, ranging from prevention of recurrence of ERU and stabilisation of vision to no great improvement and postoperative cataract formation.

General therapeutic principles in traumatic uveitis

- Medical therapy is as already described for non-traumatic uveitis, except that topical corticosteroids and, sometimes, non-steroidal anti-inflammatory drugs are usually avoided when there is corneal damage, for the reasons outlined below.
- Ulcerative keratitis is often a complication of ocular trauma and the presence of an ulcer complicates the medical therapy, as corticosteroids should not be used. Topical non-steroidal anti-inflammatory agents, if selected as an alternative, should be used with caution because their use has been associated, anecdotally, with liquefactive stromal necrosis.
- Penetrating ocular trauma (e.g. full-thickness penetrating injury to the cornea) may require microsurgical repair.
- Penetrating lens injuries may require emergency phacoemulsification ± vitrectomy to remove the lens fragments if the lens perforation does not reseal rapidly and the equipment and expertise is available. For the greatest chance of success, the surgery must be carried out as soon after the injury as possible. Adjunctive medical therapy is as already described for non-traumatic uveitis, with the addition of a broad-spectrum topical antibiotic such as ciprofloxacin.
- If there is extensive intraocular haemorrhage and/or gross disruption of the intra-ocular contents then microsurgical reconstruction may not be indicated, as the prognosis for restoration of vision is guarded at best and hopeless at worst. In such cases the eye should be removed.

UVEAL NEOPLASIA

Uveal neoplasia is rare, the commonest being melanoma. Melanomas are usually locally invasive with no cellular malignancy, and should be differentiated from cysts.

Differential diagnosis of melanomas and uveal cysts

- Melanomas will continue to enlarge, they are attached to the tissue of origin and may provoke local or more widespread reaction (including haemorrhage), they are solid and cannot be transilluminated (Figure 7.32).

- Cysts are smooth and usually spherical. They may reach a certain size and remain static, or occasionally rupture spontaneously. Cysts transilluminate with a bright light source, even when heavily pigmented. In horses they usually remain attached to their tissue of origin, but they are not infiltrative and do not provoke any inflammatory reaction.

Treatment of melanomas

Localised surgical excision is possible for small melanomas, so refer early for assessment, otherwise enucleation will be required.

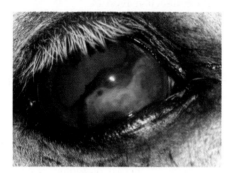

Figure 7.32 Iris melanoma. There is extensive iris involvement in this case.

GLAUCOMAS

Intraocular pressure is dependent on the balance between production and outflow of aqueous humour. Glaucoma is the result of imbalance between aqueous humour production and outflow that causes an increase of intraocular pressure above that which is compatible with normal function of the retinal ganglion cells and optic nerve. Glaucoma is rare in horses and suspected cases are best referred.

As outlined in Section 3 (pp 146–151), glaucomas in all species are usually grouped into primary, secondary and congenital types. In primary glaucoma there is no overt ocular abnormality to account for the increase in intraocular pressure (IOP), and this type has not been reliably confirmed in the horse. Secondary glaucomas are the commonest encountered in horses and have an identifiable cause, such as intraocular inflammation, neoplasia or lens luxation. Congenital glaucoma has been reported in foals and is associated with developmental anomalies of the iridocorneal angle (goniodysgenesis).

Horses older than 15 years of age and Appaloosas are at increased risk of developing glaucoma, although it has been reported in a number of other breeds including Thoroughbreds, Arabs and Welsh ponies. The presence of active or inactive uveitis appears to be a major risk factor. Anterior uveitis often leads to the formation of pre-iridal fibrovascular membranes that may limit aqueous absorption by the uvea, and cause physical and functional obstruction of the iridocorneal angle with inflammatory cells and debris.

In horses, the importance of the *conventional* pathway (whereby aqueous humour passes through the pupil, into the anterior chamber and exits via the trabecular meshwork of the iridocorneal angle and associated outflow channels) is matched by the *unconventional* pathway of uveoscleral outflow (through the iris, ciliary body and sclera). The presence of extensive outflow channels allows aqueous drainage to be maintained in the face of damage to the anterior segment pathways and may explain why glaucoma is a relatively rare sequel to uveitis in the equine eye.

Diagnosis

Glaucoma in horses is being recognised with increased frequency, although the prevalence is surprisingly low (probably less than 0.1%) given the horse's propensity for ocular injury and marked intraocular inflammatory responses. Diagnosis is made on the basis of clinical signs and measurement of the intraocular pressure.

Tonometry

- Tonometry is essential to confirm the diagnosis and to monitor the results of therapy. Sequential measurements of intraocular pressure are recommended as there are diurnal variations in normal eyes, and, in addition, horses with glaucoma have quite marked fluctuations of IOP during a 24-hour period.
- The normal equine intraocular pressure measured with a TonoPen applanation tonometer ranges from 7–37 mm Hg, with a mean IOP of approximately 23 mmHg.
- An auriculopalpebral nerve block is recommended prior to tonometry in fractious horses, as the results will be more reproducible and accurate.

Clinical signs (Figure 7.33(a,b))

- There is generally a low index of suspicion of glaucoma in horses in the early stages, the pupils are often only slightly dilated and any discomfort is subtle
- Although it is often a bilateral condition, one eye may be affected before the other, so it is common to find that the two eyes are dissimilar
- Corneal oedema may be a presenting feature, and its appearance is slightly variable, ranging from a vertical strip running from dorsal limbus to ventral limbus in the central cornea to pancorneal involvement*
- In chronic cases, subtle bullous keratopathy develops in addition to the stromal oedema, and corneal function can become compromised with eventual multiple superficial erosions and corneal decompensation
- Corneal vascularisation can also be a chronic feature
- The presence and appearance of corneal oedema may well relate to the extent and duration of IOP elevation
- Linear corneal striae (Haab's striae) indicate stretching and thinning of Descemet's membrane; the striae appear as faint, grey, parallel lines (snail tracks) and they sometimes branch*
- Mild uveitis is sometimes apparent, particularly of the anterior uvea; the *granula iridica* may have degenerated
- The pupil is more dilated than usual, and constricts poorly in bright light*
- It is sensible to compare pupil size between the two eyes and between the patient and a normal horse under the same lighting conditions
- The lens may be subluxated or luxated

---

* Readily identifiable key features

- Vision is often decreased when the IOP is high and some animals become acutely blind*
- Cupping of the optic nerve head may be observed and occasionally optic atrophy is found in eyes of horses with advanced glaucoma
- The eye may enlarge (buphthalmos)

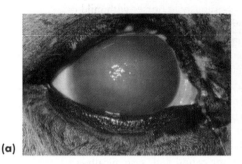 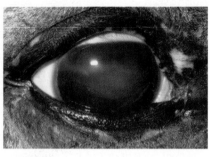

(a) **(b)**

Figure 7.33(a,b) Equine glaucoma during an acute flare up (a) with intraocular pressure of 46 mm Hg, and after treatment to reduce the intraocular pressure to normal (21 mm Hg) (b). In (a) it was possible to see that the pupil was dilated despite the panstromal oedema and bullous keratopathy. In (b) it is apparent that the pupil is of irregular shape. The left eye subsequently became affected in this Appaloosa.

Management of equine glaucoma

The underlying pathogenesis of aqueous humour outflow obstruction with consequent increased IOP is not understood, which makes it very difficult to institute effective therapy. Medical management of equine glaucoma follows the same general guidelines as that of other species, and the aims of therapy are to maintain vision and minimise ocular pain by decreasing production of aqueous humour and increasing its outflow. The response to medical therapy in equine glaucoma is usually poor, with the long-term prognosis for maintaining vision guarded, although there is some variation between individuals. Various combinations of medical therapy and surgery may be necessary to reduce the IOP to levels that are compatible with long-term preservation of vision in horses with glaucoma. Control of IOP can improve vision in equine glaucoma patients, due to resolution of marked corneal oedema and improvement of optic nerve vascular perfusion. Glaucoma is particularly aggressive and difficult to control in the Appaloosa.

Medical therapy
Reduction of aqueous humour production

Agents that reduce aqueous humour production, such as topically-administered carbonic anhydrase inhibitors and beta-adrenergic antagonists, appear to be the most successful at lowering IOP in the horse. The topically-administered carbonic anhydrase inhibitor dorzolamide 2% (three times daily), and the systemically-administered carbonic anhydrase inhibitor acetazolamide (orally 1–3 mg/kg four times daily) are useful. The topical miotic pilocarpine 2% (four times daily), and the topical beta-

---

* Readily identifiable key features

blocker timolol maleate 0.5% (twice daily) can also be used to lower IOP in horses. Combinations of dorzolamide and timolol maleate may be selected.

Miotics
Glaucoma treatment with miotics may provide varying amounts of IOP reduction in horses. Miotics and synthetic prostaglandins, such as latanoprost, can potentiate the clinical signs of uveitis and should be used cautiously in horses with mild or quiescent anterior uveitis.

Atropine
Topical atropine therapy was once thought to reduce the incidence of glaucoma in horses with uveitis, but should be used cautiously in horses with glaucoma, as it may cause IOP spikes and does not appear to have the benefit of lowering IOP previously proposed.

Anti-inflammatories
Anti-inflammatory therapy, consisting of topically- and systemically-administered corticosteroids, and/or topically and systemically administered non-steroidal anti-inflammatories, such as phenylbutazone and flunixin meglumine, also appear to be beneficial in the control of IOP. Aspirin (15 mg/kg orally once daily) may be helpful in chronic cases.

Surgical therapy
Surgical therapy is more likely to be effective for long-term retention of vision, so cases should be referred for specialist opinion as early in the course of disease as possible. The two techniques employed are ciliodestructive surgery (lowers aqueous humour production by damaging the ciliary body) and bypass surgery. Chronically painful and blind buphthalmic globes should be enucleated, or have an intrascleral prosthesis implanted.

Lasers
Laser therapy usually employs neodymium:yttrium-aluminium-garnet (Nd:YAG) laser cyclophotoablation which is probably the most effective means of controlling IOP and maintaining vision in the horse. Diode laser therapy is an alternative. Laser cyclophotoablation is particularly useful in those animals that do not respond to treatment.

Cyclocryoablation
Cyclocryoablation (e.g. with nitrous oxide) results in more diffuse and generalised damage to the ciliary body than laser cyclophotoablation and the ciliary inflammation it evokes is often difficult to control. Cyclocryoablation may produce a number of undesirable complications including severe postoperative pain, ocular hypertension, choroidal effusion, serous retinal detachment and *phthisis bulbi*.

Bypass
Bypass procedures (e.g. gonioimplantation and iridencleisis) improve aqueous humour drainage. Gonioimplantation using Ahmed gonioimplants has been reported in the horse, but is still considered experimental.

LENS

The equine lens is large, and minor imperfections are relatively easy to observe. If there is any suggestion of lens abnormality at the time of examination, a short-acting topical mydriatic (tropicamide 1%) should be applied, and the horse re-examined 20–30 minutes later. Ideally, the examination technique should utilise a focal light source, slit lamp biomicroscopy, distant direct ophthalmoscopy (some 30–60 cm from the eye) and close direct ophthalmoscopy (some 2–10 cm from the eye).

Note that if the significance of any ophthalmic finding at a pre-purchase examination is not apparent then referral should be considered.

Lens variations of no clinical significance
- Anterior (upright Y) and posterior suture lines (inverted Y) ± variations (e.g. further subdivisions of the Y sutures) are easily visualised
- 'Concentric rings', are commonly observed at the nuclear–cortical interface in horses of any age
- Nuclear sclerosis may occasionally be observed in older horses
- Mittendorf's dot, common embryonic remnant that marks the original attachment of the hyaloid artery to the posterior lens capsule
- Vacuolation (minute 'bubbles') in the lens substance is reasonably common

CONGENITAL LENS ANOMALIES AND ABNORMALITIES

- Congenital cataract is seen occasionally, sometimes in association with other ocular defects. Congenital nuclear cataracts are thought to be inherited in the Morgan horse.
- Aphakia (lens absence), microphakia (small lens), lens coloboma (section of lens missing) and imperfections of shape (e.g. lenticonus) and position (e.g. congenital lens luxation) have all been reported in foals, but they are rare.

ACQUIRED LENS DISEASES

Cataract
Aetiology of acquired equine cataract
- Uveitis is the commonest cause of secondary equine cataract
- Trauma is the next most common cause of secondary cataract
- Unknown and age-related (Figure 7.34)

Cataract surgery
- Foals less than six months of age are the best candidates for surgery. Some adult horses are also suitable, usually provided that the only ocular abnormality is cataract
- Patient selection is of crucial importance and early referral for assessment is sensible
- Many horses with cataract will not be suitable candidates for surgery because the common causes are associated with ocular inflammation

- Active ocular inflammation is a contraindication to surgery; previous inflammation may substantially reduce the success rate
- Phacoemulsification without lens implantation is the technique that is usually adopted

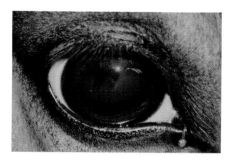

Figure 7.34 Equine cataract. In this horse the peripheral (equatorial) extent of the cataract is only apparent after the pupil has been dilated.

Lens luxation
Lens luxation is most commonly the result of trauma (e.g. blunt trauma in polo ponies) or severe inflammation (e.g. uveitis) (Figure 7.35).

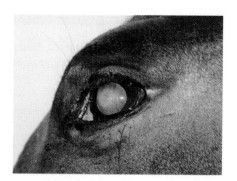

Figure 7.35 Lens luxation in a yearling following viral encephalomyelitis and panuveitis as a foal.

Lens rupture
Lens rupture is usually associated with blunt or penetrating injury and has been discussed earlier. Cases should be referred to a specialist centre as a matter of urgency.

VITREOUS

Congenital opacities
- Vitreous opacities of no significance appear as dust-like particles, filamentous and membranous structures and they are relatively common. Most variations represent remnants of the *tunica vasculosa lentis posterioris* and/or hyaloid system.
- There may be no obvious signs of the hyaloid system at birth in many foals. In others remnants of the hyaloid vasculature are present at birth, but usually regress com-

EQUINE OPHTHALMOLOGY

pletely by 3–9 months of age. Persistence of parts of the hyaloid vasculature is usually incidental, unusual and of no visual significance.
- Dense retrolental vitreal opacities suggest persistence ± hyperplasia of the primary vitreous.

Acquired opacities
- Vitritis is a very common finding in horses with uveitis, a dull or reduced fundus reflex is a helpful diagnostic feature and abnormally opaque vitreoretinal membranes and other detritus may also be apparent on ophthalmoscopic examination (Figure 7.29(b)).
- Severe inflammatory changes, such as endophthalmitis, are less common and may be associated with sepsis, for example associated with neonatal bacterial septicaemia
- Vitreal degeneration is a common feature of equine ageing. Vitreal floaters are the most likely abnormality to be encountered and should be considered as part of the differential diagnosis in 'head shakers' or in horses that 'spook' for no apparent reason. Liquefaction of the vitreous (syneresis) also tends to be associated with ageing, but can follow intraocular inflammation
- Asteroid hyalosis and *synchisis scintillans* (see Section 3, p. 157) are relatively rare in horses

OCULAR FUNDUS

Considerable variation is observed during examination of the equine fundus (Figures 7.36 and 7.37). Evaluation of vision is, inevitably, highly subjective. If the significance of any ophthalmoscopic finding at a pre-purchase examination is not apparent then referral should be considered.

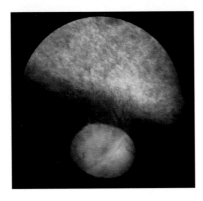

Figure 7.36 Normal equine ocular fundus in an adult horse with a normally pigmented iris. In this Thoroughbred, a blue tapetum is present and the optic nerve head is located in the non-tapetal fundus. The retinal vessels consist of a fine peripapillary halo, discontinuous ventrally at the site of the original foetal fissure. In the ocular fundus of most herbivores, choroidal vessels are also apparent as they perforate through to the choriocapillaris layer – the so-called 'stars of Winslow'. The tapetum, being collagenous, is less reflective than that of carnivores.

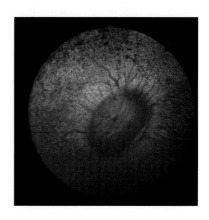

Figure 7.37 Normal equine ocular fundus. In this colour-dilute eye, including a blue iris, there is a sub-albinotic fundus and absence of the tapetum as a normal variant. The small peripapillary vessels are retinal, the larger peripapillary vessels are choroidal and are very distinct, as are other choroidal vessels seen in transverse, oblique and longitudinal section. There is a well-demarcated, peripapillary, non-pigmented 'halo' over which retinal vessels pass without distortion.

ANATOMY

The optic nerve head (ONH) or optic disc is horizontally oval, usually salmon-pink in colour and myelination can extend beyond the edge of the disc. The edge of the ONH can be smooth or scalloped depending on the amount of peripapillary myelination. The physiological pit is not obvious and the ONH often has a fasiculated appearance that relates to the contrast between the optic nerve fibres and the lamina cribrosa; the contrast becomes accentuated with age, or if there is a pathological loss of nerve fibres.

Equine retinal vasculature is described as paurangiotic. Some 30–60 fine vessels extend only a short distance from the optic nerve head and most of the retinal nutrition comes from the underlying vascular choroid. The retinal vessels most commonly originate from the periphery of the optic nerve head; central vessels are uncommon. In general, the presence of normal retinal vasculature is assumed to indicate the presence of a functional retina. It is usual to have an area ventral to the optic disc where retinal vessels are sparse or absent (original position of foetal/embryonic fissure/cleft). It is not possible to distinguish retinal arterioles and venules. Small perforating choroidal vessels appear as dark spots in transverse section (end on) and small rods in oblique or longitudinal section when viewed against the background of the tapetum. In colour-dilute animals, short or complete sections of large choroidal vessels will be apparent and choroidal veins can sometimes be seen converging to form a draining vortex vein.

In the immediate peripapillary region, especially dorsally, there is often a relative lack of pigment in the retinal pigmented epithelium and choroid, as well as tapetal thinning. In such regions a discrete choroidal vessel is sometimes apparent, or a less well defined reddish colour from the underlying choroidal vessels.

Grossly, the fundus of normally pigmented animals is divided into dorsal tapetal and ventral non-tapetal regions and the optic nerve head is usually located in the non-tapetal fundus, just ventral to the tapetal–non-tapetal junctional zone (Figure 7.1(a,b)). Tapetal colour varies with coat colour, so that light-coloured animals have a yellow tapetum, chestnut animals have variations between green and yellow, bay horses usually have a green-blue tapetum and dark bay and black animals have a blue tapetum. In colour-dilute partially albinotic or albinotic animals, which usually have

EQUINE OPHTHALMOLOGY

blue irises, the tapetum may be thin or absent and the extent to which large choroidal vessels are visible is also determined by the amount of overlying pigment. In some animals in which the tapetum is absent, the retinal vasculature and choroidal vessels can be viewed against the whitish colour of the sclera. The non-tapetal fundus is brown to dark brown in normally pigmented horses. Colour dilution allows the large choroidal vessels to be visualised.

Points to note in the assessment of the equine fundus
- Complete darkness is necessary for comprehensive examination
- Mydriasis is not always needed, but should certainly be used if fundus lesions are suspected
- Indirect and direct ophthalmoscopy should be used for examination, as the two methods are complementary rather than exclusive
- The order of examination is usually the optic nerve head, retinal and choroidal vasculature, non-tapetal fundus and tapetal fundus
- The *tapetum fibrosum* (collagen) forms a tough barrier, so pathological changes are most likely to be seen in the non-tapetal fundus and are most readily observed ventrally
- Attenuation or loss of retinal vasculature usually indicates local or generalised retinal dysfunction, possibly causing a visual deficit

CONGENITAL FUNDUS DISEASE

Colobomatous defects
Colobomatous defects are relatively common congenital, non-progressive defects (Figure 7.38).

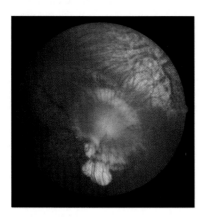

Figure 7.38 Colobomatous defects of the equine fundus. Several clearly-defined focal regions of hypoplastic retina lie ventral to the optic disc. Over these defects fine retinal vessels pass without distortion. In this old horse there is also some peripapillary pigmentary disturbance and the edge of the optic disc is not very clearly defined.

Clinical features
- Usually an incidental finding and not a cause of visual deficit
- Clearly defined round or oval reflective lesions in the tapetal and non-tapetal fundus; the papillary region is less commonly involved

- Large colobomas are sometimes associated with pigmentary disturbance
- They may be unilateral or bilateral, single or multiple

Congenital stationary night blindness

Congenital stationary night blindness is mainly a condition of the Appaloosa, but has also been recorded occasionally in other breeds including Thoroughbreds. It may be inherited as a sex-linked recessive trait in the Appaloosa and has not yet been described in the UK. There is no treatment.

Clinical features

- There is some variation in the severity of clinical signs, although the condition is usually static
- In severely-affected foals, owners note disorientation, particularly if the foal is separated from its mother; there are also stargazing and a head tilt. Closer examination may indicate a bilateral dorsomedial strabismus as the only obvious ocular abnormality
- Most commonly there is normal vision under good lighting conditions and visual impairment in dim light
- Electroretinography is required to confirm the diagnosis

Congenital retinal detachment

Congenital non-attachments of the retina and congenital retinal detachments are rare conditions; they are usually bilateral and a cause of impaired vision or blindness. Total detachment may be found as an isolated abnormality, whereas congenital non-attachment is usually associated with other ocular defects (e.g. microphthalmos, anterior segment dysgenesis, lens subluxation/luxation, cataract, colobomatous defects and retinal dysplasia). There is no treatment.

Clinical features

- The pupils are usually dilated and poorly-responsive, or unresponsive, to bright light
- Vision may be impaired or absent
- Ophthalmoscopy reveals retinal detachment. Most commonly, the dorsal retina detaches (disinserts from the *ora ciliaris retinae*), but remains attached in the region of the optic nerve head. The tapetal fundus in the affected region appears more reflective, and grey-white folds of detached retina hang ventrally, often partly obscuring the ONH

Congenital retinal haemorrhage

Multiple small retinal haemorrhages are sometimes present in normal foals, and those suffering from the neonatal maladjustment syndrome, and they resolve without treatment a few days after birth.

Optic nerve hypoplasia

As in other species, this is a very rare developmental defect in which the clinical signs can be related to the severity of the defect (i.e. the number of retinal ganglion cells). There is no treatment.

EQUINE OPHTHALMOLOGY

Clinical features
- Usually bilateral
- Most affected foals have dilated pupils and an abnormal pupillary light reflex
- Affected animals are visually impaired or blind
- The optic nerve head is smaller and usually paler than normal

ACQUIRED FUNDUS DISEASE

Pigmentary retinopathy

Pigmentary retinopathy may be a non-specific finding in older animals, of unknown cause, or may be part of the clinical presentation of equine motor neurone disease (see below) (Figure 7.39).

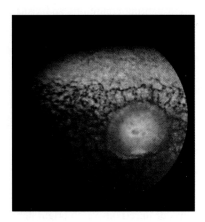

Figure 7.39 Pigmentary retinopathy with normal retinal vasculature. In this bilaterally-affected animal there was no indication of generalised disease (with acknowledgement to A.G. Matthews).

Equine motor neurone disease retinopathy

This condition is associated with neurodegenerative motor neurone disease and the fundus changes that are found in approximately one third of clinical cases are the result of accumulation of dark brownish-coloured ceroid lipofuscin in the retinal pigment epithelium.

Clinical features
- Pigmentary disturbance in an irregular mosaic pattern affecting the tapetal–non-tapetal junctional zone and the tapetal fundus
- The extent of the disturbance is variable, as is any identifiable effect on vision
- The changes are bilateral and similar

Treatment
The neurological signs of the disease can be stabilised by oral vitamin E supplementation, but treatment does not seem to reverse the retinal changes.

EQUINE OPHTHALMOLOGY

Senile retinopathy

Senile degenerative changes associated with pigmentary disturbance are not unusual in older animals, and their prevalence increases with advancing age.

Clinical features

- Affected animals are usually over 15 years of age and the fundus changes are usually bilateral
- Although vision may be reduced in some cases, owners of the majority of affected animals report no visual impairment
- Pigmentary disturbance is most obvious in the non-tapetal peripapillary region
- Subtle hyperreflectivity of the tapetal fundus and vascular attenuation are inconstant findings
- Other age-related degenerative changes involving the vitreous and lens may also be present

Inflammatory fundus lesions

In common with other species, active chorioretinitis lesions are seldom seen, but inactive chorioretinopathy lesions are reasonably common. The cause is rarely established, but active chorioretinitis has been observed in association with systemic viral and bacterial (*Streptococcus equi*) disease.

Inflammatory optic nerve lesions are most commonly seen in horses with vasculitis, chorioretinitis, panuveitis and equine recurrent uveitis. Less frequently, optic neuritis and retrobulbar neuritis are the only obvious sites of inflammation. Recognisable causes include multifocal central nervous system infections (viral, bacterial and protozoan parasites) and severe systemic problems such as septicaemia.

Clinical features

Focal or multifocal lesions

Focal or multifocal 'bullet-hole' lesions are commonest and are most readily observed in the non-tapetal fundus and peripapillary region (Figure 7.40). They are approximately circular, with a depigmented periphery and hyperpigmented centre. In the acute stage, these lesions appear as greyish-white exudative lesions. Their distribution suggests that the pathological changes are located in the choroidal vessels that perforate the tapetum to supply the choriocapillaris.

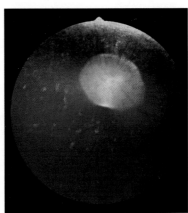

Figure 7.40 Focal (bullet-hole) chorioretinopathy as an incidental unilateral finding (with acknowledgements to A.G. Matthews).

EQUINE OPHTHALMOLOGY

Peripapillary lesions

Peripapillary lesions are also relatively common, and when they are located lateral and medial to the ONH are designated 'butterfly' lesions (Figure 7.41). The affected area often surrounds the ONH completely and the distribution of these lesions would suggest an association with blood vessels, particularly those of the choroid. Active exudative inflammation may well be accompanied by vasculitis. Putative association of these lesions with vascular pathology suggests that they are not necessarily of purely inflammatory origin; ischaemia and immune-mediated damage, for example, may be other possible causes. Infectious diseases such as leptospirosis have been linked with equine recurrent uveitis (ERU) and peripapillary lesions (see earlier under ERU).

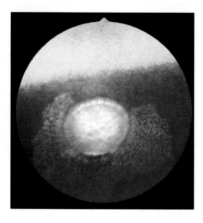

Figure 7.41 Peripapillary chorioretinopathy. This is a relatively common and non-specific finding that usually reflects previous posterior-segment inflammation. Its clinical significance is usually judged, quite empirically, by the appearance of overlying retinal vessels. If these are of normal appearance then it is assumed that there is no associated visual abnormality, but if they are attenuated then vision in the corresponding sector may be impaired (with acknowledgements to A.G. Matthews).

Diffuse lesions

Diffuse lesions are uncommon. They appear hyperreflective in the tapetal region and depigmented in the non-tapetal region. Infarction, as well as inflammation, are possible causes.

Inflammatory optic nerve lesions

Inflammatory optic nerve lesions can render the horse blind (see below). Possible causes include viral (e.g. equine herpes virus), bacterial (e.g. *Streptococcus equi*) and parasitic (e.g. protozoal) infections.

Treatment

There is no treatment for inactive chorioretinopathy, but if the cause can be established it may be possible to treat active chorioretinitis.

Fundus abnormalities associated with acute vision loss (see also
Section 2)
Aetiology
• Acute unilateral blindness can occur after direct trauma to the head or eye or severe damage to the optic nerve. Optic neuritis and retrobulbar neuritis are also causes, as is blindness caused by uveitis, glaucoma or retinal detachment. It is also possible, but rare, for such cases to be bilateral.

- Intraocular haemorrhage and generalised severe haemorrhage can cause sudden blindness. When the blood supply to the optic nerve head is severely disrupted ischaemic neuropathy ensues. Acute blindness associated with ischaemic optic neuropathy can be a complication of both primary and secondary haemorrhage, septic emboli and the surgical ligation of arteries (e.g. maxillary, greater palatine, internal and external carotid) as a treatment for epistaxis associated with guttural pouch mycosis. Such cases are usually unilateral, but not invariably so.
- Inflammation (especially that associated with infectious agents such as viruses), toxins and neoplasia should also be considered in the differential diagnosis of unilateral and bilateral visual impairment.

Clinical findings in trama-related visual loss
- The history can be of crucial importance, but on occasions is misleading, particularly when the loss of vision is the result of non-accidental injury
- External signs of damage to the head or eye may be apparent
- Partial or complete unilateral or bilateral blindness
- Normal or abnormal pupillary light reflexes (usually abnormal)
- Sub-retinal haemorrhage, retinal haemorrhage, preretinal haemorrhage and intraocular haemorrhage
- Partial or complete retinal detachment
- Optic nerve head oedema (papilloedema) ± peripapillary and retinal haemorrhage
- Ischaemic retinopathy and optic neuropathy are consequences of severe damage or disruption to the blood supply to the retina and optic nerve. Progressive retinal depigmentation and focal pigment hypertrophy are characteristic findings in the nontapetal fundus; vascular attenuation and more generalised retinal atrophy may also be apparent. Optic nerve atrophy is always present in long-standing cases

Possible treatment for suspected cerebrocortical oedema associated with trauma
- The success of treatment depends upon establishing and eliminating the cause. The damage may, however, be irreversible in some cases, as for example when there has been a fracture of the basisphenoid or basioccipital bone, shearing of the optic nerve following injury to the poll, following severe blood loss or damage from toxins
- Broad-spectrum antibiotics
- Vitamin E (20 000 units orally every 24 hours for an adult)
- If cerebral oedema or papilloedema is present then:
  ○ Dexamethasone 0.5 mg/kg intravenously every 6–8 hours for the first 24 hours after the injury
  ○ Dimethyl sulphoxide (DMSO) 1 g/kg intravenously as a 10–20% solution in saline every 12–24 hours for five days
  ○ Mannitol, but *not* if there is risk of further haemorrhage (0.5–2 g/kg of 20% solution by *slow* intravenous injection, twice daily)
- If skull fractures are present and there is gross displacement, repair should be considered

Retinal detachment
Acquired retinal detachment may be a consequence of severe inflammatory disease (e.g. ERU), intraocular surgery and trauma. In addition, some cases are idiopathic in

EQUINE OPHTHALMOLOGY

so far as there is no obvious cause, although this type is usually found in older horses and there is often accompanying vitreal degeneration. Treatment regimes that may achieve success in dogs (e.g. laser surgery and retinopexy) have not been reported in horses.

Clinical features
- Depending upon the extent of retinal detachment there may be no obvious vision loss, partial vision loss or blindness
- Clinical presentation ranges from giant retinal tears to total detachment with dis-insertion (see earlier)

Optic neuropathies
This general term covers a range of ophthalmoscopic appearances, and the lesions are described as exudative and proliferative; but common to all is the fact that they are usually incidental findings.

Exudative
The exudative type of optic neuropathy consists of delicate translucent material at the periphery of the optic nerve head, and is a common incidental finding of no clinical significance.

Proliferative
Proliferative lesions appear as raised masses at the periphery of the optic nerve head and may be focal or generalised (Figure 7.42); the latter can be large enough to obscure the optic nerve head. The origin and composition of these lesions cannot be determined from ophthalmoscopic examination.

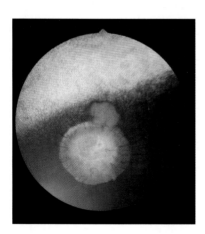

Figure 7.42 Focal proliferative optic neuropathy. This is a relatively common finding on ophthalmic examination, particularly in older horses, and is not associated with any discernible effect on vision. More florid types, especially when there are multiple proliferative lesions, may be of clinical significance (with acknowledgements to A. G. Matthews).

The *focal* type is generally benign and consists of whitish material at the periphery of the optic nerve head. Fine blood vessels are often associated with these lesions. The material may be nervous tissue ± macrophages (myelin-rich or lipid-rich).

EQUINE OPHTHALMOLOGY

The *generalised* type may be a consequence of insults such as trauma and severe acute blood loss and may represent extruded nervous tissue ± macrophages. Affected eyes are usually visually impaired or blind and there may be some indications of optic atrophy.

Optic nerve neoplasia
A number of primary tumours have been described. *Astrocytoma* of the optic nerve head resembles focal proliferative optic neuropathy and, similarly, is of no clinical significance. *Medulloepithelioma* and *neuroepithelioma* of the optic nerve are very rare tumours and both types can be locally invasive and a cause of blindness and even exophthalmos if there is orbital extension.

Optic atrophy
Optic atrophy is the end result of severe insult to the eye or the optic nerve, including the compressive effects of infiltrative neoplasia and space-occupying lesions. The effects are often a consequence of local ischaemia and Wallerian degeneration. The optic nerve head becomes pale and there is invariably profound attenuation of the retinal vessels (Figure 7.43).

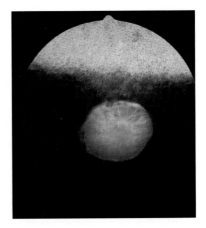

Figure 7.43 Optic atrophy. The optic disc is pale and the architecture of the *lamina cribrosa* has become more prominent because of the optic nerve atrophy. The retinal vessels were attenuated and the eye was blind. This was an incidental unilateral finding.

EQUINE OPHTHALMOLOGY

SUMMARY

Normal fundus variants
- *Partial albinism* – generalised deficiency of chorioretinal pigment; the tapetum may be thin or absent in some of these animals
- *Albinism* – complete absence of chorioretinal pigment; the tapetum is absent in these eyes
- *Lipid deposition* – localised yellow inclusions within the chorioretina
- *Peripapillary medullated nerve fibres*
- *Peripapillary pigmentation* and *hypopigmentation*

- *Absence of retinal vessels* in the ventral region of the optic nerve head
- *Focal pigment proliferation* (*ectopic pigment*) in tapetal fundus

Fundus abnormalities of no visual significance

- *Colobomas* – not uncommon; both typical (6 o'clock) and atypical (anywhere else), they may be single or multiple. The non-tapetal fundus is the commonest site, less commonly elsewhere, including the papillary and peripapillary region
- *Isolated focal chorioretinopathy* – small depigmented foci in non-tapetal fundus
- *Focal proliferative optic neuropathy* – localised proliferation of tissue from periphery of ONH, usually in older horses. They may slowly enlarge or remain the same size. Optic nerve is functionally normal
- Transient *retinal haemorrhage* may be found in normal foals and those with neonatal maladjustment syndrome

Fundus abnormalities of doubtful visual significance

- *Peripapillary chorioretinopathy with intact retinal vasculature* – so-called 'butterfly lesions'. Of unknown significance in the absence of signs of present or past uveitis, or previous intraocular inflammation
- Pigmentary disturbance associated with *senile retinopathy* and *equine motor neurone disease* does not cause obvious visual problems in the majority of cases

Fundus abnormalities of probable visual significance

- *Peripapillary chorioretinopathy with retinal vasculature abnormality*. Significant when occurring in association with signs of present or past uveitis, or other intraocular inflammation
- *Multiple focal chorioretinitis* and *chorioretinopathy* lesions – generalised focal depigmentation in non-tapetal fundus

Fundus abnormalities of certain visual significance

- *Retinal detachments* – giant retinal tears, bullous detachment, partial and total detachment
- *Extensive intraocular haemorrhage*
- *Optic neuritis* or indications of a previous optic neuritis (pathological conus)
- *Generalised proliferative optic neuropathy*
- *Ischaemic chorioretinopathy* and *optic neuropathy*
- *Panretinal inflammation* or *degeneration*
- *Optic atrophy*

APPENDIX 1

OPHTHALMIC TERMINOLOGY

GENERAL

Abiotrophy	Premature degeneration of a tissue after it has reached maturity
Adnexa	Eyelids, lacrimal apparatus, orbit and paraorbital areas
Amaurosis	Complete loss of sight in one or both eyes in the absence of ophthalmoscopic or other marked objective signs
Amblyopia	Partial loss of sight in one or both eyes in the absence of ophthalmoscopic or other marked objective signs
Anophthalmos	Absence of an eye

- Primary – optic pits fail to deepen and form outgrowths from forebrain
- Secondary – whole of forebrain fails to develop
- Degenerative – optic vesicle forms but subsequently degenerates

Aplasia	Failure of differentiation of a tissue during embryonic life
Atrophy	A diminution of size, a shrinking of cells, fibres, or tissues that previously had reached their full development
Canthus	Angle at either end of the eyelid aperture, specified as medial (nasal) and lateral (temporal)
Coloboma	An absence or defect of some ocular tissue, usually resulting from a failure of part of the embryonic cleft to close, and seen as a notch, hole, fissure or cleft. If the defect is in the line of the embryonic cleft (i.e. at approximately 6 o'clock) it is spoken of as a *typical coloboma*, other positions are referred to as *atypical*
Cyclopia	Single eye
Degeneration	A secondary phenomenon resulting from previous disease; it may be unilateral or bilateral and occurs in a tissue that has reached its full growth
Dioptre	Unit of measurement of the refractive powers of lenses, equal to the reciprocal of the focal length of the lens expressed in metres
Diplopia	Double vision
Dysplasia	Disorderly cellular proliferation during embryonic life
Dystrophy	A primary, bilateral, inherited disorder with distinct clinico-pathological findings
Ectasia	Dilation, expansion or distension
Emmetropia	Refractive condition in which no refractive error is present with accommodation at rest
Eye	Globe or eyeball
Hypermetropia	Refractive error in which the focal point for light rays from a distant object is behind the retina (long sighted)
Hyperplasia	Increase above the normal number of individual cells in a tissue
Hypertrophy	Increase above the normal size of individual cells, fibres or tissues, without an increase in the number of individual elements
Hypoplasia	Lack of differentiation because of arrested development of a tissue during embryonic life
Metaplasia	Transformation of one type of tissue into another type

OPHTHALMIC TERMINOLOGY

Microphthalmos	An eye which is smaller than normal and imperfectly developed
Miosis	Pupillary constriction
Mydriasis	Pupillary dilation
Myopia	Refractive error in which focal point for light rays from a distant object is in front of the retina (short sighted)
Nanophthalmos	An eye which is smaller than normal but perfectly formed and of normal function
Neoplasia	A continuous increase above the normal number of cells in a tissue
Nystagmus	Involuntary oscillation of the eyeballs
Ocular	Pertaining to the eye or to vision
Ocular surface	The term used to describe the continuous epithelium which begins at the eyelid margin, extends onto both surfaces of the third eyelid, the back of the upper and lower eyelids, into the fornices, and onto the globe
Ophthalmia	Inflammation of the eye, usually refers to conjunctival inflammation
Ophthalmic	Pertaining to the eye
Ophthalmoplegia	Paralysis of one or more muscles of the eye
	• External – extraocular muscles
	• Internal – intraocular muscles
	• Total – both sets of muscles
Palpebral aperture	Aperture between the eyelids
Photophobia	Abnormal sensitivity to, and discomfort from, light
Photopic	Pertaining to vision in the light, an eye which has become light adapted
Presbyopia	Physiologically blurred near vision, commonly evident soon after 40 years of age in humans
Scotopic	Pertaining to vision in the dark, an eye which has become dark adapted
Staphyloma	Protrusion (ectasia) of wall of the eye, lined with uveal tissue
Strabismus	Squint (medial squint – esotropia; lateral squint – exotropia)
Synophthalmos	Fused orbits, varying degrees of ocular fusion

GLOBE AND ORBIT

Buphthalmos	Literally 'ox eye'; used to describe enlarged globe in congenital and early-onset glaucoma
Endophthalmitis	Severe intraocular inflammation, which does not extend beyond the sclera
Enophthalmos	A recession of the globe into its socket
Enucleation of the eye	Removal of the globe
Evisceration of the eye	Removal of the contents of the eye with retention of the sclera
Exenteration of the orbit	Removal of the eyeball and all soft tissues within the bony orbit

Exophthalmos	Similar to proptosis – a forward (anterior) displacement of the globe
Globe orientation	• *Poles of the eye* – central points of the anterior and posterior curvatures of the globe
	• *Optic axis* – line connecting the poles
	• *Visual axis* – line from the object viewed to the centre of the most sensitive area of the retina (*area centralis*)
	• *Equator* – Imaginary line drawn around the eye midway between its poles
Hydrophthalmos	Enlarged globe, secondary to glaucoma
Orbital cellulitis	Inflammation of the orbit
Panophthalmitis	Severe intraocular inflammation which also involves the sclera, Tenon's capsule and even the orbital tissues themselves
Phthisis bulbi	Shrinking of the eyeball following some pathological process, the eye is blind and degenerate
Prolapse	Displacement of the eyeball from the orbit
Proptosis	A forward displacement of the eyeball/globe
Retrobulbar	Behind the eyeball (but usually within the orbit)

EYELIDS

Ablepharon	Absence of eyelid margin
Ankyloblepharon	Fused eyelids (a normal feature of neonatal carnivores)
Blepharitis	Inflammation of the eyelids
Blepharospasm	Spasm of the eyelids – typical response to ocular pain
Chalazion	Chronic, sterile, lipogranulomatous inflammatory lesion caused by blockage of meibomian gland secretions
Dermoid	A congenital growth consisting of skin and its appendages
Distichiasis	The presence of two rows of lashes on one eyelid (i.e. an extra row of eyelashes); The extra lashes (single or multiple) usually arise from hair follicles abnormally located within the meibomian glands
Ectopic cilia	Single or multiple cilia emerging from the conjunctival surface of the eyelid; the cilia commonly originate from hair follicles abnormally located within the meibomian glands
Ectropion	Eversion of one or both eyelid margins
Entropion	Inversion of one or both eyelid margins
Lagophthalmos	Inability to close eyelids completely
Meibomianitis	Inflammation (and obstruction) of the meibomian glands
Ptosis	Drooping of the upper eyelid (may be a result of damage to the oculomotor nerve, Horner's syndrome or a result of damage to the facial nerve)
Symblepharon	Fusion of cornea or bulbar conjunctiva to palpebral or nictitating conjunctiva (because of pathological denudation of epithelium and loss of stem-cell population)

OPHTHALMIC TERMINOLOGY

Trichiasis	Misdirection of one or more normal eyelashes so as to cause corneal or conjunctival irritation

LACRIMAL APPARATUS

Dacryoadenitis	Inflammation of the lacrimal gland
Dacryocystitis	Inflammation of the lacrimal drainage apparatus
Dacryops	Ductal cyst of the lacrimal gland
Epiphora	Overflow of tears, strictly speaking a consequence of poor tear drainage (but often used to denote excessive tear production, or inadequate drainage, or both)
Lacrimation	Excessive tear production
Preocular tear film (PTF)	The PTF covers the ocular surface; major components – lipid (oil), water, mucin

CONJUNCTIVA

Chemosis	Oedema of the conjunctiva
Conjunctivitis	Inflammation of the conjunctiva

LIMBUS, EPISCLERA AND SCLERA

Episcleral congestion	Usually used with reference to the congestion of the episcleral vessels that results when venous outflow is impeded as in glaucoma, or in the presence of an orbital space-occupying lesion
Episcleritis	Inflammation of the episclera
Episclerokeratitis	Inflammation of the episclera and cornea
Limbus	Junctional zone between the white of the eye and the clear cornea
Scleritis	Inflammation of the sclera

CORNEA

Corneal scars:	• *Nebula* – small, cloudy corneal opacity • *Macula* – moderate corneal scar • *Leucoma* – large, dense, white, corneal opacity
Descemetocoele	Protrusion of Descemet's membrane at the base of a deep ulcer
Dry eye	Keratoconjunctivitis sicca (KCS), consequence of deficiency of aqueous portion of PTF
Keratectomy	Excision of part of the cornea
Keratitis	Inflammation of the cornea
Keratoconus	Cone-shaped deformity of cornea; some corneal thinning will have occurred at the corneal apex
Keratoglobus	Dome-shaped protrusion of a uniformly-thin cornea

Keratoplasty	Corneal grafting (lamellar – partial thickness; penetrating – full thickness)
Megalocornea	A cornea which is larger than normal
Microcornea	A cornea which is smaller than normal
Pannus	Chronic superficial keratoconjunctivitis
Xerosis	Abnormal dryness of the cornea

UVEAL TRACT (IRIS, CILIARY BODY AND CHOROID)

Anisocoria	Inequality in pupil size, may be physiological or pathological
Choroiditis	Inflammation of the choroid, may be focal or widespread (posterior uveitis)
Chorioretinitis	Inflammation of the choroid and retina
Cyclitis	Inflammation of the ciliary body
Cyclodialysis	The establishment of a communication between the anterior chamber and the suprachoroidal space in order to relieve intraocular pressure
Cycloplegia	Paralysis of the ciliary muscle giving rise to paralysis of accommodation
Heterochromia iridis	One sector of the iris is a different colour from the remainder
Heterochromia iridum	A difference of colour between the two irises (irides)
Iridectomy	Surgical excision of part of the iris
Iridencleisis	Incarceration of a portion of the iris in a surgical incision at the limbus
Iridocyclitis	Inflammation of iris and ciliary body, hence an anterior uveitis
Iridodenesis	Trembling of the iris on movement of the eye due to lack of support behind the iris; seen in aphakia or after dislocation of the lens
Iridotomy	Incision of the iris
Iris bombé	Iris adherent to lens around whole of pupillary margin, hence non-attached parts bulge forward because of increased pressure from behind; a cause of secondary glaucoma
Iris prolapse	Prolapse of iris through a perforated cornea or corneoscleral wound
Iritis	Inflammation of the iris
Leukocoria	A white pupil
Panuveitis	Inflammation of the whole uveal tract
Pars planitis	Inflammation in the region of the *pars plana* of the ciliary body (intermediate uveitis)
Persistent pupillary membrane (PPM)	Persistence of foetal mesodermal tissue anterior to the iris; small strands may float freely or be attached to iris, lens or cornea; attachment of PPM to the anterior lens capsule is referred to as an *epicapsular star*
Synechiae	• Adhesions between iris and corneal endothelium (anterior)

OPHTHALMIC TERMINOLOGY

- Adhesions between iris root and corneoscleral tissue (peripheral anterior synechiae)
- Adhesions between iris and anterior lens capsule (posterior)

ANTERIOR CHAMBER AND AQUEOUS HUMOUR

Aqueous flare	Increased opalescence of aqueous humour due to greater than normal protein content associated with uveitis
Aqueous humour	A clear watery fluid produced by the ciliary processes of the ciliary body; aqueous clots in contact with air
Aqueous outflow	• Conventional outflow – irido-corneal angle • Unconventional outflow – uveoscleral tissue
Hyphaema	Haemorrhage in the anterior chamber
Hypopyon	Pus in the anterior chamber
Keratic precipitates (KPs)	Deposits of inflammatory cells on the posterior aspect of cornea, indicative of uveitis

GLAUCOMAS

Glaucoma	A rise in intraocular pressure which is sufficient to damage the eye and vision
	• *Primary* – no antecedent ocular disease
	  ○ *open angle*
	  ○ associated with *goniodysgenesis*
	• *Secondary* – associated with demonstrable ocular disease (e.g. inflammation, neoplasia, lens luxation)

Goniodysgenesis	Abnormal drainage angle (pectinate ligament dysplasia ± abnormal width)
Gonioscopy	Examination of the drainage angle with a special lens (goniolens)
Tonometry	Measurement of the intraocular pressure

LENS

Aphakia	The lens is absent
Aphakic crescent	The clear area between the pupil margin and lens equator which may be seen when the lens has luxated
Cataract	An opacity of the lens or its capsule
Phacodenesis	Trembling (wobbling) of the lens because it is subluxated or luxated

VITREOUS HUMOUR

Asteroid hyalosis	Calcium soaps (small yellow spheres) suspended in vitreous gel

Persistent hyperplastic primary vitreous (PHPV)	Persistent hyperplastic primary vitreous – persistence and hyperplasia of primary vitreous, which may be associated with abnormalities in neighbouring structures (e.g. lens)
Synchysis scintillans	Also known as *cholesterolosis bulbi*; cholesterol crystals present in an abnormally fluid vitreous
Vitritis	Inflammation of the vitreous (hyalitis)

RETINA

Cones	Concerned with visual acuity and colour vision in some animals; particularly concentrated in *area centralis*, which tends to be free of macroscopic blood vessels (*area centralis* approximates to the *macula* of humans)
Electroretinogram	The response of the retina to a brief flash of light; the technique of measurement is known as electroretinography (ERG); The electrical change produced by sensory stimulation is an example of an evoked response and ERG is used in the assessment of retinal function
Hemeralopia	Day blindness
Nyctalopia	Night blindness
Ora ciliaris retinae	Termination of the retina at the equator where it merges into the ciliary epithelium (known as *ora serrata* in primates)
Retinal atrophy	Loss of retinal tissue; inherited and acquired forms
Retinal dysplasia	Abnormal embryonic development of the retina (proliferation with imperfect differentiation); may be other associated ocular and systemic abnormalities
Retinitis	Inflammation of the retina
Rods	Concerned particularly with night (light/dark) vision

OPTIC NERVE HEAD (ONH) AND OPTIC NERVE

Optic atrophy	Loss of nervous elements such that the ONH appears smaller and usually paler than normal
Optic nerve aplasia	Total failure of differentiation of the optic nerve
Optic nerve head	Optic disc (papilla); ophthalmoscopically visible part of optic nerve (cranial nerve II)
Optic nerve hypoplasia	Partial failure of differentiation of the optic nerve
Optic neuritis	Inflammation of the optic nerve (bulbar and retrobulbar inflammations are distinguished)
Papillitis	Inflammation of the optic nerve head; also known as optic neuritis

OPHTHALMIC TERMINOLOGY

Papilloedema	Oedema of the ONH as a result of some pathological intracranial process
Pseudopapilloedema	The ONH looks oedematous, but both eyes are similar and the appearance is due to excessive myelination; pseudo-papilloedema is a normal feature of some breeds of dog e.g. German Shepherd Dog and Golden Retriever

OPHTHALMIC TERMINOLOGY

APPENDIX 2

TOPICAL OPHTHALMIC PREPARATIONS

TOPICAL OPHTHALMIC PREPARATIONS

GENERAL NOTES

- The drugs are listed by their non-proprietary (generic) names, as they were in the text, followed by the relevant proprietary preparations and their manufacturers. Only the proprietary preparations used in the UK are listed, and the list is not exhaustive.
- 'V' signifies a proprietary veterinary preparation and 'M' a proprietary medical preparation. The veterinary prescribing cascade should be followed.
- Topical preparations are generally instilled into the lower conjunctival sac (drops), or as a ribbon of material (ointment) across the cornea, taking care to avoid touching the eye with the nozzle of the bottle or tube, to avoid contaminating the preparation.
- The conjunctival sacs of most animals cannot accommodate a whole drop of solution, so there is no point in using more than one drop per eye for topical medication.
- If more than one agent is to be applied, an interval of at least five minutes should be allowed before the next agent is given, in order to prevent dilution and wash out of the previous preparation.

DIAGNOSTIC PREPARATIONS

- Fluorescein sodium 1% or 2% eye drops for single use: **Minims® Fluorescein Sodium** (Chauvin), M

Fluorescein is an orange dye that turns green under alkaline conditions; it may be applied topically to confirm corneal ulceration, to detect aqueous leakage (Seidel test) and to check the nasolacrimal duct for patency. It is also used in studies of ocular surface disease, either on its own or prior to rose bengal application.

- Rose bengal 1% eye drops for single use: **Minims® Rose Bengal** (Chauvin), M

Rose bengal is a red dye that is used in studies of ocular surface disease and to demonstrate subtle corneal erosions, either on its own or after topical fluorescein. As rose bengal is irritating to the eye local anaesthetic can be instilled beforehand.

LOCAL ANAESTHETICS

In addition to their diagnostic use in conscious animals, application of topical local anaesthetics prior to surgery that is to be performed under general anaesthesia may reduce the amount of general anaesthetic needed for procedures on the adnexa, ocular surface and cornea. It is important to emphasise that local anaesthetics should not be used to provide symptomatic relief or for the treatment of ocular disease.

Proxymetacaine hydrochloride

- Proxymetacaine hydrochloride 0.5% eye drops for single use: **Minims® Proxymetacaine** (Chauvin), M
- Proxymetacaine hydrochloride 0.5% and fluorescein sodium 0.25% eye drops for single use: **Minims® Proxymetacaine and Fluorescein** (Chauvin), M

Proxymetacaine hydrochloride is an excellent choice for short-acting anaesthesia (duration of 15–20 minutes) prior to corneal sampling (scrapes and swabs) and before contact tonometry and gonioscopy.

Tetracaine hydrochloride (amethocaine hydrochloride)
- Tetracaine hydrochloride 0.5% and 1% eye drops for single use: **Minims**® **Amethocaine Hydrochloride** (Chauvin), M

Provides more profound anaesthesia than proxymetacaine and can be used prior to minor surgical procedures.

TEAR-REPLACEMENT AGENTS AND OCULAR LUBRICANTS

Carbomers are more effective than aqueous tear substitutes like hypromellose (colloid) and polyvinyl alcohol (resin) as their mucinomimetic properties prolong corneal contact. Although aqueous tear substitutes are not recommended as the sole tear-replacement agent for tear-deficiency syndromes, a number of other products for topical medication of the eye usefully include hypromellose in the formulation.
Dose: Apply 6–8 times daily or more frequently if required.

Acetylcysteine
- Acetylcysteine 5% and hypromellose 0.35% eye drops: **Ilube**® (Alcon), M
Dose: Apply 3–4 times daily or more frequently if required.
Useful when there is impaired or abnormal mucus production.

Carbomers (polyacrylic acid)
- Carbomer 980 (polyacrylic acid) 0.2% gel: **Viscotears**® (Cibavision), M; **GelTears**® liquid gel (Chauvin), M
Dose: Apply 4–6 times daily or more frequently if required.
The carbomers are long-acting artificial tear preparations with mucinomimetic properties and are the most useful for tear replacement in veterinary practice.

Colloids and resins
- Hypromellose 0.3% eye drops (Non-proprietary)
- Hypromellose 0.3% and dextran '70' 0.1% eye drops: **Tears Naturale**® (Alcon), M
- Polyvinyl alcohol 1.4% eye drops: **Liquifilm**® (Allergan), M
Dose: Apply 6 times daily or more frequently if required.

Liquid paraffin
- White soft paraffin 57.3%, liquid paraffin 42.5% and wool alcohols 0.2% eye ointment: **Lacri-Lube**® (Allergan), M
- White soft paraffin 60%, liquid paraffin 30% and wool fat 10% eye ointment: **Lubri-Tears**® (Alcon), M
These preparations are ideal for overnight use in animals with tear-deficiency syndromes and corneal epithelial erosion. They can also be used to protect the eye during general anaesthesia.

Sodium chloride
- Sodium chloride 0.9% eye drops for single use: **Minims**® **Saline** (Chauvin), M

Used for irrigation, including the removal of harmful substances. It may also be used in conjunction with fluorescein to enhance staining and to flush excess fluorescein from the eye.

IMMUNOSUPPRESSANTS

Cyclosporin

Cyclosporin (ciclosporin/cyclosporine) 0.2% ointment: **Optimmune**® (Schering-Plough), V
Dose: Twice daily initially, reducing to maintenance level (occasionally to zero) according to response to therapy.
Used to treat a variety of immune-mediated disorders such as keratoconjunctivitis sicca and certain types of keratitis, including canine chronic superficial keratoconjunctivitis (pannus) and feline proliferative keratoconjunctivitis.

Tacrolimus

Tacrolimus is a macrolide lactone with potent immunonosuppressive activity, but it is not licensed for ophthalmic use in the UK. It has been used empirically at various strengths (ranging from 0.03%–0.1%) to treat ocular conditions in animals for which cyclosporin is indicated. Tacrolimus awaits scientific evaluation in controlled clinical trials.

ANTI-INFECTIVE PREPARATIONS

ANTIBACTERIALS

- The term 'broad-spectrum' denotes that the drug is effective against Gram +ve and Gram −ve bacteria.
- Preparations are manufactured as eye drops (solutions, suspensions and emulsions) and ointments. Drops need to be applied more frequently than ointments because of their lower corneal contact time. The addition of tear-replacement agents to eye drop preparations increases the corneal contact time.

Chloramphenicol

- Chloramphenicol eye drops 0.5% and ointment 1% (Non-proprietary), M
- Chloramphenicol eye drops 0.5%: **Chloromycetin V Redidrops**® (Pharmacia and Upjohn), V
Dose: Apply 3–4 times daily or more frequently if required.
A valuable drug with a broad spectrum of activity that includes a wide range of Gram +ve and Gram −ve bacteria, but not recommended for confirmed *Proteus* spp and *Pseudomonas aeruginosa* infections. Acquired resistance may be a problem in enterobacterial infections.

Ciprofloxacin

- Ciprofloxacin hydrochloride 0.3% eye drops: **Ciloxan**® (Alcon), M

Dose: Follow the manufacturer's recommendations, usually intensive application (e.g. every 15–30 minutes) throughout a 24-hour period is required for the first 2 days of treatment.

Ciprofloxacin is a new-generation broad-spectrum antibiotic, licensed for use in bacterial infections, including ulcerative keratitis. It should be reserved for complex situations, including gentamicin-resistant *Pseudomonas aeruginosa* infection. Ciprofloxacin is not always effective against *Staphylococcus* spp and *Streptococcus* spp.

Fucidic acid

- Fucidic acid 1% viscous eye drops with carbomer gel excipient: **Fucithalmic Vet**® (Leo), V

Dose: Apply 3–4 times daily or more frequently if required.

Fucidic acid is active against a number of Gram +ve bacteria, and is particularly effective against *Staphylococcus* spp. It can be used in conjunction with gentamicin sulphate to provide broad-spectrum cover.

Gentamicin sulphate

Gentamicin sulphate 0.3% and hypromellose eye drops: **Clinagel Vet**® (Janssen), V
- Gentamicin sulphate 0.3% eye drops: **Tiacil** (Virbac), V

Dose: Apply 3–4 times daily or more frequently if required.

Gentamicin sulphate is a broad-spectrum antibiotic that is effective against Gram +ve bacteria such as *Staphylococcus* spp and *Pasteurella* spp as well as a wide range of Gram –ve bacteria including *Pseudomonas aeruginosa*.

Neomycin sulphate

- Neomycin sulphate, gramicidin and polymixin B sulphate eye drops: **Neosporin**® (Dominion), M

Dose: Apply 2–4 times daily or more frequently if required.

A useful mixture of antibiotics for mixed ocular-surface infections. Spectrum of activity: neomycin sulphate (mainly Gram –ve), gramicidin (mainly Gram +ve), polymixin B (mainly Gram –ve).

Ofloxacin

- Ofloxacin 0.3% eye drops: **Exocin**® (Allergan), M

Dose: Follow the manufacturer's recommendations as outlined for ciprofloxacin.

Ofloxacin is a new-generation broad-spectrum antibiotic, licensed for use in bacterial infections. It should be used only in complex situations and is effective against *Pseudomonas aeruginosa*.

Fortified preparations

- **Fortified gentamicin** (for Gram –ve organisms): 100 mg gentamicin solution added to 5 ml bottle of topical gentamicin makes 14.3 mg/ml fortified gentamicin solution stable for 30 days (store in fridge).
- **Fortified cephazolin** (for Gram +ve organisms): 15 ml artificial tear solution added to one 500 mg vial of cephazolin makes 33 mg/ml fortified cephazolin solution stable for 48 hours (store in fridge).

Dose: Fortified solutions are reserved for serious ocular infections and are usually used every hour, day and night, in the initial period of treatment.

TOPICAL OPHTHALMIC PREPARATIONS

These antibiotics are synergistic so can be used together for mixed infections if required.

ANTIVIRALS

No topical antiviral agents for veterinary use are manufactured in the UK. Acyclovir (aciclovir) and ganciclovir are both proprietary medical preparations that are used to treat herpetic keratitis, and acyclovir is sometimes used to treat confirmed or suspected viral keratitis in animals. Trifluorothymidine is more effective than acyclovir against feline herpes virus and some hospital pharmacies will supply trifluorothymidine on request. The efficacy of acyclovir combined with human interferon-α_2 requires evaluation.

Acyclovir
• Acyclovir 3% ointment: **Zovirax**® (GSK), M
Dose: Apply 5–6 times daily or more frequently if required.

ANTIFUNGALS

No topical antifungal agents for ophthalmic use are manufactured in the UK, although a number of unlicensed preparations have been used. Moorfields Eye Hospital in the UK will compound topical antifungal preparations (e.g. miconazole) on a named-patient basis.

ANTI-INFLAMMATORIES

Although there are a number of products that contain a corticosteroid and an anti-infective, the use of these combination products is rarely indicated.

CORTICOSTEROIDS

Betamethasone
• Betamethasone sodium phosphate 0.1% eye drops: **Betsolan**® (Schering-Plough), V
• Betamethasone sodium phosphate 0.1% eye drops and ointment: **Betnesol**® (Celltech), M
• Betamethasone sodium phosphate 0.1% and neomycin sulphate 0.5% eye drops and ointment: **Betnesol-N**® (Celltech), M
Betamethasone penetrates the cornea poorly, so is best used for superficial ocular inflammation.
Dose: **Drops** are usually applied every one to two hours for up to 48 hours if the inflammation is severe, otherwise 4–6 times daily. The dose should be tapered off, reducing to zero once the eye is quiet.
  Ointment is usually applied 2–4 times daily.

TOPICAL OPHTHALMIC PREPARATIONS

Dexamethasone

- Dexamethasone 0.1% and hypromellose 1% eye drops: **Maxidex®** (Alcon), M
- Dexamethasone 0.1%, neomycin sulphate 0.35% and polymyxin B sulphate eye drops: **Maxitrol®** (Alcon), M
- Dexamethasone 0.05%, framycetin sulphate 0.5% and gramicidin 0.005% eye drops and ointment: **Sofradex®** (Florizel), M
- Dexamethasone sodium phosphate 0.1% eye drops for single use: **Minims® Dexamethasone** (Chauvin), M

Dose: **Drops** are usually applied every 1–2 hours for up to 48 hours if the inflammation is severe, otherwise 4–6 times daily. The dose should be tapered off, reducing to zero once the eye is quiet.

Ointment is usually applied 2–4 times daily.

Dexamethasone may be used to treat anterior uveitis.

Fluorometholone

- Fluorometholone 0.1% and polyvinyl alcohol (Liquifilm®) suspension (eye drops): **FML®** (Allergan), M

Dose: Drops are usually applied every 1–2 hours for the first 48 hours if the inflammation is severe, otherwise 4–6 times daily. The dose should be tapered off, reducing to zero once the eye is quiet.

Fluorometholone is the first-choice corticosteroid for ocular-surface inflammation and superficial ocular inflammations.

Hydrocortisone acetate

- Hydrocortisone acetate eye drops 1% and ointment 0.5% (Non-proprietary)

Dose: **Drops** are usually applied 4–6 times daily; the dose should be tapered off, reducing to zero once the eye is quiet.

Ointment is usually applied 2–4 times daily.

Useful for short-term treatment of superficial ocular inflammation.

Prednisolone

- Prednisolone acetate 1% eye drops: **Pred Forte®** (Allergan), M

Dose: In the treatment of uveitis, apply every 1–2 hours until the inflammation is controlled. Once the eye is quiet, the dose should be tapered off, reducing to zero.

This corticosteroid preparation offers excellent corneal penetration, combined with effective anti-inflammatory activity. It is the drug of choice for the treatment of anterior uveitis.

NON-STEROIDAL ANTI-INFLAMMATORIES

Ketorolac trometamol

- Ketorolac trometamol 0.05% eye drops: **Acular®** (Allergan), M

Dose: Apply 4 times daily.

This is a non-steroidal anti-inflammatory drug (NSAID) which can be used to treat anterior uveitis.

Flurbiprofen sodium
- Flurbiprofen sodium 0.03% eye drops: **Ocufen**® (Allergan), M

Dose: Prior to cataract surgery, apply at 30-minute intervals for 2 hours.

Flurbiprofen 0.03% is a non-steroidal anti-inflammatory drug (NSAID) which can be used alone or in conjunction with topical corticosteroids for the treatment of intraocular inflammation. In practice, however, it is mainly used to reduce intraoperative miosis and intraocular inflammation in cataract surgery.

Diclofenac sodium
- Diclofenac sodium 0.1% eye drops: **Voltarol**® **Ophtha** (Novartis), M

Dose: Prior to cataract surgery, apply at 30-minute intervals for 2 hours.

Diclofenac sodium 0.1% is a NSAID that is similar to flurbiprofen. It is similarly used to reduce intraoperative miosis and intraocular inflammation in cataract surgery.

OTHER ANTI-INFLAMMATORIES

- Antazoline sulphate 0.5% and xylometazoline hydrochloride 0.05% eye drops. **Otrivine-Antistin**® (Novartis), M
- Lodoxamide trometamol 0.1% eye drops: **Alomide**® (Alcon), M
- Sodium cromoglycate (cromoglicate) 2% eye drops (non-proprietary)

Dose: Apply 4 times daily.

These drugs are used to treat allergic conjunctivitis and lodoxamide has also been used to treat equine eosinophilic keratoconjunctivitis.

GLAUCOMA TREATMENT

MIOTICS

Pilocarpine
- Pilocarpine hydrochloride 0.5%, 1%, 2% and 3% and 4% eye drops (non-proprietary)
- Pilocarpine nitrate 1%, 2% and 4% eye drops for single use: **Minims Pilocarpine Nitrate**® (Chauvin), M

Dose for treatment of open-angle glaucoma: Pilocarpine 1% drops 2–3 times daily.

Pilocarpine is a direct-acting parasympathomimetic whose action increases aqueous outflow. It can be used to treat primary open-angle glaucoma, but, as this is a rare form of glaucoma in the dog, the most commonly-affected animal species, indications for its use in glaucoma therapy are limited.

In passing, it should be noted that some neurogenic forms of dry eye have been treated with this drug. It may also be used in the assessment of parasympathetic denervation of the pupil (e.g. Adie's syndrome) – denervation hypersensitivity is confirmed when the affected pupil constricts more rapidly than the normal pupil. Miosis usually results within ten minutes of the application of pilocarpine 1% in a normal eye.

Echiopate iodide and demacarium bromide

Echiopate iodide and demacarium bromide are long-acting anticholinesterases that are no longer commercially available in the UK. They can be obtained on the rare occasions when their use is indicated, more likely as a means of immobilising intraocular parasitic nematode larvae prior to their surgical extraction, rather than for glaucoma therapy.

CARBONIC ANHYDRASE INHIBITORS

- Brinzolamide 10 mg/ml eye drops: **Azopt**® (Alcon), M
Dose: Apply 2–4 times daily.
- Dorzolamide hydrochloride 2% eye drops: **Trusopt**® (MSD), M
Dose: Apply 3–4 times daily.

Brinzolamide and dorzolamide are topical carbonic anhydrase inhibitors which may be used to treat glaucoma. Dorzolamide is the more widely used of the two in veterinary medicine. Topical carbonic anhydrase inhibitors have all but replaced systemic preparations such as dichlorphenamide, because they have fewer systemic side effects.

PROSTAGLANDIN ANALOGUES

- Latanoprost 50 mcg/ml eye drops: **Xalatan**® (Pharamacia), M
- Travoprost 40 mcg/ml eye drops: **Travatan**® (Alcon), M
Dose: Apply once or twice daily.

Latanoprost and travoprost are prostaglandin (PGF_2alpha) analogues which increase uveoscleral outflow. Both agents are used in the same way, but latanoprost is the prostaglandin analogue that is selected most commonly in small animal glaucoma cases. Its use is associated with intense miosis, in the dog particularly, and the drug should be avoided if uveitis is present. Latanoprost and dorzolamide can be used together to treat glaucoma.

SYMPATHOMIMETICS

Brimonidine tartrate 0.2% eye drops: **Alphagan**® (Allergan), M
Dose: Apply twice daily.

Brimonidine tartrate is a selective alpha$_2$-adrenoceptor stimulant which lowers the intraocular pressure by reducing aqueous production and enhancing uveoscleral outflow. The effectiveness is receptor dependent (alpha$_2$ receptors) and therefore varies between species. It penetrates the posterior segment and has some neuroprotective effects, so that optic-nerve function is preserved. All the currently available sympathomimetic drugs require evaluation under controlled conditions for the treatment of glaucoma in animals, and drugs that exert a neuroprotective effect are desirable.

BETA-BLOCKERS

- Timolol maleate 0.25% eye drops (non-proprietary)
- Timolol maleate 0.25% eye drops: **Timoptol**® (MSD), M

- Betaxolol hydrochloride 0.5% eye drops: **Betoptic**® (Alcon), M
Dose: Apply twice daily.
The beta-blockers achieve their effect mainly by reducing aqueous production, and are sometimes used in conjunction with topical carbonic anhydrase inhibitors. Betaxolol causes fewer cardiac side effects (i.e. bradycardia) than timolol. Beta-blockers for glaucoma therapy in animals require evaluation under controlled conditions.

MYDRIATICS AND CYCLOPLEGICS

When mydriatic cycloplegics are used to break down posterior synechiae in early iris bombé, there is usually no point in prolonging treatment if the desired effect is not obtained within two hours of frequent topical application, because of the risks associated with these drugs in glaucoma patients.

ANTIMUSCARINICS

Atropine sulphate
- Atropine sulphate 0.5% eye drops and 1% ointment (non-proprietary)
- Atropine sulphate 1% eye drops for single use: **Minims Atropine Sulphate**® (Chauvin), M
Dose: Atropine sulphate takes approximately an hour to achieve maximal dilation in the normal eye, but the effects will obviously be more variable when the eye is inflamed. In the treatment of acute anterior uveitis, with intense miosis, it is usual to apply atropine initially every 15–30 minutes to dilate the pupil and relieve ciliary spasm. Once pupil dilation has been achieved, usually after only one or two applications, the treatment frequency is reduced and the drug given to effect, so as to maintain dilation. In farm animals and horses, application may not need to be as frequent as it is in dogs and cats.

Atropine sulphate is most commonly used as a mydriatic cycloplegic in the treatment of anterior uveitis. It is also used, but rarely, to try and break down posterior synechiae in early iris bombé, a potentially devastating cause of secondary glaucoma. It may be combined for both purposes with the directly-acting sympathomimetic phenylephrine 10%. It is too long acting to be used for diagnostic purposes. Cats usually tolerate ointment more readily than drops and in young animals of all species ointment may be preferable as this formulation reduces systemic absorption.

Tropicamide
- Tropicamide 0.5% and 1% eye drops: **Mydriacyl**® (Alcon), M
Dose: One drop of tropicamide 1% applied to the normal eye will be sufficient to dilate the pupil.
This agent is a short-acting and relatively weak mydriatic. Tropicamide 1% produces maximal pupillary dilation some 30 minutes after application in most species and is the most commonly used strength. It is used primarily to facilitate examination of the lens, vitreous and fundus.

TOPICAL OPHTHALMIC PREPARATIONS

SYMPATHOMIMETICS

Phenylephrine hydrochloride

• Phenylephrine hydrochloride 2.5% and 10% eye drops for single use: **Minims**®
  Phenylephrine hydrochloride (Chauvin), M

Phenylephrine 10% can be used in conjunction with atropine to dilate the pupil in anterior uveitis. It is also used to blanch superficial vessels in the differentiation of episcleritis and scleritis and as a means of attempting to establish the site of lesions in Horner's syndrome.

BASIC PRINCIPLES OF OCULAR AND ADNEXAL SURGERY

PREOPERATIVE PREPARATION AND POSTOPERATIVE CARE

- Correct positioning of the patient and the eye for the procedure to be undertaken is essential
- Standard preparation for aseptic surgery, but with great care in skin preparation (may be better not to clip)
- For skin preparation can use baby shampoo diluted 1 in 5 with water
- For ocular and periocular surfaces use 5% povidone-iodine sterile ophthalmic prep solution (Betadine 5%)
- Flush eye thoroughly with sterile saline after using baby shampoo or Betadine
- Disposable drapes are ideal for patients undergoing ophthalmic surgery
- Effective fixation of the globe, if required, can be achieved by the use of stay sutures
- Postoperatively, it is sensible to cover sharp dew claws with a light bandage; Elizabethan collars are not necessarily required but are widely used
- Healing after most types of adnexal and extraocular surgery is usually rapid and uncomplicated, so there are no special nursing requirements. Nursing care for animals undergoing intraocular surgery is beyond the remit of these notes
- Preoperative, perioperative and postoperative systemic analgesia, topical and systemic antibiotics can be provided as dictated by the type of surgery
- Prophylactic tetanus treatment is given if indicated
- Non-absorbable skin sutures are removed 7–10 days after surgery – for uncomplicated eyelid surgery the sutures can be removed within seven days because of the rapidity of healing

GENERAL ANAESTHESIA

General principles in the management of surgical patients
- Preoperative assessment should take into account pre-existing disease (e.g. diabetes mellitus) and current therapy (e.g. osmotic diuretics such as mannitol)
- Systemic analgesics are valuable as part of the management of many ocular conditions and may form part of the anaesthetic protocol for patients undergoing procedures under general anaesthesia
- Preoperatively and postoperatively a quiet environment is helpful for the patient, and dim lighting is essential if photophobia is present
- It is important to position the patient properly to provide good surgical access and to ensure that the anaesthetic equipment cannot become dislodged, blocked or kinked when hidden under drapes; armoured endotracheal tubes are very useful for patients undergoing ophthalmic procedures
- Topical local anaesthesia can be a useful adjunct if the procedure is likely to cause corneal or conjunctival pain and should be applied 1–2 minutes before surgery is to start

Basic monitoring of the anaesthetised patient
- This is more difficult in ophthalmic patients, as jaw tone, visible mucous membranes, palpebral and corneal reflexes, and pupillary size and response cannot be assessed readily
- An oesophageal stethoscope for monitoring respiratory and heart sounds and palpation of the peripheral pulse at regular intervals should be regarded as the minimum required

- In addition, the peripheral pulse and systolic blood pressure can be monitored with a Doppler flow probe and cuff and end tidal carbon dioxide can be measured by a capnograph (carbon dioxide monitor).

Anaesthetic protocol

- Pre-anaesthetic agents – may be used singly or in combination, usually a sedative (e.g. acepromazine) and analgesic (e.g. buprenorphine)
- Pre-oxygenation can be used to avoid hypoxaemia at induction, but it is important to avoid pressure on the globe from the facemask
- Induction agents – intravenous induction is preferable to minimise excitement: *thiopentone* is applicable to most species, *propofol* provides smooth induction in dogs and can also be used for maintenance
- Endotracheal intubation is usually necessary when procedures involve gaseous agents for maintenance and laryngeal reflexes can be deadened by pre-treatment with topical or intravenous lignocaine or intravenous fentanyl
- It is important to avoid stimulating the larynx when performing intubation and extubation
- Maintenance is usually achieved with a gaseous anaesthetic agent and isoflurane is an excellent choice
- Whilst neuromuscular blocking agents are useful (e.g. to immobilise the globe prior to corneal surgery and for intraocular microsurgery), their use requires that the requisite skills and equipment are available
- The use of regional and local blocks for specific procedures is outlined in the relevant parts of the main text
- All intraocular procedures require a soft eye (the intraocular pressure is slightly lower than normal), whereas adnexal and ocular surface surgery is often easier if the eye is firm (the intraocular pressure is normal). Some of the factors that modify intraocular pressure are summarised in Appendix Table 3.1 below.

Appendix Table 3.1   Factors affecting intraocular pressure

Intraocular pressure is increased by:	Intraocular pressure is decreased by:
Increased venous pressure (e.g. jugular occlusion from neck collar, choke chain, poor positioning, anything that causes airway obstruction, coughing, gagging, retching, vomiting)	Most anaesthetic agents
Systemic hypertension	Decreased central venous pressure or arterial pressure
Hypercapnia	Hypocapnia
Hypoxaemia	
Drugs (suxamethonium; ketamine)	Drugs (osmotic diuretics, carbonic anhydrase inhibitors)
External pressure (e.g. direct pressure on the globe)	Oculocentesis (release of aqueous or vitreous)

GENERAL EQUIPMENT

INSTRUMENTS

General instruments
- Surgical drapes and towel clips (NB adhesive drapes excellent for ophthalmic surgery)
- No.3 Swann Morton scalpel handle with numbers 15 and 11 blades
- Standard 1 × 2 teeth tissue forceps (e.g. Gillies)
- Stout, straight scissors (e.g. Mayo)
- Needle holders (e.g. Crile Wood)
- Mosquito artery forceps ×4 (e.g. Halstead)
- Tissue forceps ×4 (e.g. Allis)
- Swabs

Ophthalmic instruments
- Small 1 × 2 teeth tissue forceps (e.g. Lister)
- Fixation forceps ×2 (e.g. Graefe)
- Small needle holder (e.g. Castroviejo)
- Small, straight, blunt-tipped tenotomy scissors (e.g. Stevens)
- WeissCEL microspears or similar

Suture material

- For skin sutures: 4-0 to 6-0 non-absorbable braided silk, or absorbable polyglactin 910 with curved, swaged-on, spatula, micropoint needle
- For conjunctival sutures: 6-0 to 7-0 absorbable polyglactin 910 with curved, swaged-on, round-bodied or tapercut needle
- For corneal sutures: 8-0 to 9-0 absorbable polyglactin 910 with curved, swaged-on, spatula, micropoint needle or 9-0 to 10-0 nylon, with curved, swaged-on spatula, micropoint needle

OTHER EQUIPMENT

- Operating specatacles, or binocular loupe, or operating microscope (latter is essential for microsurgical techniques)
- Catholysis equipment
- Cryosurgical equipment
- Bipolar wet field cautery

INSTRUMENT SETS

Eyelids and conjunctiva
- General and ophthalmic packs of instruments

- Standard ophthalmic needleholder (e.g. Castroviejo)
- Speculum (e.g. Barraquer or Clarke)
- Entropion spatula (e.g. Jaeger)

Points to note
- For eyelids: precise apposition of skin edges with little tension on the knot is important. In general, single-layer closure with simple interrupted sutures is satisfactory for most eyelid problems. The eyelid margin is closed first and apposition should be perfect. The aim is always for primary repair.
- Buried absorbable sutures should be avoided in general, but may be required for conjunctival closure (including eyelid closure with complex blepharoplastic procedures, because more tension is needed for effective closure).

Distichiasis
- Catholysis equipment
- Cilia forceps (e.g. Whifield)

Ectopic cilia
- General pack of instruments
- Tarsal cyst forceps or chalazion clamp (e.g. Desmarre) – eyelid immobilisation is easier and haemorrhage is reduced

Lacrimal apparatus
- Ophthalmic pack of instruments
- Lacrimal cannulae, silver, non-disposable
- 5 ml or 10 ml syringe
- Balanced salt solution or distilled water for irrigation
- Lacrimal probe set
- Monofilament nylon, polyethylene tubing to catheterise the duct

Superficial keratectomy
- General and ophthalmic packs of instruments
- Speculum (e.g. Barraquer or Clarke)
- Beaver handle and blades or disposable knife with miniature edged blades

Enucleation
- General pack of instruments
- Additional artery forceps
- Stout, curved scissors (e.g. Mayo) for dissection
- Curved forceps (e.g. Wright's orbital forceps) for clamping optic nerve

Parotid-duct transposition
- General and ophthalmic packs of instruments
- Monofilament nylon (heat-blunt end to avoid trauma) to cannulate the parotid duct
- Strabismus hook (e.g. Graefe) useful for elevating the duct during dissection

Basic intraocular set
- Ophthalmic instrument tray

- Fixation forceps ×2 (e.g. Graefe)
- Wells artery forceps ×2
- Halstead's mosquito artery forceps ×2
- Balanced salt solution for intraocular use
- Viscoelastic material for intraocular use
- Range of cannulae and syringes
- Swabs
- WeissCEL® microspears or similar
- Adhesive drapes and standard drapes with towel clips
- Speculum (e.g. Barraquer or Clarke)
- Callipers
- Mayo scissors (straight)
- Standard 1 × 2 teeth tissue forceps (e.g. Gillies)
- Diamond knife or disposable knife, or razor blade and handle, or Beaver blades and handle
- Small 1 × 2 teeth tissue forceps (e.g. Lister)
- St Martin forceps
- Birks forceps
- Colibri forceps (e.g. Barraquer)
- Capsule forceps (e.g. Arruga)
- Capsulorhexis forceps (e.g. Utrata)
- Small, straight, blunt-tipped tenotomy scissors, straight and curved (e.g. Stevens)
- Left and right corneoscleral scissors (e.g. Castroviejo)
- Castroviejo corneal scissors
- Westcott tenotomy scissors
- Iris scissors
- Vannas scissors
- Iris repositor (e.g. Nettleship)
- Needle holders (e.g. Crile Wood)
- Standard needleholder (e.g. Castroviejo)
- Micro needleholder without catch (e.g. Castroviejo, Barraquer)
- Strabismus hooks (Graefe) ×2
- Vectis (Bell Taylor)

APPENDIX 4

CRANIAL NERVE INNERVATION OF THE EYE AND ADNEXA

Nerve	Function	Damage
Optic Cranial nerve II special somatic afferent (SSA)	Vision	Partial or complete blindness Dilated or completely unresponsive pupil
Oculomotor Cranial nerve III general somatic efferent (GSE) general visceral efferent (GVE)	GSE: Eyeball movement – supplies dorsal, ventral and medial recti and ventral oblique muscles; raises upper eyelid – *levator palpebrae superioris* muscle GVE: Pupil constriction and dynamic accommodation of the lens (parasympathetic)	GSE: Squint (lateral and inferior – 'down and out') GVE: Dilated pupil (mydriasis)
Trochlear Cranial nerve IV (GSE)	Eyeball movement – supplies dorsal oblique muscle	Squint (dorsal – upwards)
Trigeminal Cranial nerve V (GSE)	Sensory to globe and adnexa	Neurotrophic keratopathy (because of a loss of corneal sensitivity)
Abducens Cranial nerve VI (GSE)	Eyeball movement and retraction – supplies lateral rectus and *retractor bulbi* muscles	Squint (medial – inwards) Inability to retract globe
Facial Cranial nerve VII somatic visceral efferent (SVE) and GVE	SVE: Muscles of facial expression GVE: Lacrimal gland secretion (parasympathetic)	Inability to close lids – exposure keratopathy Corneal desiccation
Vagus Cranial nerve X (GVE)	Oculocardiac and oculorespiratory reflex (Vth nerve – afferent, to internuncial fibres in reticular formation, to vagus nerve – efferent) Stimulation produces a decrease in respiratory rate and variation of its rhythm, and slowing of heart in some species if there is manipulation of the globe +/– adnexa (e.g. the extraocular muscles)	Not applicable
Sympathetic Nerves (GVE)	Pupil dilation; supplies smooth muscle and blood vessels within orbit and eyelids	Horner's syndrome (typically ptosis, miosis, enophthalmos, prominence of third eyelid)

CRANIAL NERVE INNERVATION OF THE EYE AND ADNEXA

FURTHER READING
(Useful texts first published in English)

GENERAL OPHTHALMOLOGY

Barnett, K.C. (1996) *Veterinary Ophthalmology*. Mosby-Wolfe, London.

Gelatt, K.N. (ed) (1998) *Veterinary Ophthalmology*, 3rd edn. Lipincott, Williams & Wilkins, Philadelphia.

Gelatt, K.N. (2000) *Essentials of Veterinary Ophthalmology*. Lipincott, Williams & Wilkins, Philadelphia.

Gelatt, K.N. & Gelatt, J.P. (2001) *Small Animal Ophthalmic Surgery; Practical Techniques for the Veterinarian*. Butterworth-Heinemann, Oxford.

Grahn, B.H. Cullen, C.L. & Peiffer, R.L. (2004) *Veterinary Ophthalmology Essentials*. Butterworth-Heinemann, Philadelphia.

Rubin, L.F. (1974) *Atlas of Veterinary Ophthalmoscopy*. Lea and Febiger, Philadelphia.

Slatter, D.H. (2001) *Fundamentals of Veterinary Ophthalmology*. 3rd edn. W.B. Saunders, Philadelphia.

SMALL ANIMAL

Gelatt, K.N. & Gelatt, J.P. (2001) *Small Animal Ophthalmic Surgery: Practical Techniques for the Veterinarian*. Butterworth-Heineman, Oxford.

Peiffer, R.L. & Petersen-Jones, S.M. (eds) (2001) *Small Animal Ophthalmology: A Problem-Oriented Approach*. 3rd edn. W.B. Saunders, London.

Petersen-Jones, S.M. & Crispin, S.M. (eds) (2002) *Manual of Small Animal Ophthalmology*. 2nd edn. BSAVA Publications, Cheltenham.

Riis, R.C. (2002) *Small Animal Ophthalmology Secrets*. Hanley & Belfus, Philadelphia.

CANINE

Barnett, K.C. Heinrich, C. & Sansom, J. (2002) *Canine Ophthalmology: An Atlas and Text*. W.B. Saunders, London.

FELINE

Barnett, K.C. & Crispin, S.M. (1998) *Feline Ophthalmology: An Atlas and Text*. W.B. Saunders, London.

Ketring, K.L. & Glaze, M.B. (1994) *Atlas of Feline Ophthalmology*. Veterinary Learning Systems Co Inc, Trenton, N.J.

EQUINE

Barnett, K.C. *et al.* (eds) (1983) *Equine Ophthalmology. Equine Veterinary Journal Supplement 2*.

FURTHER READING

Barnett, K.C. *et al.* (eds) (1990) *Equine Ophthalmology II. Equine Veterinary Journal Supplement 10.*

Barnett, K.C., Crispin, S.M., Lavach, J.D. & Matthews, A.G. (2004) *Equine Ophthalmology: An Atlas and Text.* 2nd edn. Mosby-Wolfe, London.

Brooks, D.E. (2002) *Ophthalmology for the Equine Practioner.* Teton NewMedia, Jackson, Wyoming.

FARM ANIMAL

Lavach, J.D. (1990) *Large Animal Ophthalmology.* Mosby, St Louis.

TEXTS CONTAINING USEFUL MATERIAL ON THE EYE

Auer, J.A. (ed) (1999) Equine Surgery, 2nd edn. W.B. Saunders, Philadelphia.

Birchard, S.J. & Sherding, R.G. (eds) (1994) *Saunders Manual of Small Animal Practice.* W.B. Saunders Co., Philadelphia.

Bojrab, M.J. *et al.* (eds) (1997) *Current Techniques in Small Animal Surgery.* 4th edn. Williams and Wilkins, Baltimore.

Day, M.J. (1999) *Clinical Immunology of the Dog and Cat,* (second edition in preparation). Manson Publishing, London.

De Lahunta, A. *Veterinary Neuroanatomy and Clinical Neurology,* 2nd edn. W.B. Saunders, Philadelphia.

Dunn, J.K. (ed) (1999) *Textbook of Small Animal Medicine.* W.B. Saunders, Philadelphia.

Evans, S.A. (ed) (1993) *Miller's Anatomy of the Dog,* 3rd edn. W.B. Saunders, Philadelphia.

Gorman, N.T. (ed) (1998) *Canine Medicine and Therapeutics,* 4th edn. Blackwell Scientific, Oxford.

Morgan, R.V. (ed) (2002) *Handbook of Small Animal Practice,* 4th edn. W.B. Saunders, Philadelphia.

Slatter, D.H. (ed) (2003) *Textbook of Small Animal Surgery,* 3rd edn. W.B. Saunders, Philadelphia.

Smith, B.P. (ed) (2002) *Large Animal Internal Medicine,* 3rd edn. Mosby, St Louis, Missouri.

OTHER

Veterinary Clinics of North America series
Veterinary Ophthalmology (journal)

FURTHER READING

Page numbers in *italic* refer to figures.